Patient-Centred Medicine in Transition

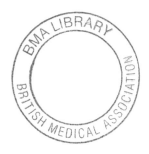

Advances in Medical Education

Volume 3

Series Editors:
Susanne Lajoie
Yvonne Steinert

For further volumes:
http://www.springer.com/series/8405

Alan Bleakley

Patient-Centred Medicine in Transition

The Heart of the Matter

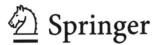 Springer

Alan Bleakley
Plymouth University Peninsula School
  of Medicine and Dentistry
Cornwall, UK

ISSN 2211-1298   ISSN 2211-1301 (electronic)
ISBN 978-3-319-02486-8   ISBN 978-3-319-02487-5 (eBook)
DOI 10.1007/978-3-319-02487-5
Springer Cham Heidelberg New York Dordrecht London

Library of Congress Control Number: 2013956606

Printed on acid-free paper

Springer is part of Springer Science+Business Media (www.springer.com)

Foreword

Reading this book is like flying over an exotic landscape at high speed. One moment, you are following the contours of Plato's Socratic dialogues; the next, you are skimming the peak of a democratic medical education of the future. Sit back and feel exhilarated—provided, that is, you can cope with the G forces. Alan Bleakley's call for medicine to be less anal, for example, will not be to every reader's liking. For those who are untroubled by gravity, this is no ordinary flight. At any moment, you can choose to stop in mid-air, hover high above the landscape to take in its startling topographical features, or come down to earth, pick up the word 'empathy' in your hands, and examine it from more facets than you would have believed a word could have. This is the writing of a polymath, a poet, a person who is deeply concerned about humanity, and a radical socialist thinker.

Here is a rough guide to the landscape: in medicine, the patient is the heart of the matter. But unsafe medical practices are causing patients to die. Practice is unsafe because doctors in general do not communicate as well as they should. They can behave autocratically towards patients and fellow professionals. They can impose their own type of reasoning and do not give patients' narratives enough space in clinical reasoning. They often communicate monologically with other health professionals in ways that maintain doctors' privileged positions within health-care teams. They can humiliate medical students when they could form caring and supportive relationships, causing students' empathy to decline. And the whole cycle repeats itself from one generation to the next.

Of course, not all doctors behave in those ways, nor do they do so all the time. But there is enough resonance between Alan Bleakley's critique of the medical profession and my own experiences as a doctor—even of my own behaviour—that I feel obliged to listen to him. Medicine needs to be democratized. Unproductive hierarchies need to be dismantled. Relationships of mutual respect between patients, doctors, other health professionals, and medical students lie at the heart of his vision for a new medical education. I have, until now, found the term 'patient-centred' troublesome because centering on any one person implicitly decentres on another and struggle must surely ensue. On the other hand, medicine must be patient-centred because there would be no medicine if there were no patients; the central ethic of medicine is to care for patients. Alan Bleakley solves my problem by putting no single person at the centre, other than in the moral imperative to be caring.

Static concept of teams, personalities, and roles are abandoned in favour of a complex, dynamic, and adaptive set of activities that focuses on communicative processes more than individual positions. Mutually enhancing conversation that tolerates and explores 'difference' makes medical science a 'warm objectivity'. Doctors develop their identities as interprofessional team workers. Whilst my heart is engaged by Alan Bleakley's warm, idealistic reframing of a relationship-centred medicine, my head is strongly engaged by the concept of knotworking that he develops from Yrjö Engeström's work in activity theory and applies to medical practice. Compared to the constraining, structural metaphor of a network, a knotwork is a process of tying, untying, and re-tying threads of team activity. It is an emergent property of the system of several teams working around a patient. It is mediated by a complex set of artefacts such as a patient's medications, records, and charts. Welcome to a 'liquid' age of team working.

If democracy is the value system that runs through this book, complexity is the logic that ties it together. Alan Bleakley applies actor-network-theory, activity theory, communities of practice, and many other conceptual orientations to medical education research and practice. The heart of the book, like the heart of medical care and education, is the point where democracy and complexity come into alignment to the benefit of patients. Medical education, the book makes clear, has to move forward from simple, authoritarian, dyadic relationships between doctors and other people to complex, emergent ones between all parties involved, in what Etienne Wenger terms 'joint enterprise'. Humanities in early medical education, Alan Bleakley argues, can democratize medical curricula. We should embrace his ideas, see the 'wonder and beauty of the life sciences', deliver medical education in 'tender-minded' cultures, and privilege no one person above another in the delivery of patient-centred education.

Maastricht, The Netherlands   Tim Dornan

Acknowledgements

I would like to thank Professor John Bligh and Ms Julie Browne for the initial stimulating conversations from which this book developed, as a partner to *Medical Education for the Future*: *Identity*, *Power and Location* (Springer 2011). I would also like to thank the doctors and medical educators who have helped me to formulate the ideas in this book by modelling inspired communication as well as clinical expertise—in particular Dr. Robert Marshall, Dr. David Levine, Dr. Adrian Hobbs, and Dr. Julie Thacker.

Contents

Part III   A Brief but Provocative Conclusion

Chapter 1
Introduction

A Health Warning

It is best to say at the outset that the book you are now reading may seriously frustrate those who are searching for a manual that teaches 'how to communicate' or provides ready-made answers to 'communication problems'. Further, I explicitly draw on debates concerning communication in medicine in 'Western' settings. I do not believe for one moment that there is a 'right' way to communicate professionally in medicine, as context will dictate styles and inflections. Hence, I am sceptical towards all-encompassing and prescriptive 'cookbook' approaches, especially where these are clearly culture specific. This is then not a book on cross-cultural issues of communication, while it does deal to some extent with medical subcultural issues—or stylistic differences across specialties.

Returning to 'how to do it' manuals, there are some very good, high-end, examples of such books that have been through more than one edition and have proven popular, such as Suzanne Kurtz, Jonathan Silverman, and Juliet Draper (2004, 2nd revised edition) *Teaching and Learning Communication Skills in Medicine* and Peter Tate (2009, 6th revised edition) *The Doctor's Communication Handbook*. Such texts focus particularly on the general practice/family doctor consultation, for example, David Pendleton, Theo Schofield, Peter Tate, and Peter Havelock (2003, 2nd revised edition) *The New Consultation: Developing doctor-patient communication* and Jonathan Silverman, Suzanne Kurtz, and Juliet Draper (2004, 2nd revised edition) *Skills for Communicating with Patients*.

It may be unfair to lump these texts together, but their approaches are remarkably similar in tone and style, as 'recipe oriented'. In this sense, they are very helpful for those who want clear frameworks and tips (such as the Calgary-Cambridge observation guide model developed by David Silverman and Suzanne Kurtz and widely used across medical schools). Note also that the same authors recur across titles. You are also likely to find that across a stable of similar books, the words 'skills', 'training' (rather than 'education'), and 'handbook' regularly appear, suggesting a

A. Bleakley, *Patient-Centred Medicine in Transition: The Heart of the Matter*,
Advances in Medical Education 3, DOI 10.1007/978-3-319-02487-5_1,
© Springer International Publishing Switzerland 2014

technical–rational or functional approach to teaching and learning communication. It is hard to escape this dominant discourse of instrumentality—with its language of 'skills', 'steps', and 'manuals'—that approaches communication a little like fixing a car engine, as a problem to be solved, and as an issue of 'training' (to acquire a skill) rather than 'education' (to think, and then act, differently).

Roger Neighbour's (2004) book *The Inner Consultation: How to Develop an Effective and Intuitive Consulting Style* was first published in 1987 and was revised thoroughly for the 2004 edition. Neighbour has explicitly and consistently pointed out that his text is not about the cumulative collection of a set of skills. Indeed, 'the inner consultation' is not about skills instruction at all, but about a release of communication abilities inherent in experienced practitioners (who should also trust their intuition). Nevertheless, when the 2004 edition appeared, it was widely reviewed in terms of the language of 'skills' and 'tools'—functional rather than aesthetic. The publishers themselves described the book as 'a sophisticated training manual'.

A retrospective review in the *British Medical Journal* (Warriner, 2008, p. a1574) recognized the radical nature of Neighbour's proposals about general practitioners trying to become part of the 'flow' of the consultation, in both a Buddhist and Taoist sense, rather than separating themselves out and worrying about what to do next, in terms of rehearsed interventions. Yet the review refers to the book as a 'self-help manual', again orienting the reader to a 'fix-it' mentality. Importantly, Neighbour's book, while highly influential, is doctor centred and, despite its sophistication in fundamental idea, reverts to 'stages' and 'checklist' thinking typical of functional approaches.

The book you are now reading explicitly avoids a cookbook, recipe-based, 'how to' approach to communication in medicine—I steer clear of checklists and stages of development of skills. Yet I am passionate about the topic of communication in medicine, and I want doctors (and surgeons particularly) to improve communication with patients and colleagues. But I argue that the functional, skills-based, toolbox approach—now the dominant method across medical schools—is misguided. I present evidence to suggest that skills-based, problem-solving approaches to communication in medical education are failing patients and colleagues, where there is serious underperformance in communication. Such underperformance would not be acceptable in the technical realm of medicine.

In response to what I see as failings in the current dominant approach to 'training' communication skills, I detail a radical overhaul of thinking and practice concerning the so-called non-technical component of medicine (communication and teamwork). The communication of doctors cannot be separated from that of other health practitioners and the patients of those practitioners, but in this book, I keep doctors' work as the focus, although many of the general points made can be generalized to other practitioners.

I am not wholly dismissing technical–rational, skills-based approaches in the education of communication in medicine. Rather, I feel that such functional approaches are seriously limited, again evidenced in the impact they have made, given that the Achilles heel of medical practice is its poor patient safety record grounded in relatively poor levels of communication with patients and between colleagues.

I suggested above that Roger Neighbour's book has been subject to a widespread misreading as a 'technical manual'. Are there any other texts that may satisfy the needs of those looking for a framework of technique as well as a deeper theoretical rationale? A new text—*Clinical Communication in Medicine*—published by the UK Council of Clinical Communication teaching in Undergraduate Medical Education will appear in 2014 (see Brown, 2008). This text promises to get away from the skills-based 'how to' approach of teaching communication skills and places current practices in a historical context. However, the text is restricted to the doctor–patient consultation and does not consider wider aspects of communication in health-care such as working in teams with colleagues, in organizations with management, and in newly emerging contexts such as online patient communities, where 'patient-centredness' is transformed to 'patient connectedness' (I owe this insight, descriptor, and its elaboration to one of my PhD students, Jules Kennedy (2013), who is researching online communities of persons with blood cancers).

I would recommend John Heron's work for those who desire structure but wish to go beyond the inevitably constraining aspects of technical–rational frameworks (and their ill fit with the messy realities of clinical practice, the latter high in uncertainty and ambiguity). Aimed at the 'helping professions' in general rather than medicine in particular, John Heron (2001) has developed a sophisticated framework for communication and professional intervention (six category intervention analysis) at the individual, team, and organizational levels that is explicitly focused on the patient, client, or service user.

What's the Point of Communication in Medicine?

I work in a self-proclaimed 'innovative' UK medical school. The majority of our first year students are 18- to 19-year-old school leavers who are highly intelligent and motivated. They mainly specialized in science subjects at school and expect that the medicine and surgery undergraduate curriculum will focus on the science behind medical practice. Even after meeting patients early in their undergraduate programme, and although they have opted to study at a progressive school, they are often resistant to, and irritated with, having to learn how to 'communicate' effectively with patients and with colleagues from other health professions.

The usual complaints are, first, that medicine is largely a technical matter and communication really does not matter to effective health prevention and intervention. The stereotypical response is: would you rather be treated by a good but rude technical doctor or surgeon or by a really nice person who is actually not a great doctor? (This, of course, is a pretty poor rhetorical strategy, as we would all like good technical doctors who can also communicate well). Second, the students often say that 'communication' is surely what everybody can do anyway, just through everyday life experience? Further, 'communication' is stereotyped as the 'pink and fluffy' stuff that takes time away from studying 'real' medicine. Again, this is in the context of an innovative and progressive medical school. I am sure that colleagues in more traditional settings hear much more corrosive remarks about having to learn about the human and professional face of medicine.

Of course this sceptical stance is not true of all of our students or our faculty, but general scepticism concerning the value of teaching and learning 'communication' remains well established in medical education. I will argue later in this book that such scepticism may be warranted where communication is, for example, learned instrumentally in simulated settings rather than with real, live patients and where communication is reduced to a set of technical skills largely for purposes of assessment.

But now I am jumping ahead. Let me first lay out briefly why we need to value communication in medicine, before outlining appropriate pedagogies for teaching and learning communication, as well as limits to those pedagogies. And by 'communication in medicine', I mean communication generally across health-care and with patients, but *focused specifically on the work of medical students and doctors*. I should add a rider here that technical medicine is progressing at an extraordinary rate and should be admired, while the non-technical face of medicine (communication and teamwork) is not faring so well. My concern in this book is wholly with the latter.

Contrary to the communication as 'pink and fluffy' stereotype, there is an informing science behind practices of communication in medicine—a body of research evidence that gives a clear indication of five main symptoms in medicine and medical education that need to be urgently addressed. Each of these is considered in detail throughout this book, and here I will briefly sketch the core of the problem concerning the five areas that can be collapsed into three main headings: (1) working in teams with colleagues, (2) communicating with patients in consultations, and (3) looking after yourself, or self-care and self-knowledge (this is important because, as psychoanalytic orthodoxy suggests, ineffective, distorted, and manipulative forms of communication can arise from unresolved personal issues):

1. *Communicating and collaborating with colleagues* about patients' medical care (including the science informing practice), to improve patient care and safety. There is an unacceptable level of medical error, and this is largely grounded in miscommunication in clinical team settings (Xyrichis & Ream, 2008). Medical errors include a variety of diagnostic errors, drug errors, results of preventable hospital-induced infections, and surgical errors.
2. *Communicating and collaborating with patients* and patient groups to improve the quality of the consultation. This is particularly important to prevent an unacceptably high rate of misdiagnoses due to not listening carefully to the patient's story (Sanders, 2010).
3. The relatively high *social and psychological element in symptom presentation*, where cure is also grounded in social and psychological, rather than medical, intervention. Twenty-five to 40 % of family physician visits are presentations of symptoms arising from chronic social deprivation and/or psychological and

psychosomatic symptoms such as mood disorders (e.g. endogenous depression and free-floating anxiety), reactive depressions (such as postnatal and post-traumatic stress), addictions, and stress-related hypertension (Buszewicz, Pistrang, Cape, & Martin, 2006). Ninety to 95 % of patients with psychological problems are seen solely by their family practitioner and associated services such as a practice counsellor or clinical psychologist (Buszewicz et al., 2006). There is increasing recognition that chronic conditions such as cardiovascular disease, type 2 diabetes, and some cancers have a high lifestyle/diet-related component and that this correlates significantly with social deprivation according to postcode (Pauli, White, & McWhinney, 2000a, 2000b).

4. *The persistent phenomenon of 'empathy decline'*, where students enter medical schools with high ideals and values, yet these are gradually eroded as the realities of doctoring kick in, and students are introduced to medical subcultures and individual doctors and surgeons advertising disillusionment and cynicism, leading to a less than optimal level of quality of communication with patients and colleagues (Neumann et al., 2011).

5. *The persistent phenomenon of poor self-care amongst doctors*, perhaps as a symptom of lack of psychological acumen. This includes relatively high incidences of suicide, depression, and substance and alcohol abuse.

Let us delve a little further into the key issues within these five areas, all bearing on the topic of communication in medicine. One of the great mysteries in medicine is why there is not greater awareness or acceptance amongst clinicians of what is now an iatrogenic epidemic—a 'disease' caused by medicine itself—that patients are dying and being harmed unnecessarily due to a variety of medical errors grounded in poor communication, half of which are probably avoidable. For those who are new to this area, it is sobering to watch the short video on *YouTube* made by an airline pilot Martin Bromiley about the death in 2005 of his wife in what was a 'routine' intubation prior to an operation that was handled so badly due to poor team communication that the patient, Elaine Bromiley, died (www.youtube.com/watch?v=JzlvgtPIof4). In this video, Bromiley says that he is not sure of the incidence of potentially avoidable medical iatrogenesis grounded in non-technical issues such as poor communication and teamwork. These figures are widely available, if contested and open to interpretation (Barron et al., 2009).

Some medical error is inevitable, but the current rate is unacceptable. Importantly, the majority of such error (estimates are consistent, at around 70 %) is grounded not in technical mistakes but in poor communication, particularly in team settings. I will not provide a long list of references here to substantiate this claim, as these are provided throughout the chapters in this book that deal specifically with the fallout from, and response to, medical error. Let us begin at the sharp end.

The UK Parliament has a number of House of Commons Committees that sit to discuss socially important and controversial topics with a variety of invited experts. Publications ensue and policy recommendations are usually made. A House of Commons Health Committee (Barron et al., 2009) sat during 2008–2009 to discuss patient safety in UK medicine and health-care. One of its briefs was to clarify comparative statistics on deaths, serious accidents, minor accidents, and 'near misses' due to medical error. Despite over a decade's worth of studies internationally in the field, this proved to be a minefield.

Reporting systems within hospitals, for example, although they are entered into a national database (the now disbanded UK National Patient Safety Agency (NPSA)), are notoriously unreliable. Under-reporting is common. Near misses (close calls) are often not reported at all. Part of the problem in obtaining reliable data is that a variety of sources can be consulted, each of which has its own inherent problems—patient records, post-mortem reports on cause of death, drug charts, insurance claims, data from observational studies, incident and accident reporting systems, and so forth. The epidemiology of medical error has become an arcane sub-specialism (Weingart, Wilson, Gibberd, & Harrison, 2000).

Experts interviewed by the Commons Health Select Committee gave a bewildering variety of responses to what seem like straightforward questions about how many people die and/or are harmed from medical error each year in the UK. In short, while the Committee was formally told that around 11,000 patients die from medical error each year, from all the evidence it accumulated, the Committee estimated the figure at closer to 72,000, largely because of chronic under-reporting and misreporting. In 2001, Charles Vincent (2001) had already published a study based in UK hospitals estimating that 40,000 people may die each year from medical error (halfway between the low and high estimates of the 2008/2009 Commons Committee).

On January 14, 2011, *The Guardian* daily newspaper in the UK published the latest (2009) UK mortality data. The figures show that the biggest killer is circulatory (cardiovascular) disease at approximately 160,000 per annum. Second is cancer at approximately 140,000. Respiratory diseases account for approximately 68,000. The fourth reported killer is digestive disease at around 25,000. What is notably absent from this list is death from medical error. Even if we take the median figure discussed above of 40,000 per annum, this would make medical error the fourth largest killer in the UK after heart, cancer, and respiratory diseases and far outstripping deaths from road traffic accidents, for example (which have fallen over the past decade from >3,000 per annum to around 2,500 per annum). If we take the Commons Committee's upper estimate of 72,000 deaths per annum from medical incidents and accidents, this would make medical error the third largest killer in the UK—truly an iatrogenic epidemic.

Starfield (2000) paints a similar picture for medical error in the USA, noting a total of up to 225,000 deaths per year from iatrogenic causes, which would rank medical error as the third largest killer. This estimate has been tempered recently, again due to lack of reliable sources, so that a US medical malpractice firm claims on its website of April 7, 2011: 'Preventable Medical Errors—sixth biggest killer in America' (http://1800nowhurt.blogspot.com/2011/04/preventable-medical-errors-sixth.html).

Butt (2010) discusses estimates of medical error in Canada following a 2004 Canadian Adverse Events study. Canada has a relatively small population (35 m) and records around 2.5 million hospital admissions per annum. Of these, 185,000 are associated with an adverse event, with 37,000 deaths per annum resulting from medical error. Of adverse events leading to death or injury, an estimated 37 % (70,000) are preventable and anything between 10,000 and 24,000 are highly preventable.

Returning to the USA, Mark Graban's blog of May 26, 2011, claims that 'Hospital errors rank between the fifth and eighth leading cause of death, killing more Americans than breast cancer, traffic accidents or AIDS'. However, as Graban notes, 'I'm once again having trouble finding a single consolidated referenced list of key health-care safety and quality statistics'. Sceptics towards the high estimated incidence of medical error will of course jump on such admissions as demonstrating that we are still a long way from accurately assessing the extent of medical error.

But, putting aside the debate about accuracy of estimated incidence of medical error, what are the sources of such error? Is this bad technical medicine? Why should these figures be of concern to those interested in communication in medicine? The medical malpractice firm's website quoted above suggests that 'Experts believe that if doctors, nurses, dentists, technicians, and other staff were simply more careful, they would make fewer errors'. This is naïve. A significant body of evidence, accumulated over more than a decade (and detailed in subsequent chapters), indicates that 70 % of medical error is due to neither technical incompetence nor personal attention by staff, but rather to systems-based miscommunications, where the basic system is the clinical team (AHRQ, 2008; HealthGrades Quality Study, 2004; Kohn, Corrigan, & Donaldson, 1999). A further 15–20 % of errors are misdiagnoses, where 70–80 % of the diagnosis is grounded in careful listening to the patient's story (Sanders, 2010). It is then vital that we take communication in medicine very seriously, to address this patient safety dilemma.

I will have much more to say about the social and psychological components of patients' presenting symptoms throughout this book and of empathy decline and its possible causes amongst medical students and junior doctors. What then of psychological acumen, self-care, and collaborative care within the profession of medicine? In short, a significant minority of doctors and surgeons do not look after themselves or care to look after themselves; and a significant minority does not appear to develop enough self-insight to know that their communication abilities are poor. Most doctors, however, show self-care and health above the norm—the majority of doctors cultivating healthier lifestyles than the average person (http://news.bbc.co.uk/1/hi/health/944503.stm). But where doctors' self-care slips, it slips badly.

Doctors are more likely to abuse drugs or alcohol, and to suffer from depression, in comparison with other professions (BMA, 2007). Suicide rates for doctors are twice as high as in other professions and more common amongst female than male doctors. While this is often blamed on overwork, high rates of stress, and easy access to drugs, there is another possible cause. This is the historical, structural condition of the culture or institution of medicine itself that applauds the values of self-help and heroic individualism and is rather suspicious of collaborative support (Ludmerer, 1999). These dominant values are archetypally masculine and may conflict with the collaborative values advertised by women physicians at a time when more women than men are entering medicine and more women than men will soon be practising medicine (Bleakley, 2013a).

In terms of viewing figures, the most successful portrayal of a doctor on television is the American series *House, M.D.*, where the British actor Hugh Laurie plays a brilliant but flawed diagnostician, who is inept at communication and interpersonal acumen and also lacks self-insight. The series has a lower profile UK equivalent, 'Monroe', where the anti-hero is a wayward brain surgeon—again a brilliant diagnostician, but flawed emotionally.

'Gregory House' is a fictional character, but is readily identifiable in a line of manipulative and arrogant physicians from Anton Mesmer in the eighteenth century through Jean Charcot in the nineteenth century (who influenced Sigmund Freud) to the quintessentially English actor James Robertson Justice's portrayal of the fictional doctor Sir Lancelot Spratt in the popular 'Doctor' film series of the 1950s and early 1960s. While these are extreme examples, offered to make a point, it is quite extraordinary that, in the twenty-first century, medical students should still be suffering at the hands of some senior doctors who teach by humiliation and who seem incapable of forming a caring and supportive relationship with those students. Readers might object to these rather extreme examples—especially as some are fictional television figures—as unrepresentative of a changing culture and one that now attracts more women students than men. However, in the contemporary world, television portrayals for public consumption are scripted for information as much as entertainment (Bleakley, Bligh, & Browne, 2011). More importantly, the individuals are secondary to the culture of medicine itself, which remains stubbornly autocratic, as the continuing evidence of 'empathy decline', 'moral decline', and 'hardening' amongst medical students and junior doctors suggests.

While these are the symptoms, what are the causes? I will argue that chronic miscommunication in medicine, shown in dysfunctional teams and individual consultations, mirrors medical culture's neurotic condition of heroic individualism. Despite the fact that medicine is fundamentally altruistic ('First, do no harm'), it is also narcissistic or self-interested, in terms of promoting heroic endeavour. This puts the individual on the line and at risk ('Physician, heal thyself'). A strong culture of self-help, grounded in the Protestant 'frontier' mentality, resists and may even scorn collaboration and team effort. Such individualism, or idiosyncrasy, pervades the styles of disciplines, subdisciplines, and units within medical settings—characterized as 'this is the way we do things around here'.

Such individualism is resistant to generalized protocols and even population-based evidence. Michael Millenson (1999) shows how difficult it has been to establish evidence-based practices against the grain of local customs and habits that have, historically, rejected accountability for autonomy. Autonomy is valued above heteronomy, and yet heteronomy or understanding of the other is essential for collaborative, patient-centred care. Kenneth Ludmerer (1999) has carefully traced the current crisis in medical autonomy, as medicine must now become transparent, accountable, and sensitive to patients' needs.

Autonomy is reflected in the desire for 'high physician control', discussed at length in subsequent chapters, where medicine's meritocracy (cultural reward for achievements such as educational attainment) is sometimes mistaken for an autocracy, as medical and surgical cultures arrange themselves hierarchically, indeed quasi-militaristically. This resists democratic structures and learning democratic literacy. The longer-term approach to communication in medicine then has a clear goal: democratizing the culture of medicine itself (Bleakley, 2012c). Medical education has the task of educating future generations of medical students into the knowledge base of democratic literacy and the activities of democratic habits. This is a complex task, but necessary for establishing an authentic patient-centred approach.

Styles of Communication

For over 40 years, I have been helping doctors, health and social care practitioners, clinical psychologists, psychotherapists, and counsellors not only to improve professional communication with patients, clients, or service users but also to improve communication between themselves in mixed professions team settings. This work has focused upon self-awareness, awareness of others, and awareness of the institutional, social, and cultural contexts for work, including historical perspectives.

Over this time, I have seen mostly positive, and often passionate, engagements with the processes of learning how to improve communication in professional helping, caring, or curing relationships. However, amongst this overall welcome response, there have always been pockets of resistance, mainly from doctors and surgeons, along the lines of 'what difference will it make to my clinical work if I also give a patient or a colleague a hug?' This is an affront to those professionals whose work is to educate others in the realm of communication—as if improving communication was not only trivial but also unnecessary. I should be able to shrug this off. The mockery part is easy to deal with, but the reduction of a substantial body of understanding to a 'hug' is difficult to stomach. Not that there is anything wrong with a hug, but this trivializes a complex arena. Not so long ago, however, such critics had a point—they would also ask 'what *evidence* is available that ways of communicating have any real effect on the care of patients or service users?' This kind of pragmatic question has always bothered me in principle, because it goes against common decency of respect for others—but the question nevertheless has to be addressed. Now, we are in a position to answer those sceptics.

Over the years, as medicine itself has committed to an evidence-based approach, research-derived evidence has accumulated to demonstrate that good communication with patients is a health intervention in its own right and not simply a supplement or value-added component to clinical interventions (Funnell & Anderson, 2004; Heisler & Resnicow, 2008). Further, good teamwork offers a health intervention, mainly because it reduces the risk of medical error. This evidence is fully documented throughout this book, but I will introduce a first layer here. As such evidence accumulates, we must ask those sceptical of the importance of communication in medicine: does turning your back on education for communication buck the opening injunction of the Hippocratic Oath—'First, Do No Harm'? Does the absence of good communication associated with particular practitioner styles, or structured within particular specialties in medicine and surgery, potentially do harm? If communication is a health intervention in its own right, then physicians have a moral responsibility to not withhold such an intervention, but to cultivate and improve communication.

Lisa Sanders (2010, p. 7) reminds us of the importance of communicating well with patients by going back to first principles—how is the patient's history received? One of Sir William Osler's most famous maxims is that the greater part of the diagnosis can be gleaned from the patient's history, but, as Sanders reminds us, first we must learn how to listen for the history. From this perspective, 'receiving' a history may be more accurate than 'taking' a history. Sanders says that 'The patient's story is … our oldest diagnostic tool. And, as it turns out, it is one of the most reliable as well. Indeed, the great majority of medical diagnoses—anywhere from 70 to 90 %—are made on the basis of the patient's story alone'. She is drawing here on work over 3 decades, by, for example, Hampton et al. (1975); Levinson, Gorawara-Bhat, and Lamb (2000); Stewart et al. (2003); and Hasnain, Bordage, Connell, and Sinacore (2001).

It might be thought that with the steep introduction of sophisticated imaging and laboratory techniques, diagnosis through the patient's history would have been eclipsed, but, as Sanders (2010, p. 7) claims 'None of our hi-tech tests has such a high batting average' as the history. Further, 'Neither does the physical exam'. As Sanders then goes on to point out, how the history is received is dependent upon how the patient's story is heard or how well the patient is listened to. And here is the rub—doctors on the whole are not particularly good at listening, if the cumulative evidence of studies is to be believed (Roter & Hall, 2006). Sanders suggests that there is a fault line running through the consultation—that doctors use an 'interrogation' method rather than a listening method, where, as she notes, if all you do is ask questions, then all you will get is answers. 'Answers' do not constitute a patient's narrative or story, but, rather, *offer a response to the doctor's narrative style and conventions.*

The interrogative method is rationalized as an efficient information-gathering style, but it may gather the wrong information. Roter and Hall (2006) have expertly summarized the evidence gleaned from over 3 decades of studies of the consultation, and a clear pattern emerges—doctors tend to interrupt patients on average 16 s into the consultation. Seventy-five per cent of doctors cut across the patient's story early in the consultation and interrupt the narrative flow, and as a consequence the patient abandons the narrative in 98 % of cases (see also Sanders, 2010, Chap. 1). The picture held of the consultation by the doctor and the patient can differ considerably, so that each can go away with a different understanding of the nature and outcomes of the visit. Typically, half of consultations end with the patient not having shared the full reason for visiting the doctor or feeling that the full extent of symptoms was not described or investigated.

A collaborative model, suggests Sanders, must replace the interrogation model, where doctor and patient work in partnership. In answer to the predictable response—but surely that will take up more time, and the consultation is short enough as it is—Mauksch, Dugdale, Dodson, and Epstein (2008) have argued that good communication and efficiency can be bedmates in the clinical encounter, where patient-centred and collaborative consultations done well actually save time. As a consequence, patient satisfaction is higher (Stewart et al., 2003). Such patient satisfaction can surely be configured as an outcome of an effective health intervention.

If diagnostic accuracy at the community practitioner stage is improved, then, clearly, referrals will improve. If patient satisfaction, including understanding of symptoms and illness, is improved, then, for example, concordance in prescribing can be achieved, where patients are not expected to comply with a doctor's wishes, but both doctor and patient are expected to understand each other's views, duties of care, moral obligations, and choices (Funnell & Anderson, 2004). This will be grounded in respect for the other.

The Democratic Encounter

Respect for another, and the collaborative engagement of views to achieve a mutually acceptable outcome, is the basis of democracy. The argument presented in this book is based on a premise—that democracy is the optimum form of political structure to inform the work of patient-centred health-care. What precisely is meant by 'democracy' is explored throughout this book. While it is understandable that medical and health-care practitioners should structure technical work through varying levels of knowledge and skills acquired through varying lengths of education and experience (a 'meritocracy'), it is hard to understand why the 'non-technical' domain of expertise (Finn, 2008) as well as the technical should typically be structured as an autocracy within surgery, medicine, and health-care. By that rather ugly descriptor 'non-technical', I mean practices that are shared by all health-care professionals: interpersonal communication and teamwork.

Paradoxically, if the non-technical domain were structured as a meritocracy, nurses may claim that they have a better working knowledge of communication and teamwork than doctors and surgeons. This book argues that democratic working conditions are a prerequisite for authentic patient-centredness, with an understanding that 'democracy' is a complex condition, and ideal to be achieved or a work in progress even in mature democracies such as North American, northern European, or Antipodean. With a differing focus for each chapter, I discuss the complexities of establishing such a democratic culture to build collaborative working partnerships between patients as persons, those who care for patients as persons, those who research the quality of care, and the numerous artifacts that mediate such collaboration, such as machines, drugs, protocols, and research publications.

The gifted clinician and clinical teacher Francis Peabody famously wrote in 1927 that 'The secret of the care of the patient is in caring for the patient' (in Ludmerer, 1999, p. 20). Nearly a century later, a technologically driven medicine may seem to be losing this human face to the consultation, where diagnoses are increasingly mediated by imaging technologies, doctors are tempted to gaze at patients' records on computer screens rather than at the patient himself or herself, and medical students are increasingly exposed to formulaic methods for taking a history and making a diagnosis and treatment plan.

There is now a well-developed movement of 'patient-centred' medicine, but this is largely described in terms of how individual doctors face individual patients. This book addresses a new concern—how do doctors learn to face patients in the multiple and fluid contemporary settings of ad hoc clinical 'teams'? (I highlight 'teams', because as discussed in depth in later chapters, 'team' is a problematic term to describe complex health-care work around patients). This approach demands that we first address the issue of how those teams are composed. How can clinical teams face patients if they cannot first face themselves? By this, I mean working democratically and caringly within and across teams. Further, how might these issues be researched to provide an evidence base for practice? In such research, how might collaboration between clinician researchers and academics be improved, and what is the place and status of patients in medical education research that claims patient benefit as its aim?

Again, research evidence—detailed in later chapters—shows that because teamwork is poor in medicine, patients suffer through avoidable incidents and accidents. It is an imperative for medical education that such patient safety issues are addressed, and I argue that this rests ultimately with democratizing medical practices through medical education. Additionally, as noted already, where between 15 and 20 % of medical errors are grounded in misdiagnoses (Sanders, 2010), we can argue that effective communication, such as careful listening to the patient's story—as introduced earlier—is a central part of good diagnostic work.

Current dominant forms of medical education, however, may be paradoxically and unintentionally undermining patient-centred practice and the practices of effective teamwork. For example, medical students are increasingly learning 'communication skills' (of the kind that I have introduced in the opening to this chapter in talking about the one-to-one consultation, but that must be extended to working collectively with colleagues), including the assessment of the use of these 'skills', through simulation. It is worrying in the first place that the highly complex arena of human communication is reduced to assessable 'skills'. I argue that communication in medicine cannot be reduced to such instrumental skills without losing the heart of the matter—the healing quality of relationship with patients that goes beyond mere skill to mindful presence.

Neither do I think that this presence is simply a gift, waiting to unfold. It is possible to learn to develop professional relationships that are deeply perceptive, caring and discriminating, but these are not the product of learned skills so much as ways of being, honed and adapted through experience and structured reflection on that experience. Development as a professional is a complex process—one of dynamic identity construction or 'becoming' that has been described in detail elsewhere (Bleakley, 2011a).

Further, I see 'teamwork' being reduced to functional strategies that do not clearly address long-standing problems such as professional insulation (often referred to as 'silos') and dysfunctional vertical hierarchies that frustrate new, horizontal ways of working such as 'networking'. Medical education may need to learn a new language for teamworking drawn from complex, adaptive systems thinking, as we move from traditional multiprofessional structures (working with others) to interprofessionalism (working with and learning from and about others), where the patient is also seen as a member of the team's activity. At this point, we might define 'patient-centredness' as 'learning with, from, and about patients' or 'learning to think *with* patients (in mind)' in order to democratize medical practice. This transition in practice has implications for identity construction. The doctor, as professional and specialist (paediatrician, oncologist, and so forth), must now also become an 'interprofessional' teamworker and a team-based, patient-centred, and colleague-centred practitioner.

The challenges for medical education run deep. Doctors are ethically committed to treat regardless of how much this stretches their humanity. Communication with patients (and colleagues) can become a limit experience, affecting the doctor emotionally. The Lithuanian philosopher Emmanuel Levinas (1969) developed a challenging philosophy of relationships as a response of a Jew to the Holocaust. Levinas suggested that the primary aim of philosophy should be the ethics of face-to-face relationships, rather than the pursuit of knowledge for its own sake. Further, we do not get to know the Other by knowing ourselves. It is only by giving up on self-knowing that the 'face' of the Other is revealed. In other words, empathy for the Other precedes self-interest. It is through mindful interest in the Other that self-knowledge emerges. As I explore in this book, this way of seeing the Other in relation to self is central to both the doctor–patient and doctor–colleague relationship.

Levinas then pushes this ethics of relationship to its limits by posing the question: 'can one forgive the ultimate enemy?' (for him, the Nazi perpetrators of the Holocaust). Levinas cannot, of course, say 'yes' or 'no' to this unanswerable question. He poses it as a dilemma for an ethical life's work, suggesting that exercising hospitality towards the Other is a way of 'facing' oneself. Medicine institutionalizes hospitality. Suggesting reversibility of roles, the Latin *hospes* means both host and visitor or guest. *Hospitalia*, the root of 'hospital', literally means a room set on one side for guests. For Levinas, philosophy is the wisdom of love rather than the love of wisdom. An ethics of responsibility precedes the objective search for truth.

Again, I am concerned that, despite the good intentions of those who design and teach communication skills within the undergraduate and postgraduate medicine curricula, the evidence demonstrates that on the whole, doctors are not as good as they could be in communicating with patients and their colleagues in clinical team settings, and this can place both the safety and the health of the patient at risk. Having said this, 'patient-centredness' is surely promised by every contemporary medical education programme. It is a given, treated as transparent. But is this rhetoric rather than reality? Has patient-centredness become a hollow mantra?

The argument for an overhaul, or reconceptualization, of medical education for the future is set out in another book (Bleakley et al., 2011) to which this book can be seen as a companion. Here, the focus is on the quality of face-to-face contact between doctors and patients, and doctors with clinical colleagues, as members of productive teams working for patient benefit. The question of what constitutes good communication with patients and with colleagues in medicine must, in my opinion, be radically reformulated.

The heart of my argument is simple in conception but complex in implementation. Those who live in fully fledged democracies—whatever the relative shortcomings of such democracies—are grateful that they can voice an opinion, engage in debate, support a minority position without fear of reprisal, see equality and equity at work, elect representatives, and help to shape policy. In the practice of medicine, many of those same people walk into the contexts where they must care for patients—clinics, community practices, operating theatres—and slot in to ready-made hierarchies and behave according to rank, where democratic citizens suddenly transform into institutional autocrats or bureaucrats. This undermines the meaning of 'hospital' as a place where hospitality is extended. Those who advocate such hierarchies rationalize them as meritocracies, based on relative levels of technical skill, but such an argument does not hold water in the realm of the 'non-technical', or shared, practices of communication, teamwork, and situation awareness (Bleakley, Allard, & Hobbs, 2013) that, as a body of research shows, have an impact on the quality of patient safety.

In Chaps. 2 and 3, I unpack this conundrum, arguing that we need to establish healthier democratic ways of working in medicine to improve patient care, patient safety, and practitioner morale and work satisfaction. I argue, realizing that this is a strong claim, that if medicine does not make a cultural shift from weak autocracy and meritocracy to full democracy, it will remain a relatively 'high-risk' culture rather than a 'high-reliability' culture. I further argue that the realization of the 'common wealth' of both the doctor–patient encounter and the encounters between colleagues in clinical team settings is often frustrated.

Chapter 2 expands the rationale for this book—based on the alarming evidence that there is a persistent iatrogenic epidemic of medical error grounded not in poor technical performance, but in poor non-technical (communication) performance. Such underachievement or underperformance is referred to as a 'hypocompetence', because it can be positively addressed or remedied to a significant extent. In brief, medical error grounded in poor communication between colleagues in teams and with patients offers a major source of risk for patients. This source of risk is, as we have seen, far higher than that of road traffic accidents and is unacceptable because such risk is in large part remediable.

In Chap. 2, I argue firstly that communication skills training in medical education is necessary, but not sufficient to address communication hypocompetence. Secondly, poor communication is a symptom of medical culture's ingrained autocracy that can be treated by culture change. Thirdly—and what may at first sight appear to be a radical recommendation—I argue that democratization of medical culture can be initiated not by more communication skills training in the narrow sense, such as instrumental clinical skills approaches, but by a humanizing of physicians through their early medical education. This can be achieved through provision of a core, integrated medical humanities in the undergraduate curriculum to provide the conditions of possibility to improve patient care and safety, an argument set out fully in Chap. 2. As noted earlier, the values and practices of such a humane medicine are not the product of learned skills so much as ways of being, honed and adapted through experience and structured reflection on that experience.

In order to set the ideas put forward in Chaps. 2 and 3 in a conceptually rigorous frame, I discuss some contemporary ideas of power, authority, legitimacy, and identity that help to explore why it is difficult for medicine to make the transition from a weak autocracy and meritocracy to a fully fledged democracy and why it is essential for optimal patient care that such a transformation does occur. More importantly, I outline the conditions of possibility for this process of transformation to occur.

In Chaps. 4–7, I argue that the patient is the heart of the matter in medicine and medical education, and critically review models of patient-centredness. Patients are central to key aspects of the clinical reasoning process, previously thought to be the primary domain of doctors based on technical knowledge. There are narrative dimensions to clinical reasoning in particular, where patients self-evidently hold expertise concerning their own symptoms and treatment.

'Patient-centredness' offers conceptual confusion, where the future of communication in medicine is not necessarily about 'centres' at all. Indeed, centres—including the traditional self-centred autonomy of physicians—afford the problem, not the solution. In the dynamic, often messy, and certainly complex settings of clinical teams, patterns and styles of teamworking (reformulated here as varieties of 'knotworking' and 'networking'—terms I explore and explain fully in Chaps. 10 and 11) offer strategies for effective patient-centred care. Importantly, drawing on terms from complexity theory (Bleakley, 2010), discussed fully in Chap. 15, 'knotworks' and 'networks' do not have 'centres', but varieties of 'attractors' or multiple hot spots permanently in transition and dynamic emergence.

In Chap. 8, written in collaboration with Dr Robert Marshall, an experienced consultant histopathologist, we investigate the status of empathy in doctor–patient relationships through a critical review of the term 'empathy'. We argue that empathy is a contemporary notion describing an instrumental skill, rather than a state of being and becoming. We return the reader to Homer's discussion of 'pity' in an attempt to restore value to this now widely abused descriptor. We alert readers to absence of conceptual rigour in discussing communication in medicine, especially in providing a historical dimension. Entertaining the idea that empathy is not a skill, but a virtue, leads us to critically explore the popular notion of 'professionalism'— the set of dispositions and practices that make up the 'non-technical' face of medicine.

Chapter 9 explores the implications for the current shift in gender in medicine, where medical schools worldwide are now matriculating more women than men. Will this gender shift permeate practice by introducing, to borrow William James' terms, a 'tender-minded' dimension to a conventionally 'tough-minded' culture, where tender-mindedness may be necessary for patient-centredness? Importantly, does medical education have literacy in gender theory, especially contemporary feminisms, to better understand these gender issues?

Chapters 10–15 explore how the landscape of teamworking in medicine, surgery, and health-care is changing, drawing on new models for analyzing work-based activity. I draw in particular on five theoretical perspectives to illustrate the rich character of current thinking about team practices, where theory itself is taken as a practice: (1) cultural–historical activity theory (CHAT), (2) Foucauldian models of resistance, (3) actor-network-theory (ANT), (4) Deleuzian rhizomatics, and (5) complexity theory. Each of these descriptors will, of course, be fully explained in these respective chapters.

Each perspective intimately ties team process to constructions of practitioner identities—or, what I do is what I become. But the 'doing' can be an explicit act of resistance, such as speaking up or speaking out against another's perceived or measured poor practice, on behalf of the patient. The coming together in 'team' settings can be less about continuity and more about adaptability, in fluid work settings where identities are also labile. Complex inter-team working around patients, perhaps the hallmark of the twenty-first-century health-care, may be best understood as initiating and maintaining networks without centres.

The notion of 'team' itself is then challenged, as a static abstraction—to be replaced by descriptions of complex, dynamic, and adaptive activities such as 'teeming', 'networking', and 'knotworking'. Here, 'team' is not a prior concept to be fulfilled, but is *performed* rather than *preformed*. 'Teams' are *achieved*—through what actor-network-theory (Bleakley, 2012a, 2012b) describes as 'forming alliances' through mediators such as dialogue, innovations in practice, and forms of resistance to unproductive, habitual, or sterile practices. Illustrative examples are given throughout, to bring these new notions alive and to help readers to deal with what may be a new vocabulary to describe seemingly familiar territory. In this, I hope to make the familiar unfamiliar, in an effort to reformulate the territory of communication in medicine.

Having argued that medical education can democratize medicine, in the penultimate Chap. 16, I argue that medical education in turn can be democratized by medical education research, developing a theme first set out in *Medical Education for the Future: Identity, Power and Location* (Bleakley et al., 2011). Here, I describe the value of an evidence-based medical education, where healthy debate about evidence should lead to less idiosyncratic and more democratically shaped practices.

While medical education research might employ collaborative practices in the pursuit of best evidence, how do researchers collaborate in environments that are framed as competitive, even cut-throat? Further, how do clinicians and academic researchers collaborate where they are grounded in differing communities of practice and show related allegiances? Finally, how is interdisciplinarity achieved for practitioner-researchers from differing professions and specialties and for academic researchers across differing disciplines?

In the final Chap. 17, I offer a provocative summary of the main arguments of the book, to plead again for learning democratic habits and literacy in democracy.

My plea is made against the background of a reminder of medicine's own (untreated) neuroses, as if putting medicine on the couch, where the suggested cure to medicine's shortcomings (communication hypocompetence) is a range of democratic habits. However tough and shifting 'democracy' and processes of 'democratization' may appear; without such literacy, we will not be able to address the structural problems that distort the potential for communication in medicine and place patients at risk through poor communication and miscommunication in various health-care settings, as detailed in Chap. 2.

This book takes a fresh look at communication, teamwork, and, to some extent, professionalism (ethical practice) in medicine. 'Professing' a medical identity, or becoming a medical practitioner, requires new forms of ethical practice in the liquid worlds of 'networking' and 'knotworking'. The first moral requirement in medicine is to take on the identity of the capable communicator in order to uphold the Hippocratic Corpus' 'First, Do No Harm'.

Professions allied to medicine and surgery share non-technical aspects of work, and these aspects overlap with lay (patient and service user) expertise. Again, as we accumulate evidence, it becomes clearer that good communication is a health intervention in its own right, supplementing the technical interventions provided by doctors and other members of the clinical team. As I suggested earlier, withholding such communication expertise is then unethical, indeed amoral as it demeans the humanity of the patient as Other.

Returning to a point made earlier, given that doctors shall 'first, do no harm', it is again unacceptable that communication in medicine is not a priority in medical education. While I argue that medical education can take a major leap in improving communication and teamwork, this will depend upon revising our conceptual understanding of what we mean by 'good' communication, professional behaviour, and 'teams'. Once the conceptual apparatus has been reformulated for understanding communication in health-care, based on contemporary thinking and associated evidence, this of course has implications for how communication and teamwork are taught and learned, particularly in the undergraduate medicine and surgery curriculum.

Such curriculum translation is of course under constant discussion and trial in medical education (Bleakley, 2009, 2012d). In short, a radical curriculum overhaul is required. Just as problem-based learning constituted the last pedagogic revolution in medical education, the next paradigm shift must be to patient-based learning, accepting that 'patient' is best understood as 'person' who is now presenting with some limiting symptom or condition—a person whose 'illness' will quickly be medicalized, as 'disease'. This is a person in a social context, and the contextual 'illness' may be 'homelessness' rather than pneumonia; domestic abuse and broken families rather than contusions and broken bones; a food disorder (such as additives, high sugar, salt, or fat content) rather than an eating disorder; or an understandable response to a manic culture and stressful job rather than depression. Further, this person will now often be well informed about his or her symptoms through Internet search and, in the case of persons suffering from multiple chronic illnesses, will be experts in their own conditions (Mol, 2008).

In summary, fundamental to change across medicine to improve patient benefit is the proper establishment of democratic participation—first, in genuinely collaborative practices that do not pay mere lip service to 'patient-centredness', and second, in the dismantling of unproductive hierarchies in clinical teams through establishing open dialogue between team members.

Part I
Communication in Medicine: Democracy and Its Discontents

Chapter 2
Communication Hypocompetence: An Iatrogenic Epidemic

Introduction

Writing in the American Medical Student Association's journal *The New Physician,* a fourth year student, Adam Carlisle (Carlisle et al. 2010), suggested that 'We train clinicians to … practice evidence-based medicine …. However, we do not train them to care'. This remark is understandable but misplaced. Carlisle opposes the science of medicine and the art of care, where these practices should not have been opposed in the first place and can be readily reconciled. 'Science' is also an art, having a wide aesthetic brief. Science can be beautiful, imaginative, and well designed and introduces both complexity and uncertainty. Indeed, as contemporary medicine becomes increasingly complex, so it must draw on complexity theory to understand the relationship between science theory and application. More importantly for the theme of this book, the 'care' aspect of medicine—with communication as the heart of the matter—has an evidence base and can be considered scientifically.

We can frame 'care' as an evidence-based practice grounded in the science of communication that turns clinical knowledge into patient benefit. Where communication skills training in medical education has failed to reverse 'empathy decline' in medical students, I will develop an argument that evidence-based care may be best learned through the medical humanities, integrated into the core, scientific medicine curriculum. In time, this curriculum intervention may serve to challenge and transform habitual autocracy in medical culture to produce democratic working patterns that, in turn, improve communication and teamwork for patient benefit and safety.

A. Bleakley, *Patient-Centred Medicine in Transition: The Heart of the Matter,* Advances in Medical Education 3, DOI 10.1007/978-3-319-02487-5_2, © Springer International Publishing Switzerland 2014

An Epidemic of Medicine's Own Making

While the power of applied technical medicine grows exponentially, this book argues that medicine's Achilles' heel is elsewhere, in the 'nontechnical' aspects of work—communication and shared decision-making with colleagues in team settings and with patients in consultations. To rehearse the argument introduced in the previous chapter and developed throughout this book, there is a cumulative evidence base detailing an iatrogenic effect that has reached epidemic proportions, where patients' health and safety are placed at risk through poor communication, making a mockery of the Hippocratic Corpus': 'First, do no harm'.

The seminal 1999 Institute of Medicine (IOM) report concluded that medical errors caused as many as 98,000 deaths annually in the USA (Kohn, Corrigan, & Donaldson, 1999). While this estimate was initially questioned on the basis of methodological rigour (Sox & Woloshin, 2000), subsequent studies suggest that the IOM study underestimated the problem. An audit of 37 million patient records doubled the IOM estimate, suggesting that as many as 195,000 Medicare patients died due to potentially preventable, hospital-based medical errors in each of the years 2000–2002 (HealthGrades Quality Study, 2004). Starfield (2000), noting that 40 million people in the USA do not have health insurance, increased the estimate to 225,000 deaths per year. If this estimate were accurate, medical error would be the third cause of death after heart disease and cancer in the USA.

The Agency for Health-care Research and Quality (2008, p. 8) produced the first US national governmental report on health-care quality, recognizing that while 'Tracking trends in patient safety is complicated by difficulties assessing and ensuring the systematic reporting of medical errors and patient safety events', nevertheless 'approximately one out of seven adult hospitalized Medicare patients experiences one or more adverse events'. Over the period of 5 years prior to the report's publication, while medical outcomes improved, quality of patient safety decreased. This is like driving a car with the brakes engaged. HealthGrades produced a further study in 2008, drawing on Medicare data from 2004 to 2006. While optimistic about an upturn in patient safety awareness, the report still found more than a million patient safety incidents in 40 million hospitalizations and a large disparity between the best and worst performing hospitals (HealthGrades Quality Study, 2008). Literally adding insult to injury, the medical profession has a poor record of apologizing to patients and their families in the wake of medical error (Truog, Browning, Johnson, & Gallagher, 2011).

What can be done to fully acknowledge and then address this iatrogenic epidemic? The AHRQ (2008, p. 5) study noted that an upturn in patient safety outcomes could be established 'by improving communication and teamwork skills among health professionals'. Xyrichis and Ream (2008, p. 232) suggested that an estimated '70–80 % of health-care errors are caused by human factors associated with poor team communication and understanding' and that 50 % of such error could be avoided through improving team-based communication. The IOM (1999) study had estimated that 72 % of hospital deaths due to medical errors were grounded in communication errors, and a 2004 US study of 2,455 patient safety events concluded that 70 % were the result of systems-based miscommunications (JCAHO, 2004), where the basic system is the clinical team. This high level of medical error with a root cause in communication may be due to what Platt (1979) called 'clinical hypocompetence' based on a 'high control style' exerted by doctors. In the context of medical education, 'hypocompetence' has been defined as a performance deficiency in clinical competence, including communication (Pilpel, Schor, & Benbassat, 1998, p. 5), but 'clinical hypocompetence' may be better termed 'communication hypocompetence'.

Gathering and reporting statistics is the prelude to explaining them. We need to know *why* poor communication is happening, to map the contributing factors so that we can intervene appropriately. Such factors centrally include doctors' styles of working that cannot be reduced to personality effects but reflect wider cultural norms in medicine. For example, Platt's (1979) early work observing over 300 clinical interviews noted 'high control style' in doctors' consultations with patients. This was not just a product of its time. Recognizing the persistence of 'high physician control', Boyle, Dwinnell, and Platt (2005, p. 29) developed the 'invite, listen, and summarize' 'patient-centred communication technique', recognizing that 'high physician control' contributes to poor communication as it frustrates information flow from the patient that may, for example, be essential to diagnosis.

Communication with colleagues can also show hypocompetence and high control styles. In a study of 444 surgical malpractice claims from four liability insurers, 60 cases involved communication breakdown leading to harm to the patient. Attending surgeons were the most common team members involved in poor communications, and 'status asymmetry' was described as the main causative factor (Greenberg et al., 2007). 'Status asymmetry' describes how differences between members of a team, such as a surgeon, anaesthetist, and nurse, are played out in terms of an unproductive hierarchy.

Differences in educational experience and subsequent technical knowledge and skill constitute a meritocracy. How these differences are expressed is important to quality of teamwork, where evidence from large-scale studies shows that collaborative teamwork can greatly improve patient outcomes (West & Borrill, 2002; Harden, 2011). 'Status asymmetry' typically describes autocratic working patterns, where those at the top exert power that is authoritarian or bullying, resisting democratic participation and collaboration.

A second factor hindering communication is that doctors generally do not listen well to patients, as a meta-review of studies of communication between doctor and patient shows (Roter & Hall, 2006). On average, doctors interrupt patients 16 s into the consultation. Seventy-five per cent of doctors cut across the patient's story early in the consultation and interrupt the narrative flow—as a consequence the patient abandons the narrative in 98 % of cases. Sanders (2010) suggests that there is a fault line running through the consultation—that doctors use an 'interrogation' method rather than a listening method, where if all you do is ask questions, then all you will get is answers. 'Answers' do not constitute a patient's narrative or story, but, rather, offer a response to the doctor's narrative style and conventions.

The interrogative method is rationalized as an efficient information-gathering style, but it may gather the wrong information. A literature review revealed only nine studies of communication with patients focusing on efficiency, but showed that patient-centred consultations not only lead to increased patient satisfaction, but also save time (Mauksch, Dugdale, Dodson, & Epstein, 2008), and a comprehensive literature review revealed that a significant result of poor communication by physicians is an increased likelihood of complaints by patients (Laidlaw & Hart, 2011).

A third area of concern linking medical error and communication is diagnostic errors, which result in an estimated 80,000 deaths annually (Winters, Aswani, & Pronovost, 2011), and where 17 % of patients in the hospital suffer from misdiagnoses (Sanders, 2010). These figures must remain estimates where there is no valid mechanism to measure diagnostic error, but a 25 % discordance between ante- and post-mortem diagnoses offers some guidance (Swaro & Adhiyaman, 2010). Graber Franklin, and Gordon (2005) conducted a retrospective study of 100 cases of diagnostic error from three medical centres over a period of 5 years to conclude that the main cause of diagnostic error is premature closure (stopping considering other possibilities once a diagnosis is reached). Norman and Eva (2010) undertook a rigorous analytic review of Graber's and others' studies to suggest that premature closure may include physicians not thinking of the correct diagnosis and then not gathering relevant data. This may suggest lack of technical skill. Sanders (2010, p. 7), however, suggests that 'anywhere from 70 to 90 percent' of the diagnosis is grounded in the patient's 'story', and 'this is well established'—although only one relevant study is cited in support (Hasnain, Bordage, Connell, & Sinacore, 2001). Sanders (2010, p. 7) further suggests that neither the physical examination nor hi-tech tests have 'such a high batting average' as the history in diagnosis.

Communication Skills Training

Evidence gleaned from the science of communication then articulates the symptoms of communication hypocompetence in medicine and also the level of the iatrogenic effect. Does appropriate treatment, based in medical education, follow? Although training in communication skills was formally established across medical schools 3 decades ago (Waitzkin, 1984), communication hypocompetence and 'empathy decline' (Pedersen, 2010) persist. 'Empathy decline' describes students gradually losing initial idealism as they meet the realities of clinical work and the 'hidden curriculum' of medical culture, including pervasive cynicism and autocracy (Hojat et al., 2009). Evidence for empathy decline has been challenged on the basis of validity of studies, including reliance on folk wisdom (Colliver, Conlee, Verhulst, & Dorsey, 2010), but a systematic review of studies shows that empathy decline is a valid and widespread phenomenon (Neumann et al., 2011). Maintaining empathy is important as it correlates with improved patient outcomes, for example, in diabetics (Hojat et al., 2011).

Where 'status asymmetry' has been identified as the main cause of poor communication in teams, this is a polite way of recognizing the communication style of many senior doctors as dysfunctional. Autocratic behaviour stifles collaboration and collective moral responsibility, producing environments that put patients at risk. Doctors continue to reinforce hierarchies, characteristically viewing 'teamwork as a form in which nurses (are) subordinate' (Xyrichis & Ream, 2008, p. 236). 'Accepting hierarchy' has been described as one of the key aspects to the hidden curriculum in medical education (Lempp & Seale, 2004). Transition from high-risk to high-reliability medicine requires culture change, a transformation of values and institutional structures—in short, a democratizing of medical culture. The iatrogenic effects of poor communication between colleagues, and between doctors and patients, may be due to the primacy of an interrogative, rather than a collaborative, model.

The Role of the Medical Humanities

What has this litany of evidence from studies of communication in medicine got to do with the medical humanities? Traditionally, the 'medical humanities' describe the study of medicine from the perspective of differing humanities, such as the history or philosophy of medicine or doctors as subject matter in literature. More recently, 'medical humanities' signify the introduction of arts and humanities *ways of thinking* into medical education—this might involve clinicians working with visual artists to improve close noticing for diagnostic acumen (Kirklin, Duncan, McBride, Hunt, & Griffin, 2007), or the use of literature scholars and writers to educate 'narrative intelligence' towards patients' stories to improve reception of the history (Charon, 2011).

Two reviews of the literature on the impact of the medical humanities in medical education reveal a catalogue of small-scale, often poorly designed studies. Ousager and Johannessen (2010, p. 988) consulted 245 articles but found only nine that gave evidence of long-term impacts of medical humanities interventions such that 'Evidence on the positive long-term impacts of integrating humanities into undergraduate medical education is sparse', and this may threaten planned provision in an evidence-based era. The review of Wershof Schwartz and colleagues (Wershof Schwartz et al., 2009, p. 377) is less comprehensive, but raises a wider set of conceptual issues. Study effects are claimed in three main areas: humanities input promotes empathy, professionalism, and self-care in medical students. Interplay of variables, biased populations of self-selecting students, and poor conceptualization confound such studies. For example, there is a strong argument that the wider values of 'humanism' may be conceptually different from, and in conflict with, the narrower confines of 'medical professionalism' in areas such as compliance. Further, the review concludes 'few data are available to support the hypothesis that humanities affects professional behaviour'.

Such outcome studies are, scientifically, focused upon proof of intervention, and it may be that there is more value in focus upon proof of concept (or principle)—a realization of an idea to demonstrate its feasibility. For example, rather than provide a humanities intervention to increase empathy and carry out a before-and-after study of changes in empathy scores on a scale, we might focus upon proof of the concept of empathy as an idea by demonstrating the conceptual feasibility of the idea in explaining a paradoxical practice dilemma.

A critical literature review of over 120 studies of empathy development through medical education concluded that persistent empathy decline might be explained as an effect of a growing polarization of the 'hard' biomedical elements and the 'soft' communication elements, leading to the perception of communication and the humanities as peripheral (Pedersen, 2010). A curriculum adjustment is needed, where 'Empathy training and the humanities should not be situated outside the hard core of medicine' (Pedersen, 2010, p. 593). By 'hard core', Pedersen means biomedical science. How science is translated into clinical practice, for example, in clinical reasoning and diagnostic work, centrally involves quality of relationship with patients and colleagues, so that the humanities may be seen as part of the process of translating science into care.

It is a short step from Pedersen's review to suggest that medicine as a 'science using' practice requires a medium for translation of scientific knowledge, and that medium is the humanities. The place of the humanities within the curriculum must then be reconsidered, with humanities as core and integrated. For Pedersen (2010, p. 599), empathy and the humanities should not provide 'soft add-ons' to the curriculum, as this 'may cloak medicine's hard edges instead of drawing attention to the systems and paradigms shaping these hard edges'. We could rephrase this as suggesting that the humanities bring a necessary tender-minded perspective to the traditionally tough-minded culture of biomedical science.

The arts and humanities, as core, integrated provision within medical schools, can provide the longer-term democratizing force necessary to change medical culture, promoting the conditions that may make safer health-care possible. Nussbaum (2010) argues for the humanities (including the arts) as the chief cultural force for promoting democracy, where the humanities diagnose social ills, such as groundless authority supporting unproductive habits, and suggest cures, such as tolerance of difference, and creative debate about quality of life. If we transpose Nussbaum's argument for the humanities as a democratizing force in wider culture to medical culture in particular, the medical humanities may play a bigger role in medical education than we imagine. *The arts and humanities may provide the contextual media through which the lessons of the science of communication in medicine are best learned and promoted.*

Drawing on the developmental psychiatry of Winnicott, Nussbaum argues that social play is essential to the development of tolerance for others and appreciation of their vulnerabilities (empathy). Where imaginative play is curtailed, children fail to learn how to collaborate and retain controlling behaviour as a means of dealing with uncertainty (the very symptom that medical culture grapples with). Transition to democratic participation as adults requires what Winnicott (1971) called 'potential space'—the arts and humanities as an adult equivalent of 'play'—where tolerance of ambiguity, as the basis to learning respect for others by resisting 'premature closure' on judgment, is reinforced. In contrast, authoritarianism, which is typical of medicine, is characterized by intolerance of ambiguity. 'Respect' for others can work within three broad social and political structures: autocracy, meritocracy, and democracy. In an autocratic structure, respect is arranged vertically and hierarchically in an upward flow, where those above have authority over those below, but this may be exerted as repression. In a meritocracy, while a vertical system may hold as an expression of merit through, say, educational achievement, such status is not wielded in an authoritarian manner. In a democracy, respect for others is equated with horizontal collaboration, sharing, and empathy—especially for those who are in need.

Luther and Crandall (2011, pp. 799–800) point out that while practising medicine demands high tolerance of ambiguity, 'the culture of medicine has little tolerance for ambiguity and uncertainty'; yet physicians who are less tolerant of ambiguity tend to order more unnecessary tests and additional treatments for patients, placing a burden upon patients and the health-care system. The purpose of the humanities is to create, and debate, uncertainty and ambiguity, which is central to the democratic experiment (Nussbaum, 2010). From a survey of 313 graduating medical students over a period of 10 years (59 % return rate), those who scored high on an intolerance of ambiguity scale were also found to show significantly greater negative attitudes towards underserved and poor patients (Wayne et al., 2011). Luther and Crandall (2011, p. 800) suggest that such tolerance of ambiguity decline can be addressed through curricular emphasis upon communication skills and professionalism through small group discussion, 'for reminding students of their own humanity and help them learn to connect with the humanity we all share'. This territory is ripe for a medical humanities intervention beyond 'communication skills', where decline in both empathy and tolerance of ambiguity offers faces of the same symptom—communication hypocompetence.

Evidence

I have set out an argument for introducing a core, integrated medical humanities provision to undergraduate medical education with a long-term aim to democratize medical culture by realizing the science behind the medical humanities. Is this a realistic goal, and is there any initial evidence for its claims? Does this argument simply constitute a manifesto, or does it have the status of a hypothesis that can be tested, or can research questions be generated from it?

A special edition of *Academic Medicine* (Albanese, Snow, Skochelak, Huggett, & Farrell, 2003) devoted to 'the humanities and medicine' attracted 'reports of 41 U.S., Canadian and International programs'. Nearly a decade on from this special edition, the New York University 'Medical Humanities' website (http://medhum.med.nyu.edu/) shows global growth in medical humanities provision.

Quantity does not of course guarantee quality, and the high number of schools providing some form of medical humanities provision disguises the fact that much of this consists of peripheral curriculum input such as short, optional study units. Further, both theoretical rationale for and well-designed evaluation of provision are lacking. The medical humanities are still habitually pitched against medical science, as compensation, rather than aligned with science. Accounts of the science behind the medical humanities are notably absent.

However, we can look forward to a new wave of scholarship aligning the humanities and medical science, resulting in curriculum reformulation such as developing the medical humanities as core, integrated provision. Riggs (2010, p. 1669) reminds us that, at the centenary of Abraham Flexner's 1910 report that revolutionized the structure of medical education, we should be ready for another, radical, wave of reform in preparing doctors of the future. Drawing on Flexner's call to produce doctors with an educated 'ethical responsibility', 'medical education could be on the cusp of another set of great advances by renewing interest in medical humanities'. Doukas, McCullough, and Wear (2010, p. 318) note that Flexner viewed a humanities education as essential to medical practice, but assumed that medical students would have already received a liberal education before embarking on medical studies.

The authors note that medical humanities education is generally not well designed and is not integrated with the scientific/clinical curriculum. They propose that medical schools could consider 'clinically relevant humanities teaching to train medical students and residents comprehensively in humane, professional patient care', to follow Pedersen's (2010) suggestion of integrating the humanities into the 'hard core of medicine'.

In an echo of Flexner, the Mount Sinai School of Medicine in New York has evaluated the impact of humanities in medical education not by evaluating a medical humanities curriculum provision, but by comparing students who enter the medicine programme as science or humanities and social sciences graduates without traditional premedical requirements requiring only a summer crash course (Muller & Kase, 2010; Wershof Schwartz et al., 2009). A carefully designed matched cohorts evaluation study over 6 years of intake shows that these 'medicine humanities' entrants perform overall as well as traditional students when compared across knowledge and performance, including basic science, by year 3. This does not demonstrate a significant advantage in bringing humanities expertise into medicine; rather, it demonstrates that medical students may not need the volume of science input that characterizes medicine programmes and that the humanities and science can settle down into productive conversation. Indeed, nearly 15 % of medical school applicants in the USA are humanities and social science majors, where the best predictor of success is overall academic ability (Wershof Schwartz et al., 2009).

Shapiro (2008) suggests that the key ethical dilemma in modern medicine is that it raises false hopes by first failing to recognize its own limits and, second, for all the good that it does in terms of cure and care, passing on false hope to patients. Students must not be drawn into a bubble of invulnerability, but must face the reality of their limits and the limits to medicine, as 'an ethics of imperfection'. Shapiro (2008, p. 11) also recognizes that current medical educational approaches introduced to promote empathy and humanistic values have limited success and that 'We must excavate more deeply to understand what interferes with learners' impulses and desires to express empathy toward patients'.

However, Shapiro chooses to not excavate medical culture for a potential fault line, but looks to the influence of wider culture—in the values of idealism inherent in modernism that promote cure and perfection, pointing to the heroic need to conquer and control illness. But this does not seem to me to be an explanation for, but a description of, symptom. We need to establish what causes the desire for perfection and control in the first place. This suggestion is not an original one and was articulated by Adorno and colleagues (1950) after the Holocaust, as they traced the psychological structure they termed 'the authoritarian personality'. At the core of authoritarianism is 'intolerance of ambiguity', where the need to control comes from a fear of being out of control. Modern medical culture does not so much have an authority problem as a fear of vulnerability or tenderness.

Conclusion

My approach in this chapter has been to shift emphasis away from potentially doomed (because riddled with confounding variables) scientific studies on specific humanities interventions to utilizing what we know from communication science to address 'communication hypocompetence' in a much wider fashion—first through proof of concept by rigorous conceptualization and second as a more encompassing and long-term curriculum-level intervention aimed at democratizing medical culture.

I also see a key role for the medical humanities as exploring the intrinsic artistry and humanity of scientific practice, and the wonder and beauty of the life sciences, on the basis that appreciation precedes, but also enhances, explanation. The place of the medical humanities in medical education currently mirrors the stage of the early history of medical ethics, once peripheral and now core. The medical humanities should follow, based not on anecdote, but on careful and caring science.

Chapter 3
Democracy in Medicine

Medicine Is by Nature a Political Domain

Aristotle famously claimed that humans are by nature political animals. Paul Cartledge (2009, p. 3) suggests that humans 'fulfil (their) potential within and only within the *polis* political framework'. The *polis* for the ancient Greeks included both the city-states, or urban centres, and a city's associated *khora*—the surrounding rural territories. Aristotle suggested that humans could not organize themselves socially without the exercise of power, and politics is the study of these forms of power. Traditionally, then, politics works at the level of kinds of cultures, nations, or states, such as 'liberal democracies', 'socialist states', and 'Islamic nations'. This is macropolitics. Politics is also employed at the level of the organization or institution, such as the United Nations, the welfare state, or a single hospital. This is mesopolitics. Finally, the political perspective can be employed to better understand a small group or a team. This is micropolitics. It is the concern of this book to better understand micropolitics in medical settings in order to inform improvements in patient care. I will argue that the patient should not be a bystander to, but an active participant in, such micropolitics.

By 'politics', I do not mean party politics, but the study of the *polis*—cultures, communities, and groups of people who are collaboratively working out ways of being. In medicine and health-care, this can be seen as professionals working together to maximize provision of care and hospitality for patients, in collaboration with those patients. As a body of potential participants in a democracy, patients may be characterized as a plurality of individuals or the 'multitude' (Hardt & Negri, 2006). Professionals such as doctors and health-care practitioners may forget that they too are part of the multitude and they too are 'patients' when they are ill (Sweeney, Toy, & Cornwell, 2009). The democracy these professionals take for granted in their everyday lives outside of work, whatever their party political persuasion, is—strangely—abandoned by many of them as they adopt their professional identities. This paradox is addressed throughout this book.

A. Bleakley, *Patient-Centred Medicine in Transition: The Heart of the Matter*,
Advances in Medical Education 3, DOI 10.1007/978-3-319-02487-5_3,
© Springer International Publishing Switzerland 2014

Talk of politics will naturally turn to talk of power. Power has traditionally been conceived as sovereign or 'power over'—the exercise of authority or leadership. Those invested with power due to birth, or sometimes those who have claimed power through force, can exert power as a 'state of exception' above and beyond the law. For example, a secular power can make autonomous decisions based on the threat of aggression by another nation; or a religious ruler can exert power based on a transcendental principle derived from religious law. In democracies, a common form of sovereign power is expert power, grounded in relative levels of skill, technique, or knowledge (French & Raven, 1959). The latter typically offers the fabric of a medical or health-care hierarchy.

Hardt and Negri (2009), amongst others, point to the decline of distant sovereign power in everyday life and the importance of a pervasive 'capillary' power that reaches, often subtly and relatively unnoticed, into individual bodies. Michel Foucault (2002) called this 'biopower'—a micropower, where primary forms of power are not used overtly to coerce or control, but power is ubiquitous, present as a force in any system, and utilized also as a form of resistance. The taken-for-granted or apparently transparent and even superficial aspects of our lives, such as the daily commerce of manners and social exchanges, the way we dress, our habits of cleanliness, and of course our self-care as far as health is concerned, are described by Foucault (1987) as regimes of 'self forming' or the shaping of selves. Such regimes not only subtly control behaviour and feelings without the presence of a finger-wagging authority figure, but also create and transform identities.

Foucault thus draws attention to the intersection of power, ethics, and aesthetics—politics as shaping of forms of becoming and being, or active, conscious and reflexive ways of making self and living a life. The beauty of Foucault's method rests in his insistence upon thinking the unthinkable paradox—that identities can be formed, unformed, and reformed within a dual process of *both* a convention-driven socialization (such as entry into the profession of medicine or the sub-professions of surgery or psychiatry) *and* patterns of resistance (challenging and reshaping of norms, including idiosyncratic self-forming).

The need to clean one's teeth, or to resist this, or to transform this into a celebrity smile through expensive cosmetic whitening, or to hope to achieve this celebrity smile in a different socio-economic group through an inexpensive one-off treatment, or to engage in preventive dentistry, or to resist the dominant flow of power through having a diamond stud embedded in a front tooth or a complete replacement set of gold teeth—all of these are examples of capillary power at work as a biopower, operating at the level of bodily function, bodily expression, and identity construction.

Clearly, medicine is implicated in such forms of power. Doctors do not simply exercise legitimate authority over patients through expert knowledge. Rather, they engage in complex forms of negotiation with patients where sovereign power is mainly displaced by capillary biopower as regimes of 'health' and bodily practices (such as 'cleanliness'). These are micropolitical acts that come to form and reform identities, define what is normal and abnormal or healthy and unhealthy, resist or comply with economic constraints or political pressures, and so forth.

As a burgeoning literature on Foucauldian approaches to medicine argues, medicine and its public health reach in particular are necessarily political at the level of capillary network, reaching into everyday behaviours such as hygiene (Bleakley & Bligh, 2009; Petersen & Bunton, 1997).

Articulating a Common Wealth

Shakespeare's *The Tempest* (1623) offers a commentary on a hotly debated issue in the early seventeenth century—the possibility of setting up utopian communities—based on reports from British settlers in Virginia, the New World. Alonso, the King of Naples, and his son Ferdinand have been shipwrecked. Ferdinand is washed up on one part of the island, while Alonso, Gonzalo (a sage and counsellor to the king), and others are washed up on another part of the island. While looking for Ferdinand, this latter group begins to engage with the island's geography and character. Shakespeare casts the island as a territory to be populated by differing ideas and ideals—a screen upon which differing models of social life can be projected and tested.

A key tension in life that is replayed on the island is that between nature and instinct represented by Caliban and culture and mind represented by Prospero. A further tension is between the island as a potential utopia or dystopia. On walking the island, Gonzalo sees utopia—an unsullied, perfumed, bountiful isle—where others see an uninhabitable and stinking wasteland. Gonzalo and another of the Lords in the shipwrecked party, Adrian, talk of the air breathing sweetly on them, while others say the air is 'rotten' and 'perfumed by a fen'. Gonzalo sees lush, green grass, where others see 'tawny' parched soil with merely 'an eye of green in it'. Gonzalo is amazed to find that, despite the shipwreck, his clothes seem fresh and unsullied, with no signs of salt stains.

For Gonzalo, this island could be the utopian 'commonwealth', where social titles—a sign of hierarchy—'should not be known'. The commonwealth would level social hierarchies and expose inequalities and inequities, where 'riches, poverty, and use of service' alike would disappear. Here, there would be 'no sovereignty'—sovereign power or ruling hierarchy—but a wealth in common, a sharing of resource. The others sarcastically rib his musings, where 'The latter end of his commonwealth forgets the beginning'. In other words, 'wealth' or use of resources will tempt and corrupt anybody and erase the idealism of the 'common'—of what may be shared capital.

This section of *The Tempest* reminds us that different players read the same world of potential capital resource in different ways. But one view will become dominant, or is legitimated, as other views are excluded, frustrating the potential or potency of a social system. In the commonwealth, all views are given an airing, and practices are compared to commonly decide the best and most productive for the common good. The commonwealth, the wealth held in common, finds its political expression in forms of democracy.

A functional way to think about the commonwealth of the clinical team (whose 'island' is their shared clinical space, such as a ward or an operating theatre) is to imagine its capital in resource terms—equipment and running costs, including salaries and overheads. What this team is producing is 'health' or 'care', as consumed by the patient. But this is a very limited view. The main capital, and production focus, of the team is subjectivities and lifestyles—primarily the subjectivity of the patient and secondarily the subjectivities of the team members. It is the production of kinds of bodies and lifestyles through a set of material, cultural, social, affective, and cognitive processes. It is never a completed work as a fixed subjectivity, but rather a work in progress, as a 'becoming', as explored later, particularly in Chap. 15. The interlinking of such subjectivities in the processes of becoming forms networks of communications, associations, friendships, and professional relations, themselves embedded in knowledge structures (cultural information and codes), values (symbols, images, and metaphors), and climates of affect or feeling.

I argue that functioning democracies offer fertile conditions for the realization of the commonwealth of clinical teams. My question in this chapter is: can democracy be established in medicine and health-care? Will we smell sweet air or the foul stench of the fen?

The prior question of course is: why should democracy be established at all in medicine and health-care? The answer is twofold. First, if doctors, surgeons, health-care practitioners, and managers expect democracy at work in their everyday lives, then why do many of them eschew democracy at work? Second, if doctors are supposed to practise evidence-based medicine, why, in the face of 3 decades of evidence that improving communication between doctors and patients and between members of clinical teams improves health outcomes and patient safety, is democracy still not the micropolitical system of choice in hospitals and community practices? Why do hospitals not predictably provide the hospitality their common name advertises? How can a house open its door to welcome strangers in an act of hospitality if that house cannot get its own relationships in order? The reader may think that I am overstating the case, but let us again examine the evidence for my claims.

In comparing the cultures of aviation and medicine, Karl (2009, p. 6) notes that 'Aviation assumes that personnel are subject to mistake making and that systems and culture need to be constructed to catch and mitigate error', where 'medicine is still focused on the perfection of each individual's performance'. In other words, medicine is still permeated by the values of heroic individualism (and this can be seen to be gendered male). It took the commercial aviation industry 2 decades to transform from a high risk to a high reliability industry, with passenger safety as the priority. Flying is now extremely safe. Medicine has yet to achieve such a cultural shift, and in comparison with flying, the intensive and high-risk areas of medicine, particularly surgery, are not as safe as they could be (Gawande, 2009).

But this is also a *political* issue—heroic individualism can be seen as a product of the Protestant–Capitalist values complex first described by the sociologist Max Weber (2002/1905) as *the* signifying feature of 'Western' culture. This values complex sees 'self' as capital, to be reinvested in self through a variety of regimes and practices of introversion (self-help, self-reflection, self-examination, self-esteem).

Such a taxis, inwards to 'self-knowing' is a continuing advert for the value of heroic individualism and insulates against political activity (again—the *polis* is the community). Medicine has thrived on such messages. But, in an age of clinical teamwork and community concerns, such a reflex seems inappropriate and outdated. If we take Aristotle's maxim—humans are by nature political animals—seriously, then heroic individualism is unnatural.

Again, it is estimated that around 70 % of medical error is grounded in poor communication in systems, where the basic system is the clinical team, and that 50 % of such errors are readily eradicated, not through a focus upon individual practitioners' mistakes or incompetence, but through improving communication within and across clinical teams (Kohn, Corrigan, & Donaldson, 1999; Pronovost & Vohr, 2010). As Karl (2009, p. 8) suggests, the 'good news is that cultural change does not require the purchase of expensive equipment or the discovery of a gene. The unfortunate news is that cultural change, especially in a profession as complex as medicine, is difficult to accomplish'.

The historically constituted culture of heroic individualism, self-help, and autonomy in medicine is, however, frustrating the realization of the commonwealth of the clinical team, described as 'collective competence' (Boreham, 2004) and 'collaborative intentionality capital' (Engeström, 2005, 2008). How—and should—the culture of medicine and its institutions such as hospitals change 'from hierarchy to networked community' (Bate, 2000)? Where medicine is slow to democratize, this may be due not only to the culture of heroic individualism, replicated in the traditional individual doctor–patient consultation (Smith, 2003), but also to a deepseated, pious culture of meritocracy (Young, 1993/1958).

Doctors logically argue that they deserve privilege in working life where their professional education is deeper, longer, and more technically demanding than the educations of their colleagues in other health professions such as nursing. However, arguments concerning meritocracies are based on differences in technical capabilities— or the capital accrued from technical education. The focus of this book is, again, on non-technical issues. Where hierarchies in medicine and health-care are, historically, grounded in meritocracies, these are expressed as the exercise of expert power, mentioned above, the legitimacy and power accrued from gaining a particular expertise. Rather, I am interested here in the *shared* human aspects of medicine and health-care—primarily interpersonal communication and teamwork. In principle, these are not subject to the exercise of expert power because they offer a commonwealth by birthright. However, professional 'communication' has also become a kind of capital gained through expertise and subject to education. How 'communication skills' should be learned is a hot topic in medical education, as the previous chapter shows.

Neither 'shared' nor 'non-technical' are accurate descriptors of communicationbased activity in clinical teams. Indeed, they are clumsy descriptors. Interpersonal communication and the ability to work in groups may be shared human capacities, a common wealth, but they are not necessarily exercised equally. It is a characteristic of medicine and surgery that communication is considered secondary to scientific knowledge, clinical reasoning ability, and clinical interventions, where skill in communication is traditionally central to nursing culture. Yet, as the previous chapter argues, this ignores the science of communication. The seemingly impersonal descriptor 'non-technical' is a rhetorical device that reminds us that there is something beyond the technical aspects of work, serving to mask the heart of 'shared' practices of communication. This heart is the emotional warmth and support that care offers—quite simply, the human(e) face of medicine. While this humane face should be appreciated before it is explained, nevertheless it can be explained and has been widely studied, as the extensive bibliography for this book demonstrates.

Two bodies of evidence suggest that, in medical education, we have never prepared doctors properly for their key work of communicating in a humane manner with patients. I draw heavily on these two bodies of evidence throughout this book. First, Roter and Hall (2006) summarize the evidence for the quality of the doctor–patient consultation across medicine, with an acknowledged bias to North American studies and an emphasis upon general, community, or family practice. Second, as introduced in Chap. 2, a growing body of evidence from patient safety studies shows that poor communication within and across clinical teams unnecessarily places patients at risk and lowers team morale especially for those who are traditionally lower on the hierarchy (Gawande, 2009; Pronovost & Vohr, 2010).

Why should doctors engage fully with the non-technical aspects of their work to become not just competent or good, but excellent, communicators with both patients and colleagues? If you want your operation done well, does it matter how the surgeon behaves as long as he or she has the appropriate technical expertise? Well, first, the surgeon is part of a wider community affecting the patient's journey, and second, how the surgeon behaves in theatre can affect the quality of the operation. I have already pointed out that it is the moral duty of a physician to not withhold an intervention that might improve patient care, and good communication is a health intervention in its own right.

Again, why should this be an either-or issue? Surgeons should be both technically excellent and interpersonally adept. Gawande (2002) also reminds us of another perspective. Surgical education, for example, has concentrated on producing individual star surgeons who excel in one area. However, this does not benefit the patient population, where the focus should be upon developing surgical procedures that can be readily replicated at a high level of expertise by numbers of practitioners.

Where democracy in medicine is most needed is where medicine mainly occurs—in chronic care in the community. General, community, or family practitioners are the first stop for patients and offer the backstop for patients with chronic multiple conditions. As urban practices in particular become multicultural and as the population balance shifts towards greater need for care for the elderly, excellent communication within a patient-centred model of care at the grassroots level of communities is a necessity.

Democracy and Its Discontents

I finished this book against the backdrop of the 'Arab Spring' revolutions in which a wave of both armed (e.g. Libya) and semi-peaceful (e.g. Tunisia and Egypt) resistance has been seen and where the future outcomes are still uncertain. I am revising the manuscript just as the supposedly democratically elected leader in Egypt has been ousted by a military coup in a second wave of revolution that may yet promise the establishment of a secular democracy. By the time you read this book, the political landscape resulting from the 'Arab Spring' revolutions will almost certainly have gone through more change, but the direction of travel will be towards working democracies. What is certain is that a first step to democratic structures has been initiated in countries such as Egypt by removing dictators and their supportive (male gendered) hierarchies. My daily newspaper recently announced that 'Women in Saudi Arabia will be given the right to vote and to stand for election within 4 years' (*The Guardian,* Monday 26 September 2011, p. 3). Only the following day, news leaked out from that a Saudi woman would be given ten lashes for driving a car (at the time of writing, it is illegal for women to drive in Saudi Arabia). The following week, after an international outcry, the King of Saudi Arabia announced that he had pardoned the woman and reminded the international community of the promise that fair and free elections would be held by 2015. Meanwhile, scores of doctors and nurses who had treated injured protesters against the political regime in Bahrain were tried and found 'guilty' of supporting insurrection and given prison sentences.

Those who live in developed democracies and seek to progress this model of social life may wonder why democracies are in a minority globally. From within democracies, there is a tendency to judge other ways of living, such as theocracies and autocracies, as undeveloped—or underdeveloped—systems that will eventually transform to democratic structures. While their critics judge such theocracies and autocracies as 'medieval' systems, they are seen as 'traditional' and worth preserving by their proponents, who see democracies as a chaotic and divisive free play of values plurality, rather than a focused ethical and moral way of life based on transcendental theological text. Those who uphold democracies live with the knowledge that forceful imposition of democracy is an oxymoron, and yet this is how the Western world has recently approached and deposed totalitarian regimes in Libya and Afghanistan in particular. Further, democracies may serve to mask or tacitly support corruption, especially where we rely on representative forms of democracy—electing representatives to a parliament where one voice supposedly speaks for a common good. Democracy is of course not beyond ideology—it is a form of ideology, but one that attempts to express the common good through collaborative effort.

We also recognize the existence of seeming paradoxes within any form of social structure. For example, what is often celebrated as the first form of democracy in the ancient Greek city-state of Athens—although this claim to origin is contested (Keane, 2009)—excluded women and slaves. In the tightly controlled social hierarchies of feudal Japan, mini democracies, or networks and circles, flourished, based on common aesthetic interests such as reading and writing poetry (Ikegami, 2005). Contemporary Japanese citizens enjoy the best health in any post-industrial nation, yet their system of medical education is feudal—traditionally hierarchical and eschewing notions of patient centredness (Bleakley, Brice, & Bligh, 2008).

An advanced or developed democracy—often referred to as a 'liberal democracy' and technically as a 'universal franchise democracy'—offers personal liberty and popular sovereignty (Mandelbaum, 2007). In other words, there is common respect for differing opinions and values within the law, where the law itself is regularly reviewed and not grounded in a transcendental religious structure. This can of course offer paradoxes—such as the right to bear arms inscribed in the American Constitution, where potential tyranny partners supposed individual liberty. A legitimate liberal democracy should satisfy the following six conditions, where I consider under each point what this implies for the passage of medicine from a weak autocracy and strong meritocracy to a fully fledged democracy:

1. A liberal democracy does not seek to offer a new form of imperialism. Local identities can still flourish within democratic structures without being subsumed under a global imperialism such as North American political interests (exploitation of natural resources) or cultural homogenization ('Coca-Cola-isation' or 'Disneyfication'). For example, in the period of the various 'colour revolutions' after the implosion of the Soviet Union, the ex-Soviet states jealously guarded their sovereignties and identities as they were rapidly supported by American interests and influences that, in principle, would undermine such identities (Carothers, 2006). In medicine, western forms (of medicine and medical education) may be exported to developing nations as a form of neocolonialism (Bleakley, Brice, & Bligh, 2008; Bleakley et al., 2008). We should then resist the type of cultural homogenization and neo-imperialism that imagines a global medical education template will fit all. The production of democracy in clinical teamwork, for example, will not come about through compulsory attendance at a standardized communication skills training course.

2. In a liberal democracy, elections must be free and fair. There should be freedom to advocate, associate, contest, and campaign; a fair and neutral administration; a credible system of dispute resolution; independent vote monitoring; and balanced access to mass media (Diamond, 2008). We cannot guarantee that the conditions of possibility for 'free and fair elections'—collaborative participation and debate—are in place in health-care until all practitioners can demonstrate fluency in dialogue rather than monologue. Clinical teams may be plagued by the inability of their leaders to engage in open and supportive dialogue where necessary (asking, open questioning, conversing, sharing information, debating, supporting, sharing emotions, supportively challenging), where the dominant pattern is monologue (prescribing, telling, demanding, closed questioning, unsupportive confrontation, resisting emotional sharing, both passive aggressive and openly hostile demeanours, blaming). The paradox remains that active citizens in the public domain can show a kind of light autism (akin to Asperger syndrome on

the autism spectrum) in professional work, where the dialogical imagination is rejected for monological communication, the latter then justified as efficient or fit for context. I am, of course, referring largely to surgical culture.

3. There should not be a desire to engage in conflict with another democracy. That fully fledged democracies do not fight each other is a given condition in politics. However, where the passage from proto-democracy to full democracy accounts for most wars, confrontation may be inevitable in this transitional stage. In order to avoid too much confrontation, democratic processes require that monitory processes be established before full elections (Owen, 2005). In medicine, we might then expect a high level of conflict in the transition from proto-democracy to full democracy (a democracy-to-come). The ongoing symptom of the inability to make this transition is the phenomenon of self-serving professional silos and the inability to engage in boundary crossings or to make a full transition from multiprofessional to interprofessional practice. As I discuss later, this can be alleviated through a range of monitory processes that offer quality assurance of the democracy-to-come. This has already happened to a large extent in medicine at the macro- and mesopolitical levels, with the recent shift from high levels of autonomy to high levels of public accountability.

   At the micropolitical level, confrontations associated with the transition to democracy can be expected where practitioners who have traditionally not had a voice are suddenly empowered, while practitioners who traditionally exerted sovereign power find that their power is no longer legitimate. This predicted confrontation might be transformed if monitory processes such as pre-briefing and debriefing of team-based work activity are implemented and well facilitated. *Con-frons* literally means 'with the forehead'. This does not have to be a head on challenge, a butting, but may be a 'but-ting' as an appropriate interruption, a call for pause, discussion, and a show of interest.

4. There will be predictable resistance to developing full democracy. The advice from politicians and negotiators is to never push too hard as this creates greater resistance from those who oppose full democracy. Thus, George Bush's (Junior) 'democracy promotion' campaign was not only misguided but also backfired, when 'promotion' became a form of zealotry (Carothers, 2006) and shadowed the ideological 'Americanization' interests of commercial global companies such as Coca Cola and McDonalds. In medicine, it is predictable that senior doctors, especially surgeons, will resist a move to democracy, and they must not be pushed too hard too soon. Practitioners must be convinced of the value of such change through evidence and through practical knowing. Ironically, as those who have been newly colonized (by managers and politicians, or policy makers), it is predictable that senior clinicians will use the same tactics that the colonized have used throughout history—not direct resistance but 'sly civility' (Bhabha, 1994) and 'civil disobedience' (Thoreau, 1995/1849). These are grudging, subtle, and mimicking forms of passive resistance.

5. A liberal democracy works where there is support for independent monitoring of elections and backing for independent civil groups including the backing of coalitions of opposition parties dedicated to promoting democracy (Carothers, 2006).

This has been a main reason for the extraordinary success of democracy in India, which challenges the idea that democracies will not root and flourish in low-income communities with poor education. The example of India shows that democracy can be established prior to the industrialization of a nation, where it serves to give hope to the disenfranchised and poor. Indeed, in India, political orthodoxy is reversed, where the poor are more likely to vote than the middle class or the rich.

For medicine, the lesson may be that, again, those practitioners lower on the hierarchy, as well as patients, may be the very groups that serve to transform medicine into a full democracy where they have the most to gain through their activism and participation. In a later chapter, I describe nurses in the operating theatre, normally downtrodden by the system and low on the hierarchy, as offering an essential service in speaking out, especially in calling for pre-briefing and debriefing as regular practice, where these are not just patient safety activities, but potentially democratic team forming activities. These previously downtrodden practitioners may exercise a moral courage (Bleakley, 2006a, 2006b; Flynn, 1987; Foucault, 2001) that the ancient Greeks called *parrhesia,* when they speak out, not only for their own art of caring, but also on behalf of patients, whose voices are silenced under anaesthesia (see Chap. 12).

In so doing, they are restoring the aesthetic, or both a common sense and sense of beauty, to a profession of nursing and caring that has long been anaesthetized or dulled by the dominance of the instrumental medical voice. There is of course a danger here of stereotyping nurses as fair and oppressed and doctors as mean and oppressive, linked to gender.

6. In outlining the prospects for the development of democracy in already democratic countries and in light of growing distrust of elected politicians and representative democracy, Tilly (2007) describes local political initiatives as 'interpersonal trust networks'. These are noncoercive, accountable, groups offering public 'think tanks' as horizontal structures that provide an alternative to, or run alongside, vertical hierarchies. While a cumbersome term, I prefer 'networks' to 'groups', because the former captures a developed fluidity and openness that 'groups' does not. Where groups go through a life history (forming, norming, storming, performing, and mourning) or develop from immaturity to maturity, the nature of teamwork in contemporary health-care suggests that we might better think of mature team practitioners creating ad hoc, ready-made teams.

Medical Education Can Democratize Medicine

Keane (2009), in a history of democracies and the ideas of democracy, describes three forms of democracy that interweave in any liberal democracy. These are assembly, representative, and monitory democracies. *Assembly democracy*, or participative democracy, is the model that we best recognize from accounts of the 'birth of democracy' in fifth century BC Athens. The populace assemble in a set place and collectively thrash out issues of social life in public debate. This has been overtaken in the information age by online assemblies (social networking sites) such as Facebook, which have served as the foundation for popular uprisings against dictatorial regimes in the Middle East during the 'Arab Spring' revolutions discussed earlier.

Tolerance is central to such a system where every voice must be heard however 'other' it may sound. Decisions are made by majority votes. As mentioned above, the Athenian form of participative or assembly democracy was flawed by contemporary standards, because it excluded women and slaves (and condoned slavery). Further, as Keane (2009) argues, archaeological evidence suggests that this system was in fact predated by a number of experiments in local assembly democracy in what is now modern-day Iran.

Assembly democracy is at the heart of a potential revolution in medicine as the landscape of health-care changes to place emphasis upon teamwork—varieties of clinical teams working around patients on a pathway of care. Evidence suggests that such clinical teams are more successful—in terms of patient safety and health outcomes—where they work democratically (Borrill et al., 2000). By this, I mean that they engage in open dialogue. I discuss this in depth in later chapters. For example, an operating theatre team is likely to have more success where it briefs before a list (Allard, Bleakley, Hobbs, & Coombes, 2011).

One of the reasons for this is that situation awareness can be set up across members of the team, where all team members, because they participate in the brief, share a common mental model of how the list will unfold and who will be doing what during the work period. Further, a pre-brief and debrief at the end of the list provide an opportunity for the operating theatre team to communicate effectively with perioperative care such as recovery teams and ward teams. Finally, assembly democracy is empowering, since it provides the condition of possibility for practitioners traditionally lower on the meritocracy hierarchy to speak out if they see poor practice. Assembly democracy can include patients in team-based discussions about their care, even in surgery pre-anaesthesia or where the patient is undergoing elective surgery under local anaesthetic.

Representative democracy places decision-making power in the hands of elected individuals. Assembly democracy is impossible where numbers become too large for effective public debate. Medicine has historically retained autonomy within a fairly tight and small assembly and representative system, but has recently undergone a radical transformation in this respect through a crisis, as public loss of confidence. Ludmerer (1999) traces this emerging rift between medicine and the public it serves for North American contexts. In the UK, the Bristol paediatric heart operations scandal, the discovery of the conspiracy of silence surrounding the mass murderer UK general practitioner Harold Shipman, and a series of organ retention fiascos have led to a call for greater public accountability of medical practice.

For many in medicine and medical education, the pendulum has now swung too far towards a representative democracy as clinical decisions become dependent upon political decisions concerning health policy, controlled primarily by economic decisions. Doctors may feel depowered rather than empowered politically as their representatives lose touch with clinical concerns.

Monitory democracy is a rather cumbersome neologism of Keane's (2009) to describe a rapidly emerging form of democratic structure that is fundamentally an audit or quality assurance culture. Being monitored is intrinsic to professional life, and doctors, as explained above, are increasingly subject to public scrutiny in a culture that was often closed, self-serving, and closed ranks in a crisis. External public accountability and internal professional, or peer, accountability, however, need not degenerate into unnecessary bureaucracies or surveillance mechanisms, but can offer peer-review-based quality assurance. The traditional example of this is the audit culture in medicine, but where mortality and morbidity meetings, for example, have often been closed affairs, this does not generate public confidence in medicine's transparency.

The best example of an attempt to create a genuine monitory democracy— monitoring practice for patient benefit and practitioner work satisfaction and morale—is the development of an appraisal culture, especially at the level of the consultant and linked with revalidation. Utilizing a combination of feedback from peers, patients, and colleagues in a multisource (360°) feedback setting is a primary model of monitory democracy in medicine. While arguments rage about veiled surveillance or managerial control, such models, based on criteria-referenced assessments and covering the range of practices necessary for contemporary medicine, offer a great opportunity for doctors to build a strong quality assurance culture.

Monitory democracy can also be closely tied with imperialist concerns, as a complex form of monitoring. The typical example is the intervention of 'mature' democracies in local political conflict that produces human rights issues (such as the American, NATO and UN interventions in the Balkans, Iraq, Afghanistan, Libya, and so forth). Here, the interventionist's speech is often with a forked tongue—on the one hand protecting human rights, on the other protecting global capitalist interests such as investment in oil resources. Those who support public accountability often treat medicine's monitory democracy as unnecessary regulation by those who support professional autonomy, but as a necessary intervention.

What, then, of democracy's discontents? I have talked as if democracy were largely unblemished and transparent—insulated from critique. Of course we are already in trouble by talking of 'democracy' rather than 'democracies'. There are varieties of democracy on a sliding scale, from proto-democracies to fully expressive liberal democracies. I note Winston Churchill's remark that all political systems are bad, but democracy is the least bad. We are hardly in a position to reflect on the maturity of democracies where women only gained the vote in Switzerland in 1971, segregation was abolished in the USA in 1964, apartheid was abolished in South Africa between 1992 and 1994, and inequalities and inequities are rife in contemporary medicine, where women doctors are still second-class citizens yet constitute the majority of students in the new era of medicine, as discussed at length in Chap. 9.

I will outline four issues that muddy democracy and serve to make the topic more complex. I do not set out to solve these four issues, but to raise them as concerns that should make us think more deeply about constituting a work democracy in medicine as a basis for and as a result of addressing 'communication' in medicine.

First, I invoke a number of loose terms in this book that we should also celebrate and encourage in medical and health-care practices, such as 'hospitality', 'friendship', and 'collaboration'. I recognize that these can become weasel words, perhaps concealing as much as they reveal. While 'democracy' itself, at root, means sovereignty or 'sovereign power' (*kratos*) held by 'the body of the people' or the 'common body' (*demos*), it is cognate with words meaning 'rich', 'yolky', and 'runny' (Hillman, 1994a). 'Runny' or 'liquid' practices (Bauman, 2000, 2007) that are adaptable, flexible, and open are at the heart of democracies and opposed by authoritarian outlooks that demand fixed perspectives.

In the wake of the Holocaust, Theodor Adorno and colleagues (1950) studied extreme autocrats as a psychological type. The fascist mentality was termed 'the authoritarian personality', whose main characteristic is intolerance of ambiguity. Such authoritarianism is alien to contemporary democratic cultures that Zygmunt Bauman (2000, 2007) describes as 'liquid' and Hardt and Negri (2009) describe as a rapidly changing 'altermodernity' of the 'Multitude'. Yet authoritarianism is still common in health-care. In subsequent chapters, I argue that authoritarianism in team structures is a burden to developing safe and effective practices. Such structures are cousins of the poor listening to patients' stories that can lead to misdiagnoses and subsequent medical error. Future health-care team practices will need to model 'liquid' democracies as a way of appreciating the common story of the clinical team, an appreciation formed from respect for each member's contribution.

Second, democracy can be a thin veneer and an unstable condition that hides the unspeakable and the abject. The harder one works at making or forming democracy— and here I describe such forming of democracy as an art, an aesthetic endeavour intersecting with politics—the more beautiful, elegant, and inspiring the democratic form, the more it seems to produce radical and ugly alternatives just below the surface. Indian democracy, held up as an example of how participative democracies can be established in industrializing nations, has also been described as a veneer. Just under the surface are fervent nationalisms and regional ethnic identifications promising strife. These run to high levels of prejudice and hankering after traditional, hierarchical caste systems. Will the exercise of democracy in medicine serve to fuel a backlash, a conservative call for return to traditional hierarchy-based values?

Third, democracies struggle with the paradox of 'free speech'. Where politics and the law intersect, in American models, using the First Amendment, 'free' speech can become prejudicial, saying what you like. This is perhaps better termed 'extreme speech' (Hare & Weinstein, 2009). In European contexts, however, extreme speech is not protected by democracy but seen as an enemy within democracy. In European settings, there is a conviction that a healthier democratic polity will emerge from punishing extreme speech such as public inflammatory racist, or sexist, comment. The paradox of a democracy in medicine is that, while the conditions of possibility may be established for speaking up or speaking out (a tradition of fearless speech discussed in later chapters), the same political climate may encourage voices of hatred or prejudice.

Fourth, as the tradition of writing on democracy from Montesquieu through Rousseau to Tocqueville suggests, there is a necessary connection between power and moral conduct. Politics and ethics are bedfellows. I suggested earlier that politics and aesthetics are also, perhaps uneasy, bedfellows. For Tocqueville, studying democracy in America in the 1830s, individualism—a particular characteristic of American democracy—frustrates the collectivism that is key to exercising democracy, and this raises an ethical dilemma. Paul Rahe (2010) fears that democracies can drift towards a 'soft despotism' exerted by stronger individuals unable to tolerate collective endeavour.

Such difficulties in a democracy-to-come plague the emergence of democracy in medicine and make more complex my assertion that medical education has the power to democratize medicine and, in turn, that medical education research can democratize medical education. Power should not dull but educate. Anaesthetic dulls and an anaesthetic power tends to control rather than educate and reveal or release potential. I then call for consideration of an aesthetic of power in medicine or power used for thoughtful 'forming' of identities. I recognize that fascism also has an (unfortunate) aesthetic, but this is impoverished, characterized by lack of an ethical perspective. For democracy to work in medicine within health-care provision, an aesthetic of power must converse with an ethical perspective (Weiss, 2005) in shaping a fair and just culture of work. Patients too must be involved in forming this aesthetic of power.

What do I mean by an aesthetic of power and communication? Let us return to an example introduced earlier. Eiko Ikegami (2005) shows how 'aesthetic networks' were established within the unyielding public social hierarchies in medieval and early modern Japan, where little distinction was made between the political and aesthetic spheres of public life. Beauty was brought into social life through the establishment of networks of, for example, poetry circles, which could include people from all walks of life.

In medicine within health-care, if we substitute the patient for poetry, this stimulates the horizontal binding of practitioners in network practices. But what if we were to equate patient care with poetry, or to see both the science and art of medicine as poetics? The practices of communication centred on patients then become aesthetic as well as political and social. These are practices that have form and beauty, elegance, and style, as well as function. Ikegami (2005) shows how both culture and identity are emergent properties of aesthetic networks. Throughout this book, I will show how new forms of work practices centred on communication in medicine—revolving around networking and knotworking (explored fully in subsequent chapters)—provide the conditions of possibility for the emergence of a new culture of communication and for new identity constructions for both practitioners and patients through establishing norms of beauty, form, propriety, and good manners.

This discussion of aesthetic networks raises another key dimension running throughout this book. As democratic structures are introduced, so the vertical is transformed into the horizontal. Vertical, hierarchical power structures are replaced by, or supplemented by, horizontal communication. This can be thought of as a shift in thinking from sovereign power to capillary power, from the influence of transcendental, abstract rules to the multiple, complex, and conflicting experiences that are immanent, concrete, and body based. Such multiple experiences demand tolerance of difference.

The shift in thinking from the vertical to the horizontal in power structures has been heralded particularly in the work of Gilles Deleuze and Felix Guattari, a philosopher and psychiatrist, respectively. This work is discussed in detail in Chap. 14, but is important to preface here. Deleuze and Guattari (2004a, 2004b) introduce two key tensions: between arborescent and rhizomatic thinking and between nomadism and settlement as metaphors for forms of power. Where a culture thinks in terms of the value of vertical hierarchies, Deleuze and Guattari refer to this as 'arborescent' thinking. Development is seen in terms of a strong root system creating healthy growth that ultimately flowers and fruits to reproduce the system. The image is of the independent practitioner. An alternative is to think of rhizomes—tangled, horizontal structures that work symbiotically with other structures and create large underground networks supporting an occasional vertical sprouting. (Yrjo Engeström (2008) has critiqued and developed this model to offer the metaphor of mycorrhizae rather than rhizomes, and this is discussed at length in Chap. 11). Deleuze and Guattari then challenge the dominance of vertical and hierarchical thinking for networked communities of practice.

Further, those committed to the independent, vertical structures are usually committed to practices of 'settlement' over 'nomadism'. The settlers build up a defensible structure and carry on pouring resources into its growth. Nomadic thinking does not place as much value in putting down roots and developing a fixed idea or ideal, but prefers fluid, adaptable thinking that can respond to changing times and has a historical sensibility that also generates predictive value. While I am cautious about such gross categories, a further extension to the tension between arborescent and rhizomatic thinking are the notions of 'territorializing' and 'deterritorializing'. Settled cultures, as they seek more resources, start to actively seed or attempt to colonize other cultures to exploit them. The deterritorializing impulse is to challenge such colonialism, to resist forcing ideas and practices on others backed by sovereign power, and to cultivate tolerance of difference.

Deleuze and Guattari do not imagine that horizontal thinking supplants vertical thinking. Rather, they suggest thinking in terms of plateaux and platforms, where vertical structures such as hierarchies are challenged by a horizontal intervention. For example, a collaborative, interprofessional, educational intervention is introduced to a previously hierarchical work team as a foundation, plateau, and platform, from which new development can occur.

In this chapter, I have introduced frameworks for democracy to help to build a challenge to what has traditionally been a less than democratic culture of medical work within wider health-care. In the next chapter, collaboration between medical and health-care professionals, as colleagues, is extended to include patients.

Chapter 4
Patient-Centredness Without a Centre

Mutuality as a Model of Care

How shall we put patients at the heart of medical education? I will argue, paradoxically, for a patient-centredness without a centre. This initially strange notion will become familiar as I develop an argument for a collaborative model of both patient care and medical education, progressing the established model of 'mutuality' in communication (Roter & Hall, 2006, pp. 34–37), generated from the *differences* between patient and doctor. To this dyad we shall add the medical student, to form the basic triad of communication in medical education: patient–medical student–doctor, as teachers and learners (Bleakley & Bligh, 2008; Bleakley, Bligh, & Browne, 2011).

In 1970, the medical sociologist Friedson (1970) published a groundbreaking work, *Profession of Medicine*, in which he argued that, in return for the high level of autonomy that the profession of medicine enjoys, doctors have a responsibility for social accountability. Over 30 years later, Sir Donald Irvine (2003) described a 'new professionalism' that meets the conditions of Freidson's critique, to include 'partnerships with patients, and accountability rather than professional autonomy … teamwork, rather than individualism, collective as well as personal responsibility, transparency rather than secrecy, empathetic communication and above all respect for others'.

In a commonly used rhetorical gesture, Irvine opposes the 'old' and the 'new', but we should not throw out the baby with the bathwater. We cannot call for 'self-directed' learning in students and at the same time ban 'self-regulation' in medicine. Rather, key elements of self-regulation of the profession can be retained, but must be accompanied by a transparent social contract. One way in which this can be achieved is not just through more open dialogue with patients, but more thoughtful and *formed* dialogue. If talking with others, particularly in a professional context, is an art, then doctors need to be both inventive practitioners and connoisseurs of this art. Communication is not simply technical, but an aesthetic and an ethical activity. Further, patients can educate doctors if doctors will listen, and close listening is vital for doctors to develop a diagnosis and treatment plan—echoing Osler's famous

A. Bleakley, *Patient-Centred Medicine in Transition: The Heart of the Matter,*
Advances in Medical Education 3, DOI 10.1007/978-3-319-02487-5_4,
© Springer International Publishing Switzerland 2014

dictum that the diagnosis is in the history. Close listening is the most difficult aspect of communication's repertoire and something that doctors in general, according to a body of evidence (Roter & Hall, 2006), do not do well.

Where the quality of relationship between doctor and patient has been shown to be a significant factor in positively shaping the outcomes of care (Roter & Hall, 2006; Stewart, 1995), the anatomy and dynamics of this relationship also delineate an educational model for how medical students can learn from contact with patients, properly supported by experienced clinical educators. 'Relationship' is an ambiguous term. Through a critical review of key literature, I will articulate a theoretical basis for a positive *educational* relationship between doctors and patients and between medical students and patients.

Drawing on patients' expertise in medical education is, of course, not new. The celebrated nineteenth century Canadian medical educator, William Osler, referred to above, said that 'the best teaching is that taught by the patient'. John Spencer and colleagues (2000) have expertly reviewed the literature demonstrating that experienced doctors can orient today's students, as tomorrow's doctors, to successfully learn from patients.

Imagine what medical students might learn from participating in one of the ward rounds described by the American doctor Joshua Horn (in Taussig, 1992, p. 96), working in Chinese hospitals between 1954 and 1969: 'The patients often select representatives to convey their opinions and suggestions to teams of doctors, nurses and orderlies who have day-to-day responsibility in relation to specific groups of patients'. Horn goes on to describe how 'ambulant patients play an active part in ward affairs', not only by getting to know and supporting other patients, but also by attending clinical team meetings and ward rounds, where 'a retinue of patients … look and listen and often volunteer information'.

Accountability of doctors is first to their patients—to be technically good, but also to create dialogue for understanding, insight, and care. This may be framed as a working collaboration, but can deepen into mutuality, based on respect. Where collaboration can still work with minimum input from one partner, 'mutuality' describes a reciprocal, or symbiotic, relationship between doctor and patient that is primarily educative and is grounded in the difference between doctors and patients as a potentially positive, rather than divisive, condition.

There is a necessary paradox in this model of 'mutuality'. Pauli, White, and McWhinney (2000a, p. 178) suggest that the *therapeutic* aspect of the extended medical encounter is neither 'merely an expression of a humanistic attitude' nor 'an invocation of the "be kind to patients" movement'. Rather, it progresses the humanistic view to a greater-than-persons model: the mutual creation of a complex, dynamic ecology or environment in which a common reality is negotiated. Indeed, as evolution by natural selection suggests, just as larger, natural ecologies are established through generation of variety and complexity, so a local ecology is richer for differences between its constituent parts. However, a dyad is not a meaningful system until the two parts interact dynamically.

The doctor and poet Dannie Abse (2008, p. 20) notes that 'A physician or surgeon needs to be alert and objective and not to be at one with the patient, to judge the clinical condition from a little distance—a sympathetic and sensitive distance certainly, but still a distance'. In that subtle descriptive and poetic phrase, 'a little distance', Abse describes the paradox we refer to at the beginning of this paragraph—professional mutuality in medical care is a warm objectivity. It is clinical science, but an engaging, warm science. 'Objectivity' does not have to be cold, detached, and inhumane. Indeed, Freud taught that the therapeutic encounter is not a blind personal entanglement, but requires understanding and management of the dynamics of intimacy—transference and countertransference and resistance and counter-resistance, as well as the dynamics of ego defences such as projection, displacement, repression, and denial.

In *The Second Coming*, the poet W.B. Yeats famously says:

…
Turning and turning in the widening gyre
The falcon cannot hear the falconer;
Things fall apart; the centre cannot hold;
Mere anarchy is loosed upon the world
…

Let us turn Yeats against himself. This fragment of the poem described Yeats' fear, after the Russian Revolution in 1917, that the common people, the multitude, would displace the aristocracy. Yeats was highly conservative in his politics. Conservative medicine, favouring paternalism, may feel that things will fall apart in the current 'marketplace' culture of patient-as-consumer (or customer) and the emerging climate of clinical care as democratic teamwork, where the traditional centre of authority cannot hold.

In the move from hierarchical teams based on traditional authority structures, to flat hierarchies and democracies ('meshworks' and 'networks') based on shared capabilities, there is a fear that this may lead to a leadership crisis or leadership vacuum. However, ask any good doctor: 'who leads the team?', and they will almost certainly answer 'the patient'. The patient is a kind of absent, or fluctuating, centre.

We suggest that it is fruitless to concentrate on 'centres' as loci of control— either the 'soft' centre as the patient in 'patient-centredness', 'patient autonomy', or 'patient-as-consumer'; or the 'hard' centre as the autonomous, self-regulating doctor in traditional paternalism. What is important is the quality of *relationship* between doctors, patients, and medical students, necessarily involving negotiation and some positive friction. I disagree with Yeats that when centres cannot hold, anarchy is loosed. In fact, as I suggest here, the notion and status of 'centre' can be reconsidered. Again, what if there were nothing at the centre, but the primary issue were to do with the 'difference' between doctors and patients (and in teams, doc-tors, and other health-care professions)? And what if that difference is an engine of production of knowledge and not indifference?

Doctors are experts in medicine, and patients are experts in knowledge of what Mishler (1984) termed their 'lifeworlds'. These two kinds of specialist knowledge may produce some friction or awkwardness as they meet, but such awkwardness is productive and can offer a powerful combination, making a unit with differing components, such as a lock and key. As patient and doctor enter into dialogue, so they can constructively build a relationship of care and education that transcends the excesses of either medical paternalism or aggressive patient autonomy.

Such dialogue is not easy. Nor does it follow a philosophy of 'presence', in which what matters is what is visible (or audible). What matters just as much is what is absent, or unspoken, in the encounter—communication is often tortuous and must be studied in depth to reveal its treasures. The anthropologist Michael Taussig (1992, p. 89) discusses a medical case—which he deliberately calls a 'situation'—first written up by him in an essay in 1978. The *situation* is a 'forty-nine year-old white working class woman with a history of multiple hospital admissions over the past 8 years with a diagnosis of polymyositis—inflammation of many muscles'. Taussig describes this as a fatal rheumatoid disease whose cause is unknown and whose palliative treatment consists of large doses of steroids.

Where the doctors treating this patient had no idea of cause (and 30+ years later, the causes of polymyositis are still unknown or remain vague—as a possible autoimmune disorder or a viral condition), the patient herself, a deeply religious woman, had a complex and highly personal narrative explanation that offers a moral rationale for her condition. Despite objections from her mother, the woman married at 15, had five children in quick succession, and followed by six miscarriages. Her husband was an alcoholic and unable to support the family. She developed a deep guilt about her life and saw her condition as a punishment. More importantly, a deeply religious woman, she felt that God had chosen her as a subject for medicine, so that, through her, doctors would find a cure for her disease and then be able to help others.

How will the scientific mind of the doctor deal with this premodern patient narrative without dismissing it as naïve or primitive, where it is precisely this narrative that offers meaning and hope for the patient in the absence of a medical explanation? We see now why Taussig prefers to call this patient's 'case' a 'situation', for both patient and doctor are 'situated' by their main belief systems, values, or what the psychoanalyst Alfred Adler perceptively called 'guiding fictions' (Hillman, 1994b). This situating—in the case of doctors within a science narrative that paradoxically promises, but has not yet delivered, an answer, and in the case of the patient within a prescientific narrative that is one of faith rather than evidence or proof—produces what seem like incompatible identities. How then will a doctor set up a relationship with such a patient? How will the doctor hold the tension of offering the best evidence-based scientific practice as the patient's prescientific belief system is simultaneously mobilized?

Sir Kenneth Calman (2007, p. 382) quotes from Glenn Colquhoun's (2007) *Playing God: Poems About Medicine*, where the author exacts some humorous revenge on the formal 'medical encounter', set as a fragile meeting of the specialist language of the doctor and the native world of the patient:

> She asked me if she took one pill for her heart and one pill/for her hips and one pill for her chest and one pill for her/blood how come they would all know which part of her body/they should go to.
>
> I explained to her that active metabolites in each/pharmaceutical would adopt a spatial configuration leading/to an exact interface with receptor molecules on the cellular/surfaces of the target structures involved.
>
> She told me not to bullshit her.
>
> I told her that each pill had a different shape and that each/part of her body has a different shape and that her pills/could only work when both these shapes could fit together.
>
> She said I had no right to talk about the shape of her body.
>
> I said that each pill was a key and that her body was ten/thousand locks.
>
> She said she was not going to swallow that.
>
> I told her that they worked by magic.
>
> She asked me why I didn't say that in the first place.

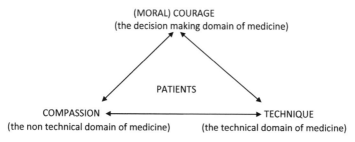

Fig. 4.1 The heart of the matter

Seeing the patient as 'the heart of the matter' in contemporary medical education is not an empty metaphor, but a way of expressing a patient-centred medicine. We can put heart back into medical education in three ways, tracking the broad historical discourses of 'heart' (Hillman, 1981). First, there is the heart as locus of love, passion, and feeling. Medical education focused on patients should be a passionate affair without literal entanglements—an exercise in compassion. Compassion is a quality that medical education should nourish, not extinguish, whether it appears as a modern 'professionalism' competency (Stern, 2006a, 2006b) or a timeless heart-felt response to suffering (Szczeklik, 2005).

Second, there is the heart as the seat of courage, and we see a sensitive and humane medical education as both grounded in the courage of patients and a spur to the moral courage (that the ancient Greeks called *parrhesia*) of practitioners (Bleakley, 2006b)—to speak up on behalf of good patient care and safety in the face of perceived poor practice.

Third, there is the functional heart of Harvey, the muscle as pump and the engine for circulation of the blood. Medical education must be technically advanced, and we wish to see doctors who know their clinical science and the practices or techniques that follow—who can expertly read the heart and its pulses as they offer a practice of the heart. It is a bonus if medical students are also interested to know that the normal heartbeat is the basis of iambic pentameter in poetry and of syncopation in jazz. Science, however, should also be taught with syncopation or artistry and have poetic value. It must be arresting, calling on both passion and the courage to teach and learn in new ways, such as translating problem-based learning into patient-based learning (Fig. 4.1).

Communication and Clinical Reasoning

As John Bunker (2001) details in *Medicine Matters After All*, medical interventions at the level of the *technical* relationships between doctors and patients now make a significant difference to health outcomes. Cumulative evidence from a couple of decades of study of preventive clinical interventions and related health outcomes—in areas as diverse as screening for hypertension and immunization for influenza and in curative clinical services (such as interventions for ischaemic heart disease and diabetes)—show that medical interventions count significantly amongst other contributing factors such as environment, education, housing, and employment. The epidemiologist Thomas McKeown (1979) has shown that in the three centuries up to the mid-twentieth century, clinical medicine's contribution to life expectancy and prevention of death had been smaller than other factors such as environment and standard of living.

This is the technical face of medicine. The depth and breadth of this technical knowledge is what delineates a *medical* education from an education in other health professions. It is then thought of as 'vertical' knowledge that gives a doctor a certain status and a prominent role of clinical leadership within a mixed professions team and offers a significant marker of difference from laypersons. Such expertise may be translated into a meritocracy—a structuring of society based on 'merit' as educational capital and technical skill. The technical face of medicine also includes complex decision-making (such as diagnostic problem solving) that is grounded in, or dependent upon, technical knowledge, even, *or especially*, where this knowledge is 'hidden' as expertise, such as the doctor making a rapid diagnosis on the basis of pattern recognition (Eva, 2005).

But of what importance is the 'non-technical' face of medicine, often termed 'shared' skills and knowledge (shared, of course, not only with other medical colleagues and health professionals, but also with patients)? These shared capabilities include the ill-defined and overlapping areas of communication, teamwork, and interpersonal skills. And where do the desired personal virtues, such as altruism (Quirk, 2006), fit with these areas? Are such virtues spin offs from a 'deep' learning in the technical realm, or do they automatically sit with the narrative and ethical face of medicine that can be characterized as purposefully humane communication with patients and colleagues?

Mark Quirk's (2006) model of medical education is grounded in the development of clinical reasoning expertise. The model integrates clinical reasoning with communication and the doctor–patient relationship, which support and inform each other (the reality of clinical practice). Drawing on evidence from the cognitive psychology literature, Quirk argues that the primary way of developing clinical expertise is through a set of conscious, deliberate cognitive and metacognitive abilities that come to organize, retrieve, and utilize biomedical science information. The cognitive abilities encompass a cycle of planning, as 'defining the problem', 'mental representation', and 'planning how to proceed', while the metacognitive ability is a reflection on this cycle of planning, as 'evaluation'. These are capabilities needed for lifelong learning. Without these, learning is reproductive and stilted, rather than productive and transformative.

At the same time, the doctor is mobilizing metacognitive 'relationship' capabilities such as 'perspective taking' (empathy), 'emotional intelligence', 'self-assessment', 'self-care', and 'cultural awareness', filtered through a set of virtues including 'integrity', 'respect', and 'altruism' (as the highest level of perspective taking).

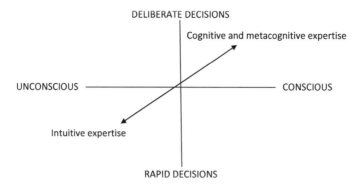

Fig. 4.2 Clinical reasoning in the technical domain (after Quirk, 2006, p. 9)

With repeated exposure to patients, doctors gradually replace conscious deliberation and metacognition with rapid, unconscious intuition. This is mainly pattern recognition. However, pattern recognition, or clinical intuition, is vulnerable to a variety of judgment biases and breeds overconfidence that may lead to misdiagnoses. In uncertain contexts, experts check their initial pattern recognition with a deliberate, reflective judgment, working through alternatives. Intuition and metacognition feed each other. Quirk (2006, p. 55) suggests that 'in many respects, intuition is reliance on clinical experience to modify the findings of evidence based medicine'. Medical students, as novices, rely on more deliberative cognition, using protocols, evidence, and information from tests. As junior doctors, they characteristically tend to order too many tests and investigations as they rely on decision analysis tools and algorithms for fear of judgment error or bias.

With experience, expertise and confidence develop through greater exposure to patients, where doctors tend to rely more on intuition and pattern recognition. This is summarized in Fig. 4.2 above, adapted from Quirk (2006), where gaining *technical* expertise is seen as a dialogue between deliberate, conscious decisions (cognitive and metacognitive) and rapid, unconscious decisions (pattern recognition). In cases of uncertainty, experts go back to deliberation. In cases of certainty, pattern recognition is trusted.

Such a model is widely recognized as a broad description of how *technical* clinical expertise is developed early in a medical education. However, it does not explain how expertise is gained in the *non-technical* arena of communication, interpersonal skills, and teamwork (again, capabilities that are, importantly, shared by other health-care professions and with patients). To encompass this area, we must redraw Quirk's quadrants for the non-technical realm of practice.

If we separate out the non-technical realm from the technical (although this black-and-white abstract division does not reflect the messy, concrete reality of the clinical context), we reveal a rather alarming state of affairs as far as gaining expertise is concerned. It is clear from the research evidence that doctors generally have not gained the level of expertise in the non-technical realm that they have in the technical. While conscious deliberation (cognition and metacognition) shapes the non-technical realm, particularly through problem solving and post hoc reflective evaluation, communication is assumed, as an intuitive ability. As Pauli and colleagues (2000a, p. 19) suggest, 'psychological and social domains (of medicine) are considered to be a matter of intuition on the part of health professionals—usually consigned to the rubric: "the art of medicine"'.

Hilliard Jason (2000, pp. 157–9) suggests that 'There are many paradoxes in our traditional approaches to educating health professionals. None is more striking than the contrast between the level of need for communication skills and the amount of time that is actually spent reinforcing these skills'. Evidence from studies of communication between doctors and patients and between doctors and other health-care professionals in teams suggests that metacognitive positions such as perspective taking, which characterize expert communicators, are not widely achieved (Lipkin, Putnam, & Lazare, 1995; Waitzkin & Stoeckle, 1972). Platt (1979), as described in Chap. 2, then refer to these widespread communication inabilities as 'hypocompetences'. Such hypocompetence is reflected in poor or underachieving teamwork through widespread resistance in health-care to adopting what Quirk (2006) calls 'collective perspective taking', described in the patient safety literature as 'situation awareness' achieved through practices such as team briefing (Bleakley, Allard, & Hobbs, 2013).

The evidence on quality of communication that I have referred to in the previous chapters, while it has largely been gleaned from North American studies, reveals a chronic pattern of poor communication. For example, we have seen that doctors, on average, interrupt within 18 s of the consultation starting. On average, two-thirds of patients do not complete the agenda that they brought to the consultation, and on average, communication is more often through closed questions and statements (monological) rather than open questions promoting dialogue. Further, 70 % of medical errors are grounded in systemic miscommunications, where the basic system is the clinical team. Poor communication is putting patients at risk, where doctors hover in the lower, left-hand quadrant of intuitive practice in the interpersonal medical encounter, in the diagram below (Fig. 4.3).

It is therefore vital that we understand more about the non-technical realm of doctors' work so that appropriate educational interventions can be made. The nature of such a complex intervention is, however, debatable. It is not as easy as simply saying that medical students should 'learn communication skills'. Even the normally pragmatic 'can do' *Oxford Handbook of Clinical Examination and Practical Skills* (Thomas & Monaghan, 2007, p. 2) suggests that 'Communication skills are notoriously hard to teach and describe'. It is not just *how* we educate in the non-technical dimensions of medicine, but the prior conceptual conception question of *what* it is that we are educating when we talk about 'patient-centredness', 'empathy', 'virtues', 'professionalism', 'teamwork', and so forth. Treating communication as a set of 'skills' itself offers a *value* position—instrumentality—that is open to critique. Further, there are wide cultural and individual differences in habits of

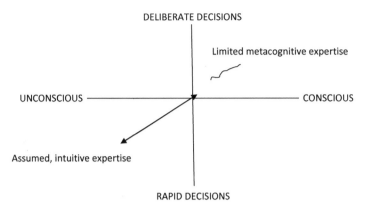

Fig. 4.3 Expertise in the non-technical domain (communication)

communication so that, however, medical students are prepared through standard-ized practices of communication; such standardization will never cover the spec-trum of cultural and individual styles of communication presented by patients. Finally, as Cumming (2002) notes, there is no point in educating doctors who are excellent communicators but otherwise deficient in their technical medical expertise.

I have already mentioned cultural awareness as a metacognitive capability of both communication and professionalism. There is a large anthropological and soci-ological literature describing potential and actual mismatches between doctors edu-cated in one cultural sphere and patients presenting with another cultural background (Fadiman, 1997; Helman, 2006). I have already shown, in the case study above drawn from Michael Taussig's (1992) work, that *sub*cultural variations in outlook can also produce wide differences of meaning for the medical encounter between doctor and patient.

Here, one further illustration will suffice. There is, historically, a significant difference between Western and Chinese cultures in the way that people think (Jullien, 2007). For Westerners, thinking is usually direct, going to the heart of the problem, clarifying, analyzing, and testing. For Chinese culture, this kind of thinking is alien, although it can be imitated. The cultural style is rather to suggest, glance off, hint, and circumnavigate, without stating a direction, a goal, or a 'centre'. This carries through to debate, which is combative in the West, but all about deflection in Chinese thought; and to the personal encounter, in which eye contact and direct gaze is expected in the West (and where it does not occur, is thought of as unskilled or symptomatic of a dysfunction), whereas the dropped gaze is the norm for Chinese culture and direct eye contact is thought to be disrespectful.

How do we then proceed in preparing students for the medical encounter, where the evidence suggests that the non-technical side of doctors' work is assumed and is treated less reflectively than the technical side? This must be challenged—there *is* substantial content to learn, and we know that expert application of such content has positive effects on patient outcomes (Stewart, 1995). This is best learned from patients (Kelly & Wykurz, 1998; Salter, 1996) and from the experience of being a patient (Klitzman, 2006). Experienced medical educators who are good communicators can creatively support medical students in this process in the work setting (Ashley, Rhodes, Sari-Kouzel, Mukherjee, & Dornan, 2009) and through well-facilitated, small-group reflection on critical incidents (Branch, 2001).

We should be more sceptical about engineered communication 'skills' teaching that is sometimes divorced from context and relies on formulae and prescriptions (such as a tick-box list of set outcomes) (Bligh & Bleakley, 2006; Marshall & Bleakley, 2009). Parallel with this pedagogical work, we must work harder on conceptual issues in the field of communication. It is to this area that we turn in the following chapters, to consider 'patient-centredness', 'relationship-centredness', and 'empathy', to offer a conceptual critique of these taken-for-granted notions.

I will retain the term 'patient-centredness' as necessary for describing a form of medicine that moves beyond technique-centredness and doctor-centredness as paternalism. However, 'patient-centredness' is not sufficient for describing an ideal of the democratic medical encounter, which, while centred on the patient, has more to do with the space of difference between patients and doctors. It is in this space of difference that the quality of the medical encounter is grounded, as an expression of a guiding value—tolerance of difference or tolerance for what is different from both self and the 'known'. Cultivating tolerance of difference is the basic educational challenge for teaching and learning non-technical capabilities in medicine. In the following five chapters, I explore this space between self and other that must be consciously and expertly inhabited and neither abandoned as alien nor conquered through paternalism.

Chapter 5
How Physicians Think Can Be Judged from How They Listen and Speak

For the Hardened Students of Communication Only

It is vital to set up experiences for medical students that involve learning with, from, and about patients, so that the patient becomes *a focus for collaborative learning* and not an object of inquiry. However, this does not divorce doctors or medical students from their expertise, or developing expertise, as clinicians and diagnosticians. It is not just that doctors must communicate well, but what we now know is that the quality of communication of doctors is intimately linked with the quality of how doctors *reason*, as noted above (Quirk, 2006). This is important, because it grounds abstract cognitive principles of reasoning (often delineated from psychological experiments) in actual cases and shifts the focus of interest from the cognitive process of the doctor to the meaning of the *transaction* between doctors, patients, clinical colleagues, and artifacts, as a total activity system (Bleakley, 2006c).

Jerome Groopman (2007, p. 17) suggests that 'How a doctor thinks can first be discerned by how he speaks and how he listens'. Establishing rapport with the patient, gaining his or her confidence, and pacing the dialogue are all key to gleaning the knowledge that the doctor needs to make, confirm, or progress diagnoses (Sanders, 2010). Having an offhand manner; failing to make eye contact; asking closed, rather than open-ended, questions; and making statements rather than asking questions—all of these typically close down consultations and then frustrate clinical reasoning.

Thomas and Monaghan (2007, p. 2) suggest that in teaching and learning communication skills, 'The rule is: there are no rules'. There is no recipe for good communication, as context is all important, and there would be nothing worse than a standard approach to communication. Idiosyncratic differences between doctors are welcome as long as they do not disadvantage, but help, patients. This is again to celebrate 'difference'. However, I do not follow Thomas and Monaghan's (2007, p. 2)

A. Bleakley, *Patient-Centred Medicine in Transition: The Heart of the Matter*, Advances in Medical Education 3, DOI 10.1007/978-3-319-02487-5_5, © Springer International Publishing Switzerland 2014

further suggestion that 'There are many models of the doctor–patient encounter which have been argued over at great length for years. *These are for the hardened students of communication only*' (my emphasis). This is a throwaway remark that only adds to the anti-intellectual reputation of medical education. It is important for doctors to consider basic theoretical elements that inform communication, just as they would for clinical reasoning based on knowledge of science. For example, assessors on an Objective Structured Clinical Examination (OSCE) station should be aware of Brian Hodges' (2003) argument that the OSCE can be read as a 'performance' and that its validity as an assessment tool is made more complicated (and perhaps more interesting) because of this.

Clinical reasoning cannot be divorced from the contexts of communicating the results of that reasoning (to both patients and colleagues). Patients and their families need to know clearly and precisely the meanings and possible consequences of their symptoms. Returning to our example in Chap. 2 of the most famous television (anti) hero in medical soap operas, Gregory House, Hugh Laurie expertly portrays a brilliant diagnostician who fails to translate insight into decent human encounter, blighted by a kind of autism. Where the reasoning is divorced from the human touch, it remains sterile. Brilliant insights require careful translation, especially if they carry serious consequences for future health or illness.

Taking a theoretical perspective, three general principles can be drawn from the growing body of research on doctor–patient communication, summarized in the meta-analysis of Roter and Hall (2006), as discussed earlier. First, doctors interrupt patients too early in the clinical encounter (on average, within the first 18 s). Second, communication is more often through directives, prescriptive language, statements, and closed question, rather than through open questions. Monologue then prevails over dialogue. Indeed, this pattern may be repeated in communication between the professions in a clinical team, such as a surgical team, where the surgeon sets the tone, and this is often prescriptive (Bleakley, Allard & Hobbs 2013). Third, in two-thirds of one-to-one consultations, the patient does not actually generate 'closure' or successfully complete the cycle of questions and issues that they came with, within the timescale of the consultation. The first two issues, premature closure or interruption and monologue rather than dialogue, contribute to the third issue, failure to satisfy the agenda you came with as a patient. Addressing these three research findings alone would provide a good structure for a communication skills component in the undergraduate curriculum.

However, we must expand this curriculum to include a fourth issue raised above—that of the need to educate doctors, medical students, and patients in tolerating the ambiguity of initial messy encounters that may, through patience, open up a deeper dialogue. This approach progresses 'patient-centredness' from its current instrumental, skills-centred model of 'presence' (what is said matters) to a model of 'absence' (what is not said, hinted at, just below the surface, is of vital importance). Drawing on both psychoanalysis and literary studies can develop this framework. Psychoanalysis suggests that unconscious desires frame what we see on the outer, and such desires can be made conscious. Indeed, what is called the 'ego', or self, is paradoxically where the unconscious rests. Or—we are most unconscious when we claim stubbornly or dogmatically that 'this is the way to do things around here'. We are then driven by habit and unquestioned cultural values. But such habits may be distorted and values biased.

This is not a controversial view. The heart of the argument of Michael Millenson's (1999) book supporting evidence-based medicine is that practitioners are stuck in habitual, self-centred (and sometimes institutionally centred) practices that are ingrained and unquestioned (again, 'this is the way we do things around here'). Millenson argues that many of these habitual practices have not taken into account the evidence accrued from large-scale studies, not because doctors are unaware of evidence-based medicine, but because of resistance to change habitual practices.

A further example is the resistance of clinical teams—especially in highly conservative areas of medicine and surgery, such as the operating theatre and accident and emergency departments—to respond to the evidence referred to several times previously that 70 % of medical errors are grounded in systemic communication issues, particularly miscommunications within and across clinical teams. Teams resist adopting simple practices, such as briefing and debriefing, because this challenges habit (Gawande, 2009). The power of habit to create a blind spot can be seen as an ego being unconscious.

In the USA, as opportunity for extended and intensive patient contact for medical students has eroded, there has been what Roter and Hall (2006, p. xi) call 'unprecedented reforms in medical education' as far as teaching and learning communication skills are concerned. Institute of Medicine (IOM) reports in 1999 (Kohn, Corrigan, & Donaldson, 1999), 2001 (Richardson et al., 2001), and 2003 (Tang et al., 2003) had all called for improving the quality of communication in medicine, especially in relationship to patient safety. In 2002, the AAMC and the Accreditation Council for Graduate Medical Education (ACGME) set out competency requirements for graduates from medical schools in six key areas, one of which is interpersonal communication (ACGME, 2005).

There has been exponential growth in researching the medical dialogue, and this has revealed undesired consequences of communication skills training, where both undergraduate and postgraduate medicine paradoxically cultivate *negative* attitudes towards patients, professionalism, and caring or humane behaviour that extend beyond patients to colleagues from other health-care professions. This distressing story was first broken in detail by the studies of Becker, Geer, Hughes, and Strauss (1980) and Lief and Fox (1963). Half a century later, we still recognize the story of socialization into medicine leading to a gradual increase in cynicism and emotional detachment on the part of medical students and junior doctors (Neumann et al., 2011). These studies suggested that in the non-technical realm, medical education 'works' *in spite of*, rather than *because of*, the way that it is structured.

Contemporary work suggests that problems of 'empathy decline' persist and are not being reversed by current approaches to communication skills training (that favour simulation methods). In American settings, Arno Kumagai (2008, 2009) describes how medical students may have both 'idealism' and 'compassion' 'trained out' of them by their medical education. Albanese, Snow, Skochelak, Huggett, and Farrell (2003) show that, as medical students progress through their education, they harden attitudes towards patients. They lose the idealism they came to medical school with and become noticeably (and measurably) more cynical and less patient-centred. Again, mainly in the North American context, studies show that the same process of disillusionment continues into early medical practice. Worryingly, Roter and Hall (2006, p. 87) note that 'no investigators credit the medical training process with inspiring or furthering anything that could be considered even close to idealism or humanism'. This is a terrible indictment—can there be an explanation?

Roter and Hall (2006, pp. 87–88) note four reasons. Each of these, I suggest, can be addressed. First is a key and infamous structural factor: junior doctors (interns) have been subject to a notoriously 'antisocial' socialization regime based on a military model. This combines intensive, stressful experience with sleep deprivation, supposedly to build character and test commitment. As the rationale for this method of socialization, not to mention the personal and patient safety issues, have been questioned for modern times, so legislation has been introduced to combat the severity of the initiation.

In the USA, the ACGME introduced rules in 2003 limiting the number of hours and length of shifts that junior doctors should work. In Europe, the European Working Time Directive (EWTD) has produced an even more stringent trimming of hours and shift lengths. In the UK, for example, surgical training hours have been more than halved overnight, producing what some see as a crisis in surgical education and others see as an opportunity to streamline such educational provision, trimming redundancy in 'socialization' experience and focusing upon intensive structuring or design of learning (de Cossart & Fish, 2005). Liberals in the field see such changes in surgical education as offering women an opportunity for a career in surgery previously denied through structural commitments.

Inevitably, the tough minded (often also conservative) bemoan the loss of a socialization process that they saw as producing character and sorting out the wheat from the chaff—the committed from the less committed. The initial research evidence into the effects of the restructuring of postgraduate medical education—as removal of the kind of intense sleep deprivation and stress that used to characterize a junior doctor's (intern's) life—is encouraging. For example, Jagsi, Shapiro, and Weinstein (2005) compared American medical students' views on work placements over the transition period to shorter hours, as a before-and-after measure. Students said that they valued the new work structure as this allowed their teaching physicians to spend more quality time with them (as they were less stressed at work), and students who previously had thought that they might leave medicine were now inclined to stay in the profession.

Second, students are said to lose their idealism because of increasing pressures to learn science and the fundamental dehumanizing that an intensive science education may bring as this translates into focus on biomedical issues with patients, rather than addressing the patient holistically. However, science need not be dull or dehumanizing. Science teaching can both be grounded in patient examples to make it relevant, and the intrinsic artistry and creativity in science can be taught as standard. This should be addressed by how medical schools recruit, develop, and support faculty.

Third, a knock-on effect of a science focus may be that while contact with patients is enjoyed in the early stages of a medical education simply for meeting a variety of interesting people, this may transform into reductive 'hypothesis testing' encounters, as students try out their emerging clinical reasoning skills. However, I have discussed above how patients are central to clinical reasoning, and students' learning opportunities should be structured to make the best of the dialogue with patients in this respect.

Fourth, and finally, through the informal curriculum, students will meet experienced doctors who are hardened to patients and who may appear harassed, overworked, and stressed. This is seen as a norm. The less entanglement with patients' 'personal' problems, rather than simply diagnosing and treating symptoms, the easier the job may seem. This is then a problem of recruitment, selection, education, and continuing support of clinical teaching faculty, but more, an inoculation of students against the well-documented 'hardening' effects of medicine, particularly hospital medicine and surgery.

Technically, this does not make sense. As discussed, the stereotype of the brilliant diagnostician who is emotionally detached from his patients offered in the most successful medical television series of all time, 'House, M.D.', does not reflect reality. Ironically, the programme scripts are based on the physician Lisa Sanders' monthly 'Diagnosis' column in the *New York Times* magazine. It is Sanders (2010, p. 7) who reminds us, as we described in the Introduction, that 'the great majority of medical diagnoses—anywhere from 70 to 90 %—are made on the basis of the patient's story alone'.

A fifth reason, which Roter and Hall do not discuss, has long been recognized and may be the most powerful—that over-identification with patients can be emotionally overwhelming and lead to potential burnout. Students therefore resort to classic psychodynamic defence mechanisms, such as 'emotional insulation' (not allowing themselves to be deeply touched by suffering), that become externalized and ritualized in black humour and negative stereotyping of patients. Typically, these defences become chronic and institutionalized, so that medicine as a whole can operate through repression and denial, rather than the softer protective ego defence patterns of displacement and projection.

Paradoxically, the energy needed to maintain the defence mechanism itself becomes the symptom—as exhaustion and burnout, sometimes leading to suicide, or as drug or alcohol dependency amongst a minority of doctors leading to exhaustive means of masking the addiction. Discussion of these issues would not be meaningful without a basic psychodynamic intellectual and theoretical framework, discussed in more depth in the following chapter.

Communication Is (Necessarily) Ambiguous

In the current climate of medical education, in which instrumental or technical–rational values are dominant (evidenced in the competence movement), there is a tendency to reduce the complex to the simple. This mirrors a primary characteristic of medicine, first described in depth by Renée Fox (1957), of an inability to tolerate uncertainty. This is in part driven by the desire of patients to have answers to their questions.

However, uncertainty, or ambiguity, is common to doctor (and medical student)/patient encounters and is a primary source of what doctors may see as patient 'noncompliance', including passive and active forms of resistance. For example, Tarkan (2008, p.6) reports that in the USA, 'A majority of emergency room patients are discharged without understanding the treatment they received or how to care for themselves once they get home'. What was once labelled 'noncompliant' is often now termed 'health illiteracy', where 'as many as half of all patients are considered to lack the ability to process and understand basic health information that they need to make decisions'. However, 'doctors are notoriously inept at communicating (such information) to patients'.

Again, where doctors are able to make clinical judgments and to reason clinically, it is imperative that they not only pass on the outcomes of this reasoning to patients (diagnosis, prognosis), but also, they *communicate the process of clinical reasoning and judgment itself in language that the patient can understand, to create dialogue*. Indeed, if patients' narratives and styles of communication offer a basis to, and for, diagnosis, doctors must reciprocate through democratizing their own more technical narrative styles. Importantly, content of a message is often secondary to delivery of that message. Patients should not be left confused about what is being conveyed to them because of poor communication. Doctors should recognize that while the clinical reasoning process itself may be largely cognitive, delivery of its outcomes might be loaded with affect. Importantly, where the clinical encounter may engage a good deal of uncertainty and ambiguity, the level of ambiguity can be discussed and opened up with patients, rather than prematurely closed by the doctor who either cannot tolerate the level of uncertainty himself or herself or feels (perhaps unwisely) that the patient should be protected from such uncertainty.

Rather than target either doctors' poor communication and/or patients' 'health illiteracy', we should recognize that much communication works at the level of a 'subtext', including unspoken, or unspeakable, issues; and effectiveness of communication can be all about *timing*. For example, a study by White, Levinson, and Roter (1994) showed that in approximately 20 % of routine primary care visits, the patient introduces a new and significant problem during the visit's closing moments. Where at least 25 % of such visits are motivated not by clear physical symptoms that are readily diagnosed, but by complex and ill-defined, perhaps unconsciously motivated, psychological or psychosomatic symptoms, then the subtext or the *absent*—not the spoken encounter or what is *present*—is the issue.

Where Roter and Hall (2006, p. 3) say that 'most of what occurs is talk' in the clinical encounter, their own major text refutes this, as they go on to discuss the importance of non-verbal communication. We know, for example, that positive non-verbal behaviours by practitioners—such as smiling, warmth, and appropriate contact—lead to better health outcomes when compared to poor non-verbal communication such as 'distancing' (Ambady, Koo, Rosenthal, & Winograd, 2002). What Roter and Hall (2006) do not account for are the 'surplus' grey areas of communication: ambiguities such as conscious or unconscious indirection, misdirection, simulation and dissimulation, and the ubiquitous *rhetorical purposes* of communication, which are unstated but evident and whose purpose is to persuade the recipient of the veracity of the communicator's message. The reader need look no further than the extensive body of work by the Canadian medical educator Lorelei Lingard (e.g. 2007) to appreciate the value of the application of study of rhetoric to communication in medicine.

We can add to this mix of uncertainties the disconcerting evidence of the common practice of 'thin slicing' in communication (Quirk, 2006, pp. 77–79). Thin slicing refers to the rapid (within the first 30 s of meeting) summing up of another that becomes the basis for later judgment. These are 'snap' decisions based on first impressions. Quirk (2006, p. 78) suggests that medical students should learn about this intuitive tendency and balance it with the metacognitive act of deliberation and reflection based on challenging first impressions: 'Intuition alone may not be the most effective way to make decisions about patients and their care. Studies and common sense tell us that intuitive impressions that underlie decisions don't always pan out'.

Where communication exchanges between doctor and patient are highly ritualized, such rituals include tactics of avoidance, navigating possible loss of 'face' or potential embarrassment and so forth. Communication is, above all, purposefully ambiguous to allow for interpretation of readings, masking, and a variety of other tactics to 'save face'. Across a lifetime's work, the sociologist Erving Goffman (1971, 1991) studied the subtleties of interpersonal encounters and came to the conclusion that interaction is best understood through the metaphors of theatre and drama. Goffman developed the work of the American pragmatist George Herbert Mead, who saw human communication as performance and 'mind' as a consequence of that social performance. For example, doctors put on carefully scripted and rehearsed performances, especially to appear 'professional'. Such a dramaturgical model is openly embodied in medicine's most famous 'theatre', the operating room, where literal and metaphorical 'masks' and predictable scripts are the communication norm.

As noted earlier, Brian Hodges (2003) in particular has employed Goffman's framework to make sense of students' performances in highly artificial, yet high stakes, settings, such as the OSCE. 'Unmasking' performances (e.g. where students may simulate what they do not know, or dissimulate what they do know, for purposes of passing the assessment) is not based on the premise that there is a 'right' and a 'wrong' way to perform (a truth claim) or possibly even that there are authentic and inauthentic performances. Rather, through study and interrogation, medical educators may gain deeper insight into the *meanings* of performance.

Taking into account the evidence base discussed above, that there are shortfalls in capability in the body of practising physicians in communicating effectively with patients and colleagues, medical students should gain some expertise in what is bread and butter practice in psychiatry (Hodges is a psychiatrist)—sensitivity to the unspoken, to nuances, and to hints. Patients typically offer 'exit' remarks, apparently offhand but loaded with significance: 'by the way doctor, I didn't mention that I am going through a pretty difficult divorce and I haven't slept properly for weeks now'. Medical students need to become familiar not just with the frequency of such patient 'bombs', but should also be aware of the evidence that what may be unspoken by the patient, or left to the critical 'leaving remark', may be a *product* of the doctor's style.

For example, a study by Beckman and Frankel (1984) looked at the first 90 s of the consultation. Typically, doctors ask an opening question such as 'what is the matter?' or 'what can I do for you?' (note that the first question focuses on the patient, where the second focuses upon the doctor). In two-thirds of visits, doctors interrupted patients' responses to this opening question after only 15 s, and the patient did not actually complete, or even return to, their opening statement. For the third of patients allowed to continue with their stories, the patient, on average, only took 3–4 min to get the story out to their satisfaction, where the average length of a consultation for general practitioners in Europe is 11–12 min and for the USA, 17 min (a notable increase since studies in the 1990s) (Mechanic, McAlpine, & Rosenthal, 2001). Marvel, Epstein, Flowers, and Beckman (1999) replicated the original Beckham and Frankel study and found strikingly similar results.

Thus, allowing patients to tell their stories may be more efficient in time terms in the long run, as well as offering plain human(e) consideration. But, importantly, how will more accurate diagnoses be made if the patient's story is habitually interrupted, curtailed, or even distorted, or if it is not complete? Again, the technical work of clinical reasoning is intimately bound with the non-technical work of communication—close listening, entering into dialogue, and close observation of non-verbal cues such as mismatch between what a patient says and how she presents herself.

Doctors typically ask closed, rather than open-ended, questions or worse make statements, where questions would have opened up dialogue with the patient. These endemic, chronic, and fundamental communication patterns are repeated throughout medical encounters (Roter & Hall, 2006). Clearly, they serve a purpose. Consciously or unconsciously, the doctor appears to want to maintain control and authority in most cases, repeating the commonly noted pattern of avoidance of uncertainty (Montgomery, 2006). (Of course, patients may be asking for certainty from their doctors that the latter are often not able to provide.) This not only restricts patients from pursuing their legitimate aims in seeking a consultation with a doctor, but it frustrates deeper kinds of collaborative or mutual consultations with patients that focus on emergence of new issues.

Patients should not leave medical encounters feeling that their needs have not been addressed, or only partially addressed, so that what was talked about was peripheral or tangential to their needs, or they felt inhibited and could not discuss what they really wanted to discuss. Psychotherapists are familiar with consultations where clients only come out with what is really on their mind 10 min before the end of the 50-min sessions (UK and American General/Family practitioners, as noted above, have on average about a quarter of an hour). The psychoanalyst Jacques Lacan infamously used (or abused) this knowledge by booking his clients for a 50-min session but making them wait 40 min before seeing him, forcing them (in his view) to get straight to the point! which is also a cue for me to draw this chapter to a close.

In this chapter, I have described how cognitive clinical reasoning process and communication of the outcomes of that reasoning are necessarily and intimately entangled. Subsequent chapters will formulate ways to address this entanglement. I begin this process by attempting to clear the ground of conceptual confusion concerning terms such as 'patient-centredness' and 'empathy'. What, precisely, might such terms mean?

Chapter 6
A New Wave of Patient-Centredness

Introduction

In the next three chapters, I look closely at the two key conceptual frames that inform contemporary communication between doctors and patients: first, 'patient-centredness' and second, 'empathy'. The fact that these conceptual notions have gained a foothold in medical practice shows how far medicine and medical education have moved towards the 'patient' as the subject, rather than the object, of activity. As Sir Donald Irvine (2003) suggests, the patient has become the focus of the new professionalism, and the new medical education, to the point, argues Moira Stewart that 'The patient should be the judge of patient centred care' (2001).

Not only has the patient's status shifted from object to subject but the 'abject' or most suffering patient has now become the test case for a new humane, inclusive medicine, which has learned much from nursing practice, so that medicine is now facing the challenge to be as much about 'care' as 'cure'. In saying this, I am not rejecting the long tradition of caring doctors, especially in family medicine, who would claim that perhaps the nursing profession has learned from them about bed-side manner. Rather, I am thinking about doctors now being embedded in wider networks of practice such as sets of clinical teams that are likely to be fluid. In this wider care model of networked and 'open' teams, discussed in depth in Chaps. 10–15, technical capability must be supplemented by nontechnical capability. Medical educators, in deciding how best to support the learning of patient-centred communication across the spectrum of medical education, must now put more effort into conceptual clarification of the nontechnical realm of practice, as they mount programmatic research agendas.

A. Bleakley, *Patient-Centred Medicine in Transition: The Heart of the Matter*,
Advances in Medical Education 3, DOI 10.1007/978-3-319-02487-5_6,
© Springer International Publishing Switzerland 2014

Journeys Without Maps

Consider the adaptability in communication that, for example, a community-based practitioner must develop: in multicultural settings, with children, with the elderly and confused, and with persons across a spectrum of disabilities, including mental health issues. This same doctor will also engage with the 'autonomous patient' (Coulter, 2002) who rejects paternalism, with patients' advocates including family members and with the savvy, Internet-informed patient. How shall we best prepare medical students for such intense and contrasting work of *relationship*? How can we develop a 'relationship centred' medicine? (Beach & Inui, 2006; Tresolini, 2000)

Breaking bad news, dealing with an aggressive patient, talking with family members, explaining something to a person with learning difficulties, second-guessing what is on a patient's mind, and so forth are everyday events in medicine. Traditionally, such communication was learned on the job or assumed. Now, such 'transferable skills' are formally taught and learned, indeed 'trained'. While communication skills are included in learning outcomes (ACGME, 2005; GMC, 2007) across the spectrum of medicine curricula globally and are at the heart of recommendations concerning good medical practice (GMC, 2009), just how to best teach and learn such 'skills' is hotly debated. Indeed, communication with patients goes far beyond the limited notions of 'skills' and 'training' to embrace *ways of being* ('Training', while habitually present in medical education, has always seemed to me to be a misnomer. The root of 'training' is 'to drag behind', where the root of 'education' is to 'draw out from'. The latter—'education'—seems to me to be a more appropriate descriptor for what we do in facilitating learning).

There is an emerging trend of learning communication in medicine in 'safe' simulated settings with both actor-patients and expert patients, involving video-taped encounters and direct feedback in custom-built clinical skills laboratories or communication suites. Proponents argue that this offers both 'standardization' of experience and possibility of standardized assessment (Klamen & Williams, 2006). But do we need a standardized communication? Is there such a person as a standard 'patient'? How can one 'be', and 'become', existentially, if outcomes are known and practices are standardized? This turns 'being', or reflective existence, into robotics. It is a condition of authoritarian regimes and personalities that activity becomes robotic or mechanical, detached from feeling and pity (Weiss, 2005).

Standardized patients of course are usually utilized in medical education not to present a standard face to symptom, but to present a uniform problem for all students in order to make assessment equitable and fair. But this approach may be misguided where it aims for homogeneity where patient presentations in real life display heterogeneity. Assessment of communication skills in undergraduate medicine is usually through a station of an Objective Structured Clinical Examination (OSCE). In such contexts, typically, a set of skills such as 'shows empathy', 'maintains eye contact', and 'communicates information clearly and precisely' are atomized as 'competences', serve as learning outcomes, and offer assessment criteria. This instrumental approach is now seamless with postgraduate education (Ryan et al., 2010).

For example, the UK General Medical Council's *The New Doctor* (2007, p. 86) specifically lists competences to be achieved for a Foundation (Junior) doctor to progress to registration, including demonstrating *'empathy and the ability to form constructive therapeutic relationships with patients'* (my emphasis).

Before we engage on a journey, it is vital that we have a map. Conceptual maps help enormously with journeys of learning, and conceptual maps are both derived from evidence (inductive research) and tested by gaining evidence (deductive research). It is strange, then, that in medical education we feel confident—as the quote above from *The New Doctor* suggests—in accompanying medical students upon journeys of learning without detailed maps. In this case, I refer to conceptual maps. To return to the recommendation from *The New Doctor* above, both 'empathy' and 'therapeutic relationships' are conceptually complex, historically and culturally contingent notions. Yet they have established themselves firmly in the vocabulary of the nontechnical face of medical education, seemingly beyond critique, as transparent practices.

Also, as 'the new doctor' implies a new kind of identity construction, what might a 'new' patient-centred and empathic doctor look like in comparison with an 'old' doctor? Is this new doctor one who draws on new technologies (such as imaging) and new sciences (such as genetics) but applied neither in a way that reduces the person to object or information? Surely this new doctor is one who can utilize the new medicine in a humane manner, bridging traditional bedside manner and diagnostic acumen with scientific expertise and insight?

The Many Faces of Patient-Centredness

Within the 'relationship', or nontechnical, aspects of medicine, 'patient-centredness' is a term that needs to be carefully unpicked. In this section I examine key literature on patient-centredness. While patient-centredness has been discussed for over half a century, its conceptual basis remains contested and its implementation has then been haphazard.

The philosopher Hegel's dictum that there is no master without slave and no slave without master offers a model of both identity and power (Singer, 1983). The master may have authority over the slave, but paradoxically, *without the slave there is no master*. Identity is created from the *difference* between the two, rather than some intrinsic characteristic of either 'master' or 'slave'. In the ancient Roman rite of 'carnival', masters and slaves would swap roles for a day, reminding us that we can step into the identity of the 'other', if only temporarily and in a ritualized manner (e.g. wearing a mask). In the contemporary world, 'identity theft', first coined in 1964, is now a common crime. This sometimes goes beyond fraudulent access to private information (e.g. through online hacking), to taking on a complete persona. Examples include persons pretending to be doctors without having qualifications ('quacks').

There are no doctors without patients. It is through difference from patients that doctors can be said to gain an identity, so patients are the heart of the matter as far as medical education is concerned. To ground the identity of the doctor in this difference challenges the orthodox model that doctors gain identity from socialization into the profession of medicine, where key influences are professional guidelines (the explicit curriculum) and role modelling from seniors (the hidden or informal curriculum) that shape character (Hafferty, 2006). The key work of the doctor–patient relationship may happen in the gap between the two identities (i.e. in the difference). For Tresolini (2000) and Beach and Inui (2006), *patient*-centred approaches in health-care should be recast as *relationship* centred. Tresolini (2000) insists that in health-care organizations, 'relationship' must be 'the bottom line'.

There are styles of managing this gap. For example, the doctor who is indifferent, or insensitive to difference (who judges the patient, or communicates poorly), is creating an identity out of a negative reading of difference, such as the exercise of paternalism (unquestioned authority). This echoes a master–slave relationship based on intolerance of the 'other' shown in a clear power relationship of control. On the other hand, a doctor who is sensitive to difference shows respect for the Other, and the identity construction of the doctor is then born out of a positive relationship of difference (tolerance, understanding, valuing diversity). This doctor makes a conscious effort to see the world from the perspective of the patient as the Other.

It is through mutual perspective taking that the doctor–patient relationship may develop as one that is grounded in difference but which seeks to exploit such difference as a positive resource. Such a relationship of difference characterizes what we now think of as tolerant, multicultural, multifaith societies. A key characteristic of, and tension within, the late modern or postmodern cultural condition is the simultaneous presence of positive multiculturalism and a return to 'identity' politics. Identity politics includes separatist feminism (women who see no value in masculine ideals) and single faith outlooks that can become zealous or fundamentalist (such as radical Judaism, Islam, and 'born-again' Christianity). The equivalent in medicine is zealous paternalism and resistance to social accountability.

Patient-centredness can then be understood in terms of the positive *difference* between doctor and patient. Szasz and Hollender (1956) first coined the term 'patient-centred' (with or without the hyphen), and this was echoed in 'client-centred' or 'person-centred' counselling and psychotherapy, a descriptor first coined by Carl Rogers (1957). Patient-centredness is a core principle in the biopsychosocial model of medicine proposed by Engel (1977), developed in particular by McWhinney (1988), and later refined by Pauli, White, and McWhinney (2000b, p. 169—a significant 'think tank' that included McWhinney). Pauli's group extended the awkward descriptor 'bio-psychosocial' to the impossibly cumbersome 'psychosomatosociosemiotic' to describe how Engel's term must be expanded to accommodate medicine entering the 'information age' (late modernism, or postmodernism), where medical education can be characterized as a complex, adaptive system. For Paul, White, and McWhinney (2000a, 2000b), the question of 'what' we teach in medical schools is, for the first time in the history of medical education, now formed by the prior question of *how we relate in a society*. This is a radical notion, redefining what we mean by a medical education.

In brief, Pauli puts emphasis upon the ways that doctors come to understand symptom presentations as characteristics of a cultural age. It is clear that many of our medical conditions expressing as *soma* (such as hypertension) are grounded in *psyche* (stress, anxiety, work ethic, cultural performance pressures). As Pauli et al. (2000b, p. 174) note 'There is growing recognition of the importance for health of socially based life conditions' such as 'organ system breakdown, degenerative, neurological, arteriosclerotic, and neoplastic chronic illnesses under conditions of mal- and overnutrition, alcoholism, AIDS, drug addiction, family violence, work stress, unemployment, poverty and environmental poisoning', where the 'traditional conceptual separation of the mental from the physical domain has become increasingly anomalous'. The future of medicine is in prevention and health education and in the understanding of the complex relationship between psyche, soma, and environment.

While recognizing the relationship between symptom and society, Pauli and colleagues do not consider political positions as issues of health or symptom. For example, should we not consider collaborative behaviour and tolerance towards others as healthy and deviations from this as symptom? Surely authoritarianism and the desire to control others is a chronic symptom? My primary concern in this book, introduced earlier, is to ask why the institution of medicine refuses the full democracy that Western post-industrial societies enjoy and now expect? Why are many doctors 'citizens' in everyday life, but unable to become 'medical citizens' within their profession, and why are patients not automatically treated as equal citizens in a community of health? Patient-centredness in medicine and health-care should offer a genuine democracy, inviting participation by all stakeholders as appropriate. The kind of democracy depends, as outlined in Chap. 3, on the mix of three kinds in any given context—assembly (participative), representative (elected), and monitory (quality assured) democracies. In other words, contexts will shape the form of democracy as well as the particular identity of the 'citizen'.

A Brief History of Patient-Centredness

Despite, as we have seen, a coining of the term 'patient-centredness' in the mid-1950s, Jolly and Rees (1998, p. 264) note that 'the concept of patient-centred care was virtually non-existent in UK medical education in the 1980s', while a report from the American Association of Medical Colleges (AAMC), in contrast, had placed patients and their families at the heart of medical education as early as 1984. In 1968, a family practitioner from the UK, Ian MacWhinney, introduced a patient-centred approach to the department of family medicine in London, Ontario. This followed Carl Rogers' method of 'client-centred' therapy and 'learner-centred' pedagogy. MacWhinney thought about patient-centredness not just as 'communication', but also as a *clinical* method going beyond therapeutic technique. Through acting as learners in a medical education context, doctors could learn how to empathize with patients, so that patient-centred technique was intimately tied with lifelong professional education. MacWhinney emphasized that forming a relationship with patients was a moral imperative in medicine, not simply a technical requirement.

Moira Stewart et al. (2005) championed MacWhinney's work, and the patient-centred consultation has been systematized into six steps: (1) assessment, (2) integration of the assessment into the whole person (including the patient's lifestyle and lifeworld), (3) finding common ground between patient and doctor, (4) educating about prevention, (5) building a long-term relationship, and (6) allocating resources realistically and equitably.

The distinguished medical historian Kenneth Ludmerer (1999, p. 293), however, does not recognize such initiatives in medicine as generally being sustainable, where, in his view 'In the molecular era, patients were bypassed'. By the era of managed care in the 1990s, students were spending less time with patients in the developed nations because hospitals were being forced to increase efficiency and throughput. Indeed, Ludmerer argues that by the 1990s, American medicine had lost public confidence, resulting in a pressing need for medical education to restore the traditional 'social contract between medicine and society' (Ludmerer, 1999, p. 399).

Authors seem to position themselves in relationship to patient-centredness without the long view, or the benefit of a historical perspective, leading to conflicting claims. Thus, while Salter (1996) describes learning from patients already as 'unfashionable' by 1996, 2 years later Kelly and Wykurz (1998) describe 'patients as teachers' as a 'new perspective' in medical education. As we enter further into the new millennium, there is certainly recognition of the enormous scale of institutional culture change required to shift from a 'traditional' to a 'patient-centred' curriculum that promotes the learning of 'professionalism' (Christianson et al, 2007). The problem is—and this is a healthy problem, stimulating debate—while we do not necessarily need to have agreement on concepts such as 'patient-centredness', or 'professionalism', we do need an educated *literacy* in the field, to critically compare different readings. We need to interrogate the quality of theoretical models and carefully review research evidence supporting models.

Patient-centredness has become naturalized in medical education, immune from critique because it is self-evidently 'good'. But it is a confused and contested term and is invoked on behalf of different, sometimes conflicting, interests. Further, there is, worryingly, still a relative paucity of high-quality evidence linking positive patient outcomes with varieties of patient-centred medical interventions (Stewart et al., 2003). Patient-centredness is invoked as desirable largely as a moral assumption— that to act humanely is intrinsically good or virtuous.

Kathryn Montgomery (2006, p. 192) approaches the problem of efficacy from another perspective where she, properly, asks: what are the alternatives to patient-centredness and are they viable? She frames a patient-centred approach in terms of its antagonism to 'numbers' (test results, statistics), where the latter can distort the ethical encounter with a flesh and blood individual. In contrast, Michael Millenson (1999) argues for a model of patient-centredness that begins with the numbers and the significance of population studies. Ethical practice equates to evidence-based clinical decisions, talking through the significance of the numbers (evidence from large scale studies) with, and for, individual patients. The point for Millenson (1999, pp. 318–320), following the advice of the ethicist Howard Brody, is 'responsible use of power' by the doctor to bring about patient-centredness. This may seem like paternalism in disguise, but, as Millenson explains, is actually a shift from 'good quality care from the physician's view ("Quality of care is what I provide") to the patient's perspective ("Quality of care is what I receive")'.

Montgomery's and Millenson's approaches both offer a tension, respectively, between narrative-based medicine and evidence-based medicine, although there is no reason why the two approaches cannot be in productive dialogue rather than unproductive opposition. Oppositionalism—as a strategy not just for thinking and arguing, but also for activity and practice—is not interested in the qualities of difference between approaches or persons, but tends to get bogged down in promoting one approach at the expense of the other. One identity is then privileged over another in a support of 'selfsame' rather than 'difference'.

Narrative-based approaches listen from the perspective of the patient's story and how the patient makes meaning of his or her illness. Treatment follows this trajectory, shaped by patient autonomy. Evidence-based approaches follow what population studies have found, where treatment follows the best available evidence. This may cross the patient's wishes and lead to 'noncompliance', but the doctor is acting ethically, in good faith, according to the best science.

As two legitimate ways of sense making (Bruner, 2002), or 'worldmaking' (Goodman, 1978), narrative- and evidence-based approaches can work in tandem. Indeed, Mark Quirk (2006) claims that authentic realization of this tandem would offer a 'new paradigm' for contemporary medical education. However, as argued earlier, if we separate the technical and the nontechnical realms of medicine and medical education, we find that Quirk's model works well for the technical realm of clinical practice, but has shortcomings in the nontechnical realm, where communication proceeds largely on assumption and intuitive response rather than evidence.

What is now called 'health illiteracy', rather than 'noncompliance', may not be a result of patients consciously choosing autonomy, but of a misunderstanding between patients and doctors arising from poor, or hasty, communication (Tarkan, 2008). Jerome Groopman (2007, pp. 91–92) gives an example of where doctors need more than sensitivity to the individual patient—they need to be aware that a diagnosis can occur at the social and cultural levels, so that 'patient'-centredness must also be social awareness. A 74-year-old African-American woman was labelled 'noncompliant' by several doctors for not taking several medications that had been prescribed for multiple chronic illnesses: diabetes, rheumatoid arthritis, coronary artery disease, and hypertension. She appeared, after hospital admissions, to be not reliably taking her medications, leading to readmissions. What doctors had missed was that she could not read or write, common for African-American women of her generation from the Deep South. She simply could not read the labels on the medicines, but was too embarrassed to admit this.

In the sophisticated model of 'professionalism' developed by Louise Arnold and David Stern (2006, p. 23), paradoxically, patient-centredness is not centred on patients or on quality of the relationship between patient and doctor, but on attributes of the doctor. Patient-centredness is a set of values at the heart of professionalism, expressed particularly through 'humanism', which in turn is characterized as demonstrating fundamental respect, or 'regard for another person with esteem, deference, and dignity'. Empathy and compassion are key traits defining modern patient-centredness. While the authors acknowledge that this 'presents physicians with a special challenge since signs of respect may vary across cultures', the challenge is deeper and wider. Where patient-centredness is based on what appears to be fixed traits, or essential virtues, the approach is ahistorical, insensitive to context and denies the possibility of plural identities (Bauman, 2004).

Although Arnold and Stern warn that we should be cautious about setting 'professionalism' in stone and that there will be local variants, their project is to operationalize patient-centredness in terms of 'professionalism', as a reasonably stable set of traits that can be assessed. Again, patient-centredness is expressed not as an act of collaboration with patients but as a stable (or stabilizing) identity construction for doctors. This is not simply slippery semantics, a reversal of terms. Rather, it is a choice concerning identity as 'selfsame' (begin with the doctor, in the socialization of the doctor and within the medical community and work outwards to the patient) or, in contrast, as based in 'difference' (begin with the place between two terms— the 'other' who is the patient and the self who is the doctor).

Mark Quirk (2006) offers similar epistemological slippage to that of Arnold and Stern. In discussing how 'perspective taking' is vital to developing both clinical reasoning and communication skills, Quirk argues for a medical education that includes learning 'metacognitive' capabilities. These are core, transferable skills that any professional should learn, that should be in a core curriculum, and that offer the basis for lifelong learning: 'planning', 'reflection', 'self-assessment', and 'perspective taking'. Perspective taking is a reflective process that allows one to understand what it is like to be another, such as the patient, from which both cognitive empathy and affective compassion are generated.

First, the evidence suggests that such metacognitive abilities are largely not achieved by doctors, who resort to the intuitive in the nontechnical realm of practice. Second, slippage occurs where such metacognitive capabilities are reduced to competences expressed as learning outcomes. In this move, the skill (or rather, an apprehension) of 'perspective taking' that is 'patient-centredness' is located in the personality of the medical student, so that as a quality held by the student (and then the doctor), patient-centredness is again not located in the activity of the doctor– patient relationship (in the place of difference between the two) or in transactions— activities of collaboration and mutuality.

Let me stress again that if patient-centredness is located in the doctor, even if it is a positive virtue, paradoxically we encourage the familiar refrain of doctors calling the tune—medical paternalism. If patient-centredness is located in the patient, as radical autonomy, then we are in danger of losing the opportunity to realize the full technical expertise of doctors. Patient-centredness may be better realized as mutuality—as the quality of relationship *between* doctor and patient. This also turns patient-centredness into an activity, moving away from trait models, where patient-centredness is characteristically a personality expression of doctors.

Quirk (2006, pp. 369–380) elegantly links the power of clinical reasoning with the quality of the doctor–patient relationship, but clinical reasoning is returned to the doctor as an individualized and internalized cognitive activity, repeating the bias of 30 years' worth of psychologically based (and biased) research in the field (Norman & Eva, 2010). Such bias fails to account for clinical reasoning as a *transaction* between doctor and patient, or an effect of distributed cognition across a clinical team or within a community of practice (Gao & Bleakley, 2008). In a single paragraph tucked away in a chapter on the relationship between clinical reasoning and doctor–patient communication, Quirk (2006, p. 76) does, however, refer to Scardamalia's (2002) notion of 'collective cognitive responsibility' as the 'ideal functioning of expert teams'. More could be made of this insight.

There is, in fact, an extensive literature on the notion of 'situation awareness' in teams (Bleakley, Allard, & Hobbs, 2013), which echoes similar ideas of distributed cognition (Clark 1997, 2009). The point is that Quirk, like many other North American medical educators, predictably tends to reproduce the dominant cultural model of individualism in a bias towards psychological models of internal cognition rather than sociological, anthropological, or systems models of shared, distributed, and negotiated thinking—a cognition of *mutuality*.

In contrast to both Arnold and Stern's and Quirk's, models, for Angela Coulter (2002, xii), patient-centredness begins not with the doctor, but with empowerment of patients and is necessarily political: 'paternalism … has had its day. Instead, we must redefine the patient's role to emphasize autonomy, emancipation and self-reliance rather than passivity and dependence'. This rhetoric of liberation is couched in both paradoxical imperatives and prescriptive economic and management metaphors: 'patients *must* be treated as *co-producers* of their own health and *care-managers* when they are ill' and '*must* be encouraged to see themselves as decision-makers, evaluator, and stakeholders with a key role in shaping health policy' (my emphases). Thus, patients not only have a right, but a *duty*, to shape healthcare through informed decisions as 'active citizens'. The rhetoric is combative, urging us to muster forces to challenge the enemy of 'paternalism'. Indeed Coulter's (2002) subtitle 'Ending Paternalism in Medical Care' calls not for a dialogue with paternalism (even in its generous form, such as Millenson's model above), but for its demise.

Laine and Davidoff (1996) define patient-centred care as 'health-care that is closely congruent with and responsive to patients' wants, needs, and preferences'. While this challenges paternalism, it is psychoanalytically naïve. I argue in more depth later in this chapter that it may be the case that neither patients nor doctors (and, particularly, medical students) always consciously know what they 'want' out of a consultation. First, the consultation may be driven by what is not made explicit, is not voiced, or remains unconscious. Second, what may be of significance in the consultation is what emerges as a consequence of the consultation. Such emergent properties are, by definition, not known in advance.

Jerome Groopman (2007) offers an illustration of a woman with a chronic illness who had been misdiagnosed and then offered inappropriate treatment for many years for what turned out to be celiac disease, an autoimmune disorder. Groopman focuses upon the quality of the communication exchange she has with a sensitive specialist, who was able to build rapport and collaboratively explore possibilities of a new diagnosis as these unfolded in the moment, or were emergent properties of an intense, high-quality consultation. What looks at first to be a brilliant diagnosis turns out to be a revelation made possible by the quality of collaboration between the technical interests of the specialist, the expertise gained by the patient into her own suffering, and the mutual trust developed in the formal consultation. What is surprising in this account is that the patient had not previously experienced such mutuality in the clinical consultation, over a long history of treatment. Differences were respected and utilized as points where relevant information or insight would be generated. But such insight could not be predicted in advance.

In contrast to a focus upon either medical autonomy (paternalism) or patient autonomy (and the unproductive opposing of these positions), Atkins and Ersser (2008, pp. 377–387) read patient-centredness in the context of potential collaborative decision-making—focusing on the activity of health-care rather than the identities of either practitioner or patient (although identities are shaped by such activities). They identify four theories informing patient-centredness: (1) exchange, dialogue, and negotiation, as a sociocultural model (focusing upon power differences); (2) humanistic (focusing upon the quality of relationship); (3) ethical (focusing upon moral obligations of practitioners); and (4) professional (focusing upon the contexts of care and the particular ways in which collaboration can be supported in differing contexts).

Patient-centredness as mutuality must be learned early in a medical student's career, but hazards appear along the way—the most pressing being 'empathy decline' and 'moral decline', discussed in earlier chapters. Here, students' ideals are gradually eroded in the face of various challenges, tensions, and inappropriate role modelling as they are gradually socialized into medical culture. Students 'harden' through excessive work pressure; the institutionalized expectation to act autonomously rather than to seek help; disappointment at the realization that practising medicine includes management, paperwork, teaching, and other duties; and meeting unfortunately infectious cynicism in seniors. How then will mutuality be developed in the face of such pressures?

Mutuality between medical students and patients can only develop if the patient first consents to the student's presence (Price, Spencer, & Walker, 2008). There is a significant literature on patients' attitudes towards medical students' presence in consultations and other clinical activities (Yardley et al., 2010). Students may be actively involved, for example, in examining the patient or passive observers. Locations vary, such as general practice, hospital wards, outpatient clinics, and hospices. At one end of the scale is the Linkoping model (Savage and Brommels 2008) of both extensive and intensive student–patient interaction: a student-run, multiprofessional teaching ward with real patients, supervised by a senior doctor and nurse but planned on a daily basis by medical, nursing, and other health-care profession students. At the other end of the scale, medical students tag along as peripheral observers on a ward round and may not even be introduced to patients as a courtesy. The Linkoping model offers central, legitimate participation in a team setting and promises a high yield of learning; the ward example offers marginalization without participation and promises a low yield of learning. Somewhere in-between is the usual state of affairs, with 'legitimate', but 'peripheral', participation in a team (Lave & Wenger, 1990) giving the student some sense of worth and identity.

That medical students should benefit from patients is a given—they must learn the job. However, patients may generally see themselves as passive recipients of care and not active teachers. One would think that there is no better learning situation in medical education than structured work with an expert patient who has also had some education in how to teach students. In a literature review of 23 papers focusing upon the effect of patients as teachers in non-simulated settings, where this role was explicitly formulated, Wykurz and Kelly (2002) report consistently positive reactions from learners, some of whom preferred being taught by the patient rather than a supervising doctor. In particular, this was considered by students to be a good format for learning communication skills, especially where patients were involved in feedback and assessment.

Gruppen, Branch, and Laing (1996) studied rheumatoid arthritis patients trained as educators of second year students, where the focus was upon integration of basic science and clinical examination. Using a pre/post-evaluation format, they showed significant changes in attitudes and knowledge in students after exposure to patient teaching. Follow-up evaluations showed that the learning persisted. Knowledge was then co-produced by patients and students. The student's role, as in the Linkoping model, can be extended to provide care to, as well as learning from, patients. For example, Black and Church (1998) used a questionnaire to evaluate the views of psychiatric inpatients concerning medical students as care providers and found the patients' reactions to be positive.

It is important that patients feel that they benefit from the presence of students—otherwise mutuality in both learning and care is compromised. Patients say, predictably, that they want students who will listen well, in settings as diverse as palliative care (Franks & Rudd, 1997) and severely deprived communities (Jackson, Blaxter, & Lewando-Hundt, 2003). The dignity of patients must be respected. In a study of patients' views towards the presence of students in obstetrics–gynaecology outpatient clinics, women patients understandably felt most uncomfortable about intimate examination—undergoing a pelvic examination with a student present—and consent issues were seen as important. Nevertheless, 75 % of patients were willing to have students present during the consultation, including non-intimate examination (Hartz & Beal, 2000).

Patients in general practice settings have generally welcomed students, and when planned well, this has been shown to not be disruptive to the flow of practice. O'Flynn, Spencer, and Jones (1997) offer some caution, however, since 30 % of patients found the presence of students constraining when it came to discussing personal matters. Findings such as this mean that we cannot simply assume that generating volume of work-based learning experiences on an ad hoc basis is the way forward for undergraduate medical education—such experiences must be designed: planned and structured. Current thinking suggests that a core, work-based, educational practice could allow students to follow a panel of chronic patients in the community (and then in acute settings where necessary) longitudinally (Cooke, Irby, & O'Brien, 2010). Students then build a relationship of some depth and, in following the patient, rather than being attached to teams in locations, they get to understand what patient pathway care means on the ground.

In the following chapter, I distil the discussion above into a variety of models of patient-centredness, recognizing that the descriptor 'patient-centredness' generates multiple legitimate possibilities.

Chapter 7
Models of Patient-Centred Care

Where Is 'Patient-Centredness' Centred?

In the previous chapter, I outlined three main differences in approach to patient-centredness: first, as a characteristic of doctors (with its archetype as *paternalism*); second, as empowered activities by patients (with its archetype as *patient autonomy*); and third, as the relationship between doctor and patient in action (with its archetype as *collaboration*, leading to *mutuality*).

Conceptually, and paradoxically, patient-*centredness* is not formally centred on patients (although it may be in spirit and intention) since it is, first, centred on doctor's professional identities and personalities (following the values of individualism); second, on political and economic values that inform emancipation and empowerment approaches; and third, on educational values informing collaborative activities between doctors and patients. We need, however, to refine these rather stark categories where there is a good deal of conceptual confusion around them. For example, Annemarie Mol's (2008) research work on care for persons with diabetes problematizes the notion of patient-centredness in arguing that the current political drive for 'patient choice' is misguided if this issue comes to overshadow patient *care*. Mol suggests that even in a collaborative model, patient 'choice' may compromise good medical advice, where such advice should always be based on 'logic of care' rather than 'logic of choice'.

There is a further paradox at play. Critics of patient-centredness point out that some patients may not want doctors to adopt a patient-centred approach, but may prefer a more instrumental, disease-centred approach and may not mind impersonality. However, where Moira Stewart (2001) claims that 'The patient should be the judge of patient centred care' (strictly, a 'person-centred' view), then if patients *prefer* to see doctors who are not patient-centred and that view is honoured, we are still being 'patient-centred' in Stewart's definition.

A. Bleakley, *Patient-Centred Medicine in Transition: The Heart of the Matter*,
Advances in Medical Education 3, DOI 10.1007/978-3-319-02487-5_7,
© Springer International Publishing Switzerland 2014

I describe below 12 models of patient-centredness that can be derived from the historical literature. 'Historical' is important because the first model—paternalism—has become the antithesis to contemporary views on what constitutes a patient-centred approach and is often seen as promoting a dysfunctional relationship to patients, although it can still be regarded as the default position. There was a time, as explained below, when paternalism was seen as good for patients and resistance to paternalism was seen as unhelpful to the healing process. Historically, paternalism is then an example of 'patient-centredness' but dictated entirely by the doctor, in good faith, in the patient's supposed best interests. Times, of course, have changed. What was once considered legitimate practice is now frowned upon, while, ironically, paternalism—albeit 'softened'—may still be the norm in the institution of medicine.

The models can be grouped broadly into four themes (expanded below) and further collapsed into three sets of tensions: (1) paternalism versus patient autonomy (Coulter, 2002), (2) collaboration/mutuality versus dysfunctional 'care' (Beach & Inui, 2006), and (3) 'naturalistic' versus virtual.

Paternalism in tension with patient autonomy is a long-standing issue in medicine and often centres on compliance/noncompliance of patients in taking prescribed courses of medicines. Patient autonomy is sometimes referred to as 'consumerism' (Haug & Lavin, 1983). This grounds patient autonomy in economic rather than interpersonal values, with doctor as producer and patient as customer. Autonomy can be seen as a more open category, where patients can be producers of *knowledge* (and co-producers with doctors).

Collaborative models are clearly in tension with those of dysfunctional 'care'. The former are rich, productive, and caring; the latter are manipulative and uncaring—where, for example, the doctor is consciously unprofessional or unethical in behaviour. This includes acting out sexual relationships with patients, treating patients while under the influence of alcohol or drugs, treating patients entirely with an economic profit motive in mind, treating patients without gaining prior consent, or treating (and/or refusing to treat) patients from a religious or cultural perspective (e.g., women seeking a termination of pregnancy or families forcing a young girl to undergo clitorodectomy performed by a doctor).

'Naturalistic' doctor–patient relationships include all encounters that are not online or virtual. An explosion has occurred in medicine and health-care facilitated by the development of the Internet. New patient behaviours are emerging such as self-diagnosis, enhanced diagnosis, self-treatment (buying pharmaceuticals online without prescriptions), and collaborative patient groups. The latter includes a variety of online communities, usually centred on one chronic illness, who exchange information, support and empower one another, and form pressure groups related to issues such as research, availability of treatments, and behaviour of the medical community.

Classification of Types of Patient-Centredness

1. *Paternalism*

    (a) Paternalism

2. *Varieties of patient autonomy*:

    (b) Empowerment
    (c) Advocacy

3. *Varieties of collaboration and mutuality between doctors and patients*:

    (d) Patient as catalyst for interprofessional activity
    (e) Mutuality/relationship-centred care
    (f) Deeper mutuality: psychodynamics and the therapeutic alliance
    (g) Local ecosystem
    (h) Clinical reasoning
    (i) Pedagogical
    (j) 'Difference'
    (k) Intertextual

4. *Collaboration and mutuality between patients* (*where doctors also assume the roles of patients*)

    (l) Patient-centredness as patient connectedness in online communities

Paternalism as Patient-Centredness

As suggested above, this model may seem to offer a paradox, now that 'paternalism' has taken on a negative connotation. However, as first set out by the sociologist Talcott Parsons (1991/1951) in the 1950s, 'paternalism' was originally conceived within a model of legitimate authority and power based on professional duty grounded in expertise. Parsons argued that the doctor–patient relationship is one of consensual agreement or accommodation of the patient to the legitimate authority of the doctor. While the patient is allowed to legitimately claim absence from the productive workforce during periods of illness, he or she must recognize the legitimate authority vested in the doctor by his or her expertise (to which the lay patient has no real access) as the means by which the patient will be legitimately restored to the workforce. Questioning the doctor's judgment is then a breach of the privilege of care. Paternalism is for the good of the patient as he or she is returned as rapidly as possible to a productive role in the social order.

Eliot Friedson (1970) and Ivan Illich (1975), in different ways, both saw medical paternalism and the medical profession's self-regulation as means of avoiding social accountability. This view leads to a direct challenge of Talcott Parsons' model.

Medicine, however, has changed greatly since these critiques, prompted not just by high profile ethics cases in the UK such as the Bristol paediatric heart surgery cases, serial murderer Harold Shipman, and organ retention scandals, but, importantly, by the work of medical educators offering a vision of collaborative care. The rhetoric of contemporary medicine is diametrically opposed to paternalism. Yet the historical paternalistic authority structures of medical power and dominance linger, so that the democratizing of medicine is still a challenge rather than inevitable.

Patient-Centredness as Varieties of Patient Autonomy

Empowerment

We have already referred to Angela Coulter's work that is explicitly political, seeking to empower patients. Nicky Britten (2003, 2008) has focused upon a variety of subtle ways in which patients manage their prescribed drugs. These range from collaborative decisions with their doctors through to the types of independent decisions that doctors may call 'noncompliance', but that can be read as 'reduced adherence' from the patient's viewpoint. The rhetoric of the work—delicately avoiding apparent bias or blame—in revealing communication shortcomings on the side of the doctor explicitly persuades the reader into accepting the legitimacy of patients' acts of resistance in a power relationship.

Such sociological research can be read as expressly empowering where it reveals patient-led strategies that lead to satisfactory outcomes for the patient. The 'trail' for such empowerment is not, of course, direct. Members of the lay public do not generally read sociology of medicine papers. Rather, the empowerment comes through the supportive activities of informed health-care professionals and academics working with expert patient groups. These activities may then address the wider community or lay public through translation into health education and promotion.

Such activities are now subject to media representations of medicine and patient care through television 'medi-soaps'—medical soap operas such as *Holby City*, *Casualty*, *Bodies*, and *Monroe* in the UK and *ER*, *House, M.D.*, and *Grey's Anatomy*, amongst others, in the USA. Some of these television programmes inform viewers of helpline numbers they can call if any issues portrayed have affected them, turning medi-soaps from 'medutainment' to 'infotainment'. Such medi-soaps are supplemented by reality television series of real medical life, such as *Junior Doctors: Your Life in Their Hands* in the UK. These follow in a tradition of soap operas (*Dr. Finlay's Casebook*, *Dr. Kildare*) and reality television (*Your Life in Their Hands*), where the significant historical shift is from portrayal of doctors as paternalistic to portrayals of patient empowerment. Yet, the rhetoric of medical dominance lingers—'your life in their hands', where 'lifestyle' (the patient's choice of diet, alcohol consumption, and so forth; or the life circumstance of poverty, deprivation, domestic violence, work stress, environmental pollution, and so forth) is not the focus. Rather, we see chronic illness and system breakdown as medical conditions open to medical interventions—'your life in their hands'—surely reinforcing paternalism.

The sociological research shows a range of examples of self-empowerment through strategies of resistance to conforming to doctors' prescriptions. Benson and Britten (2003) report qualitative data gathered from interviews of patients on self-management of prescribed antihypertensive medications. Patients reported a wide range of strategies that can be read as acts of resistance against doctors' prescriptions that clearly led to self-empowerment. In discussing how patients reacted to, and learned how to manage, side effects through self-education about their prescribed drugs, Benson and Britten (2003, p. 8) report '(that) coping with unwelcome effects goes on without medical involvement supports the notion that many patients actively manage their medicines themselves'. The following sentence reveals the researchers' act of empowering patients, and in the gentle invitation to doctors to change their behaviours, the act of writing up research also becomes a form of advocacy: 'If clinicians wish to take these experiences and patients' consequent actions into account when planning treatment, they are likely to have to explore them actively'.

This does raise a contradiction: if the researchers use their work to get the doctors to change their behaviours, how is that evidence that they are empowering the patient? It might be argued that researchers are just another group of professionals taking a paternal or parental view by claiming that they know what patients want. It may be that this group speaks more authoritatively on behalf of the patient, but that would be arguable. However, the final paragraph in the Benson and Britten (2003) study subtly promotes the model of concordance in prescribing ('in which patients are involved in decision making'), where it is framed as an invitation, thoughtfully avoiding alignment with the overly (and literally) prescriptive behaviours of some doctors that the article brings into focus and gently questions. This subtler rhetorical tactic in writing up research offers a sharp contrast to the more combative and insistent tone of Angela Coulter's nevertheless admirably passionate views on patient autonomy.

Britten's subtle patient empowerment model can be compared with Homi Bhabha's (1994) notions of 'sly civility' and 'mimicry' as typical forms of resistance in colonialism. Where a country is colonized, for example, India at the height of the British Empire, resistance to the colonizers is inevitable. This usually takes two forms. First is an active or hostile resistance such as an uprising or an underground resistance movement (Fanon, 2001/1961). A second, more common, form is subtler. This is to outwardly take on the imported customs of the colonizer, but to slightly distort them, to mock them, to engage in comic mimicry, and to be apparently civil but with a sly edge of disobedience. Patients may choose outright disobedience or active resistance to doctors' prescriptions and will then be labelled 'noncompliant'. Or, they may engage in a variety of subtle forms of resistance as 'reduced adherence' with a twist (civil disobedience, creative mimicry, gentle mocking).

Advocacy

Advocacy and empowerment could be collapsed into one category, but advocacy usually involves speaking on behalf of patients who may not be able to speak for themselves rather than helping patients to find their own voices. Advocacy is common for children; for persons who are physically or mentally challenged, or in a temporary state of challenge such as a psychotic episode; where patients do not possess specialist language or expertise; where translation between languages is necessary; and/or where the patient is legally protected or in a vulnerable state.

Advocacy does not have to be overtly political—it may simply speak on behalf of patients when they are compromised, such as when they are under general anaesthetic. For example, Klemola and Norros (1997, 2001) point to two 'habits of action'—styles—of anaesthesiologists. One is oriented more towards monitoring machines while the patient is anaesthetized and undergoing surgery, while the other group 'treats' the patient even when anaesthetized and undergoing surgery, moving back and forth between monitors and bodily signs and checking with the surgical team about the patient's condition. Klemola and Norros claim that the latter anaesthetists, those who are overtly advocates of the temporarily disadvantaged patient, are the better clinicians, although they have no patient outcome data to support this claim. Rather, the judgment is based on descriptive observations.

Advocacy is key to the report from the University of British Columbia, *Where's the Patient's Voice in Health Professional Education?*, the product of an international conference on the topic (Farrell, Towle, & Godolphin, 2006). This approach can also be linked to the pedagogical model of patient-centredness. Medical educators who set up patients as teachers and co-researchers automatically promote advocacy. Key to this movement is good preparation of patients for their roles as teachers and researchers and building an infrastructure that supports and develops these roles. Such an infrastructure involves medical schools making long-standing arrangements with patient advocate groups and with the lay public to build collaborative practices, and to educate patients as educators and researchers, to act as agents of change within academia and health services. A key issue is induction of patient educators and researchers into ethical obligations that come with the role and shape an identity: a 'patient' identity for a proactive, informed patient educator is quite different to that of a reactive, passive consumer of services.

Patient-Centredness as Varieties of Collaboration and Mutuality

Patient as Catalyst for Interprofessional Activity

How do colleagues work together effectively for both best patient care and patient safety? 'Patient involvement in health professions education' (see section 'Advocacy' above) has been a major force in the field of interprofessional education (Warne & McAndrew, 2005; Wykurz & Kelly, 2002). The patient, as focus for the clinical team (or a number of teams working around a patient in a patient pathway model), can act as a catalyst for interprofessionalism (Royal Pharmaceutical Society, 2000).

A working definition of patient-centredness—doctors learning with, from, and about patients—is borrowed from the UK Centre for the Advancement of Interprofessional Education's (CAIPE) (http://www.caipe.org.uk/about-us/defining-ipe/) definition of 'interprofessionalism'—'when two or more professions learn with, from, and about each other to improve collaboration and the quality of care', where patients are catalysts for such learning. If there is one obvious paradigm change in contemporary medical education, it is the focus upon how clinical teams can work more effectively for patient care and safety. The literature on teamwork consistently shows that a shift from 'multiprofessionalism' to 'interprofessionalism' improves the working climate for patient care and safety (Bleakley, Boyden, Hobbs, Walsh, & Allard, 2006). Multiprofessionalism describes occasions when health professionals work together, but make no explicit effort to learn with, from, and about each other.

Good practices in interprofessional teamwork, such as briefing and debriefing, are not primarily focused upon how the team works (which seems the obvious focus), but rather, on how well the team works around the patient. Again, the particular requirements of the patient offer the catalyst for the interprofessionalism of the team in meeting those requirements. In terms of complexity theory, where individual patients present unique problems, this moves the system of care (a number of teams, such as the ward, anaesthetic, operating theatre, and recovery teams in a surgical care pathway) further from equilibrium into greater complexity. In order to prevent the system from falling into chaos, the new level of complexity must be accommodated. The system must be adaptive.

Mutuality: Relationship-Centred Care Model

Sir Kenneth Calman (2007, p. 415), to make the point about the changing culture of communication in medicine, quotes from the section on how to take a history from a patient in a 1956 handbook on clinical methods that was used by Calman himself as a student. This frames history taking as 'interrogation' (perhaps not surprising in the shadow of the Second World War). While the advice is to listen closely to what patients say, the medical student is warned that some give 'poor' histories, so that the reluctant patient has to 'have the history of his illness dragged out of him by methods of slow extortion'. Today, these militaristic interrogation and torture metaphors feel wholly inappropriate, where we are more comfortable with communication as support rather than confrontation.

The Pew-Fetzer Task Force on Advancing Psychosocial Health Education published an influential report in 1994, reprinted in 2000 (Tresolini, 2000), that reframes patient-centred care as 'relationship-centred care', in recognition of the potentially therapeutic power of the relationship. Beach and Inui (2006) describe the Relationship-Centred Care Research Network that has subsequently evolved. With its more psychotherapeutic orientation, relationship-centred care particularly stresses the importance of the emotional dimensions of the medical encounter.

The emotional dimension to communication, often reframed as the more technical and neutral term 'affective', tends to be instrumentalized in the literature on communication skills, especially through contemporary accounts of 'professionalism' (Stern, 2006a, 2006b). Once placed in opposition to 'cognition', or in tandem with the cognitively charged word 'intelligence' ('emotional intelligence'), 'emotion', that previously uncontrollable demon, becomes subject to control. Quirk (2006) provides an illustrative example, where emotional intelligence (EI) is configured as a metacognitive ability. Now we seem far from the messy and spontaneous business of catharsis: grief, sadness, anger, joy, desire, and so forth. However, controlling emotions can also be seen as a duty of the doctor, and my remarks should not be read as invitations to indulgent emotional expression.

The activity focus of the Pew-Fetzer Task Force could readily have been placed within the category above of 'Advocacy', where its aim is to challenge wider changes to health-care *structures* that diminish the quality of patient/health-care practitioner therapeutic relationships, including the option for patients to explore their feelings. However, its theoretical framework is very much centred on the one-to-one relationship.

Deeper Mutuality: Psychodynamics and the Therapeutic Alliance

Medical students need to know the basics of the psychodynamics of professional relationships, such as how patients may set up transference and resistance dynamics with a doctor and how the doctor may set up countertransference and counter-resistance relationships with the patient (Guggenbuhl-Craig, 1983). This can be summarized as a therapeutic alliance. The UK General Medical Council's *The New Doctor* (2007) thus calls for the doctor to *demonstrate* 'empathy and the ability to form constructive therapeutic relationships with patients' (strangely, and regrettably, the updated, 2009, version of *The New Doctor* omits this call).

Such dynamics are essential to management of any long-term relationship with a patient where they have both productive and counterproductive consequences. While we should not expect medical students to explore these dynamics in the depth that, say, clinical psychology students will (unless they develop an early interest in psychiatry), this model of patient-centredness has a great deal to offer.

A symptom of the intensity of medicine is the relatively high rate of work-related suicide, burnout, depression, and drug and alcohol dependency associated with the profession. One recent estimate from North America suggests that about 15 % of physicians 'will be impaired at some point in their careers, which means that they will be unable to meet professional obligations, in some cases due to mental illness, drug dependency, or alcoholism' (Cole & Carlin, 2009, p. 1414). It is a poor reflection on medical education that it does not extend fully to professional and regulated supervision, rather than simply support structures, for doctors in postgraduate education. A therapeutic model of patient-centredness in medicine would also see 'relationship' as the 'bottom line' (see section 'Mutuality: Relationship-Centred Care Model' above). This, however, would extend this from a humanistic model that privileges empathy to a more sophisticated psychodynamic reading that extends relationship to a therapeutic alliance—a complex transaction grounded not in ideals (such as 'unconditional positive regard') but in the realities of personal and cultural psychological histories, where unacknowledged and/or unresolved patterns continue to distort current behaviour. An example might be 'I am a man who has always had difficult personal relationships with women. How will I continue to work effectively with female patients and colleagues?'

The bottom line here is not simply 'relationship' as the necessary complement to science-based medical care, but active understanding of the complexities of relationship so that personal and cultural distress is not acted out to distort interventions, but is actively worked through in educational or therapeutic settings such as supervision.

Local Ecosystem

Pauli, White, and McWhinney (2000a, 2000b, p. 174) suggest that 'augmented by the alienating effects of technology, we seem to have produced a generation of detached health professionals (especially physicians) who cannot communicate effectively with patients'. However, this cannot be fixed by instrumental communication skills courses, which are at best cosmetic. Rather, this is a structural problem, where the structure at stake is each idiosyncratic relationship dyad between a doctor and a patient. The *meaning* of this structure is the meaning of illness to each patient, and the therapeutic issue is 'mutual appreciation of the experience and its meaning'.

Importantly, Pauli et al. (2000b, p. 178) describe 'relationship' in terms of a biological environment, as a local ecosystem. We can develop this into a model of patient-centredness that avoids the more sentimental pitfalls of 'identification' with the patient, but more importantly (from section 'Deeper Mutuality: Psychodynamics and the Therapeutic Alliance' above) notes the dangers of psychodynamic issues of over-identification, as an effect of countertransference. I have already mentioned Dannie Abse's (2008, p. 20) perceptive remarks that a doctor needs to create 'a little distance—a sympathetic and sensitive distance certainly, but still a distance' from the patient, to avoid 'identification' (or, strictly, over-identification).

This 'ecological' model also grounds patient-centredness in the biology, rather than the psychology, of relationships—again in the unique ecosystem of the relationship rather than in the characters of the persons involved. A relationship, beginning with a dyad, can be seen as an ecological phenomenon. An ecology, local or global, is a product of difference between elements, such as persons, in an environment. A number of elements interact to form an adaptive, complex system that operates at maximum complexity this side of chaos (i.e. not slipping in to chaos, where a system that falls into chaos has lost its *logos* or internal meaning). Where a meaningful, adaptive, and developing relationship is established ('mutuality'), the whole is greater than the sum of its parts. This characterizes all ecosystems, whatever their size. The lesson for medical education is that the patient–student encounter cannot be learned as—or be reduced to—an instrumental skill or competency. Such encounters are far more complex and inherently unstable.

Clinical Reasoning Model

Atkins and Ersser (2008) remind us that the *activity* of collaborative and mutual care may be more important than the conventional foci upon what is 'in' either the doctor or the patient. This is supplemented by the patient being embedded in multi- or interprofessional clinical team settings in which clinical reasoning can be modelled as a collaborative activity between health-care providers, including doctors (Shaw, 2008). Atkins and Ersser then suggest five strategies for promoting patient involvement in clinical reasoning, as a key form of patient-centredness:

- Enhancing professionals' communication
- Improving patient education
- Developing patient decision aids such as pamphlets and online packages
- Advocacy
- Creating a humane health-care environment

For a clinical reasoning model of patient-centredness (see Chap. 5) to be effective, doctors have to gain the dual capability of clinical science-based reasoning and narrative-based judgments that Rita Charon (2011) calls 'the novelization of the body'. Charon properly asks how physicians will gain the second sensitivity, a narrative intelligence, if they do not read and appreciate literature beyond the confines of the medical narrative. The latter is restricted to one genre—objectivism or minimalism (Marshall & Bleakley, 2011). Patients' stories cross genres (characteristically epic and tragic, sometimes comical and lyrical) and draw on a variety of rhetorical devices (Marshall & Bleakley, 2009, 2011). Physicians draw on a range of visual and verbal metaphors (Bleakley, Farrow, Gould, & Marshall, 2003a, 2003b) and aphorisms and maxims (Levine & Bleakley, 2012) that may not be consciously utilized or reflexively accounted for. This is one reason for incorporating the medical humanities into an undergraduate medicine and surgery curriculum as a patient-centred pedagogy (Bleakley, Marshall, & Brömer, 2006).

Pedagogical (Learning and Teaching) Model

Although all the models of patient-centredness I consider may have implications for learning and teaching, there are approaches that are explicitly pedagogical. Such approaches are generally grounded in the translation of student-centred learning principles to patient-centred learning (Howe, 2001). The more patients take part in educational roles—as teachers, on selection and admission panels, for curriculum development, on appeals committees, and as assessors and appraisers—the less medical educators may think in terms of the 'great divide' (doctors–patients) and more in terms of the medicine curriculum as a 'conversation' (Applebee, 1996), or better as a 'complicated conversation' (Pinar, 2004, 2006), between doctors, medical students, and patients.

Evidence for students learning positively from patients in ambulatory consultations is provided by Ashley and colleagues (2009), who progress the dyadic models of patient as teacher in relationship to medical student as learner, to a triadic model where the role of the supervising doctor-educator is 'now reframed as a leader who helped patients and students find ways of relating to one another effectively rather than conveyor of subject matter'. Excellent teachers help students to overcome perceived inadequacies by setting up situations in which patients act as teachers and students play active, rather than passive, roles as learners. Importantly, students are then offered legitimate *central* participation in a community of practice forming an identity in which learning to think as a doctor, rather than as a student, is central.

A pedagogical model, which comprehensively explores the role of the patient as the fulcrum of a learning process in medical education, is activity theory. Yrjo Engeström and colleagues (2008) have carried out an intensive, longitudinal study of a small number of care teams working around chronic patients in the community in Helsinki, Finland. Through an educational intervention, teams gradually built better ways of coordinating complex care arrangements, with the patient as catalyst and educator. Formally, in an activity system, the patient is the 'object' of the system. 'Object' is an unfortunate term where it can be read as 'objectification' of the patient, but in the activity system model, object means the outcome of a learning system—an objective.

The authors of the British Medical Association's (BMA, 2008) report on patient-centredness stress that it is vital that patient-centredness continues to be developed through postgraduate and continuing education, whatever the level of expertise of the doctor. Without ever fully conceptualizing patient-centredness, the BMA report nevertheless sets out the evidence for its effects: patient-centredness helps to develop clinical reasoning, encourages valuing of cultural diversity, and fosters empathy and the development of professional skills, including communication. We have already seen that not only is patient-centredness a contested and complex notion, but, as illustrated in the following chapter, 'empathy' is a modern and contested term. Conceptual frameworks should precede and inform practice interventions, and the lack of a conceptual framework or even clear definitions of terms already weakens the potential impact of such reports.

Importantly, it is not clear that patient-centredness will necessarily develop simply from greater contact with patients. Rather, quality and structuring of patient contact as a designed educational experience is more important than quantity or frequency of contact. It does not help that the majority of studies of patient–doctor communications offer frequency count, quantitative data such as length of talk. This does not account for quality of interaction or subtleties of the unspoken and tacit dimensions of interaction. The BMA report does not untangle the issue of quality versus frequency, implying that frequency of contact for medical students will lead to development of patient-centred values or at least attitudes. This, of course, was always the argument of traditional apprenticeship—quantity of activity (exposure) would ultimately lead to (over)learning or skills acquisition in 'getting to know the ropes'. The 'new apprenticeship' (Ainley & Rainbird, 1999) model is focused on quality rather than quantity of learning and appropriate structuring of cognition, where learning is 'deep' or has lasting impact on shaping performance.

Thus, learning experiences must be properly designed—structured, focused, and paced as a form of 'scaffolding' (presenting new opportunities to learners that challenge them, but are anchored in previous learning)—where expertise is 'hothoused' or accelerated. Formative feedback is essential to this process. Learning from patients is necessarily risky, since meaningful contact is often opportunistic rather than designed and structured. The BMA report quite rightly points out that preparation for getting the best out of patient contacts for students and using a mix of expert, actor, and ad hoc patients will be necessary to overcome some of the structural problems. Unfortunately, the report does not set out the most powerful theories of learning that may inform optimal structuring of work-based experiences to develop patient-centredness. For example, there is no reference to contemporary cognitive apprenticeship models.

The report properly, and expertly, details challenges to patient involvement in medical education, but does not address these. In principle, and in many cases in practice, each of these challenges can be addressed. First is the inherent resistance of the medical community itself, where medicine, rather than medical education, is structurally resistant to change as an institution. The clinical teaching community would surely welcome greater emphasis upon practical, work-based experience, and medical schools have a responsibility to attract, educate, and support faculty.

Second is lack of interest in the topic. This is another strange objection. If we think that medical educators are not interested in educating students with patients in mind, we have a serious fault line running through the culture. Third is competition across curriculum content. This is understandable. Faculty of medical schools may resist developing work-based learning around patients where they see that the basic informing science for getting the best out of such experience is not in place. This calls for integrated curriculum thinking, drawing on learning experiences that combine science with practice.

Much of the best of problem-based and case-based learning follows this integrated model. It is not simply hollow semantics to switch from 'problems' and 'cases' to *patient*-based learning within an activity system model of education. Further, learning content in its own right is always a poor educational strategy.

Content must be contextualized and applied, or made meaningful, for it to be learned. Often, too much content is learned, or content is over-learned, at the expense of strategic application of content.

Fourth are service pressures. This is also understandable and the most pressing of the challenges. Working with students potentially takes supervising doctors' (and clinical teams') time and energy that may take them away from patients. However, research on students learning with patients in a number of clinical settings consistently suggests that students can be accommodated without undue pressure on services (Ashley, Rhodes, Sari-Kouzel, Mukherjee, & Dornan, 2009). Fifth is insufficient evidence of effectiveness. This is a strange objection as there is a reasonable evidence base for effectiveness of students learning with patients at the level of satisfaction, but this can of course be improved with greater focus upon clinical outcomes.

Sixth is a lack of an effective mechanism to spread good practice. This is a key role for academies—professional organizations such as the UK *Academy of Medical Educators* (http://www.medicaleducators.org/)—within a wider continuing medical education framework. Seventh are organizational and practical difficulties. These are key, including administrative issues such as timetabling, linking students with availability of patients, with the added problems of unpredictability of consent. However, students may be attached both to teams and to a panel of patients from the community. While providing greater administrative challenges, medical students might work in pairs or in manageable combinations with students from other health-care professions, forming 'buddy groups' as contexts for small group reflection on learning from and about patients. Such buddy groups may serve academic/intellectual and pastoral functions and could be facilitated by interprofessional faculty.

Eighth, and finally, are issues of patient consent and confidentiality. There are challenges on the ground, and a number of studies address these, such as O'Flynn, Spencer, and Jones (1997); Branch (2006); and Price, Spencer, and Walker (2008). Addressing such challenges in medical schools could turn into an opportunity, taking ethics and law lectures out of the classroom and into the clinic, while integrating curriculum content.

'Difference' Model

There is a little more to be said beyond the account given so far and repeated throughout this book as a refrain, describing the doctor–patient relationship in terms of Hegel's master/slave dialectic, where the identity of one is dependent upon the presence of the 'other'. Or, self-identity (selfsame) is only realized in the mirror of the Other.

Drawing on the ideas of Emmanuel Levinas (1969), who, perhaps, more than any other writer has articulated what it means to offer a hand of friendship to the Other who may be hard to reach or may even be 'intolerable', I have developed a model of education as 'hospitality' (Bleakley, 2002). Here, the 'gift' of education is offered freely from teacher to student, where the student is a welcome guest in the 'house' of the teacher. I have extended this argument to consider how operating theatre personnel may act professionally by extending hospitality to the patient, who, even when anaesthetized, is an equal and welcome guest in the houses of anaesthetic room plus operating theatre and recovery room (Bleakley, 2006b).

Intertextuality Model

Patients and medical students can be said to engage in collaborative 'readings' of the patient's condition, where the patient is both the first author and reader of his or her condition (as 'text'). This collaborative, or intertextual, reading (Orr, 2003) is supported and illuminated by the sensitive interventions of an expert educator-clinician (Bleakley, Bligh, & Browne 2011). In such textual readings, students can be alerted to:

- The *context* of the patient's expression of symptom.
- The *subtext* that is, for example, the unspoken narrative of suffering or hidden symptom and hidden cause of symptom.
- The *pretext* for symptom presentation, where the patient's presenting narrative may in fact be a pretext for another, deeper, or more significant symptom.
- The *paratext*—where the medicalized (doctor's) narrative is privileged; the patient's narrative may be displaced or frustrated. The two texts run side by side (as paratexts) and can be brought into creative conversation. While the medicalized text is given functional legitimacy because of the medical context, it can also be legitimated aesthetically, as a form of minimalism. The case study is a stripped-back, 'less is more' narrative, following the literary examples of William Carlos Williams' later poetry, the stories of Raymond Carver, or the 'flash fiction' of Lydia Davis. For example, Williams' poem *The Red Wheelbarrow* describes what the eye sees, nothing more or less, just as the doctor (Williams himself was a paediatrician) may describe one of his patient's expression of symptoms:

The red wheelbarrow
so much depends
upon
a red wheel
barrow
glazed with rain
water
beside the white
chickens

The point is that medical students can be taught to be reflexive about the stylistic approach of framing the case history—as a reminder that other approaches exist to telling the patient's story. While the medical student and doctor may listen with a minimalist ear, they can still, in parallel (as paratext), appreciate the style or genre in which the patient's narrative is delivered.

Patient-Centredness as Patient Connectedness in Online Communities Model

I noted above that an explosion has occurred in medicine and health-care facilitated by the development of information technologies and the Internet. This can be seen throughout medicine, such as doctors carrying prescription formulary apps for smartphones, but also in patient empowerment. Through the Internet, service users can self-diagnose and enhance diagnoses given by professionals, self-treat (such as buying pharmaceuticals online without prescriptions), and join or engage with collaborative patient support and pressure groups. Such online communities are usually centred on one chronic illness, where information is exchanged, and people support and empower each other, often forming pressure groups related to issues such as availability of treatments and current research. Through such activities, patients may become experts in their own conditions, more knowledgeable certainly than their family doctor.

This development has radically altered the landscape of 'patient-centredness', transforming this notion to what Julia Kennedy (2013) calls 'patient connectedness'. In patient connected online communities, doctors also may engage as patients, suffering from the same illness as other members of the community. They may or may not bring specialist knowledge, but are treated as co-participants within the community. Kennedy (2013) shows that such online communities are not without their problems, encountering the same issues of democratic participation as 'naturalistic' communities. (The distinction between 'naturalistic' and 'virtual' is somewhat false as all activity can be seen to be socially and culturally mediated and constructed, and the act of going online is itself a naturalistic act of sitting in front of a computer and engaging with a keyboard).

Dysfunctional: Default Care

In contrast to these models of patient-centredness is the most distressing kind of encounter found in medicine. Here, doctor and patient collude, to engage in negative mutuality, a dysfunctional collaboration in which both doctor and patient inputs are underachieved, misguided, or misinformed. Distorted dynamics of relationship may be played out, with (mis)consent in a potentially mutually abusive relationship. The doctor's unprofessional behaviour is supported or confirmed by the patient, and colleagues may be involved in collusive support. What is important about such encounters is that, where possible, positive intervention and remediation are offered. In chronic cases, structural or institutional remediation may be needed. The fact that such dysfunctional encounters are not uncommon in medicine alerts us to the importance of incorporating 'deeper' mutuality models in a medical education curriculum, such as psychodynamic approaches focusing upon the therapeutic alliance.

Dysfunctional relationships are perhaps more common in medicine than has been acknowledged, where such relationships include reinforcing patient dependencies and supporting, rather than treating, chronic habits such as unhealthy lifestyles. Patient dependencies may reflect doctor dependencies—these are unresolved countertransference issues. Patently dysfunctional professional relationships include acting out inappropriate sexual relationships and clear abuse of patients' trust.

Responses to a colleague's dysfunctional behaviour may itself be dysfunctional, such as brushing it under the carpet or piety, finger-wagging, and tut-tutting. Rather, a more psychotherapeutic approach may be taken, where doctors actively mentor and support to help to remediate. A good model for this is provided by Abraham Verghese's (1998) 'factional' novel *The Tennis Partner*, in which Verghese, as a senior clinician, struggles with issues of mentorship, guidance, and support for a junior doctor who has also become a friend and tennis partner, but increasingly exhibits unprofessional and then dysfunctional behaviour. What is compelling about the novel is the refreshing honesty with which Verghese admits to moral dilemmas that have no straightforward answer, but must be addressed. The account at one level is a deep engagement with issues of empathy and concern.

I recognize particularly in this chapter that I may be feeding in to the paternalistic model of medical work by continuing to use the word 'patient' rather than 'service user' (or even 'person'). Service user has become the politically correct term to describe health-care users and challenges the passivity of 'patient'. However, the Oxford Dictionary says that a patient is 'a person receiving or registered to receive medical treatment'. This definition does not indicate inferiority or subordination, and I will continue to use 'patient' for clarity throughout this book.

In the next chapter, written in collaboration with Dr. Robert Marshall, an experienced consultant histopathologist, medical educator, and champion of the medical humanities, we critically discuss what is often seen as the essential interpersonal glue for patient-centredness: 'empathy'.

Chapter 8
What Is Meant by 'Empathy'?

Education for Communication Must Go Deeper Than 'Skills'

Chapter 2 described 'empathy decline' as a significant undesired effect of a technical medical education and as contributing factor to the overall problem of communication hypocompetence in medicine. But 'empathy' is a complex notion that needs to be further discussed and unravelled. Debates surrounding what we mean by 'empathy' can coalesce to form a case study for progressing our thinking about communication beyond the current, dominant reductive models of instrumental skills or competences.

If we reduced our complex, aesthetic, and ethical everyday communications to instrumental 'competences', there would be no need for literature, cinema, opera, and drama; no need for character studies, television soap operas, or reality television shows to provide a mirror showing how inventive, subtle, and complex (and far from equilibrium) much of our communication is—whether everyday or in professional settings. There would be no need for comedians—especially satirists—or media commentary in such an instrumental world; no need for actor patients, dramaturgical or depth-psychological models of interaction. Why then do we not see professional relationships as equally complex, unstable issues in need of a complex response, including a complex educational response?

We will not make a case *for* empathy, but use 'empathy' as a case study for illustrating the demise of serious thinking about communication in professional relationships. While a body of research evidence highlights areas for intensive attention in doctor–patient communication, just *how* we educate such ability is contested. In undergraduate education, as already noted, focus has developed on 'training' communication as a set of atomized skills. For example, Rider and Keefer (2006) describe a defined set of 'communication skills competencies' linked to a 'teaching toolbox'—the toolbox metaphor sitting comfortably within the technical–rational approach—as if instrumentalizing communication 'solves' the 'problem' of how we teach communication.

A. Bleakley, *Patient-Centred Medicine in Transition: The Heart of the Matter*, 95
Advances in Medical Education 3, DOI 10.1007/978-3-319-02487-5_8,
© Springer International Publishing Switzerland 2014

The argument is circular. If we frame communication as a 'problem' to be solved and as a set of competences to be performed, then we *produce* communication within the parameters of our definition and we produce conforming identities of 'communicators' who follow this pattern. When things go wrong, we fix them, our toolbox at the ready. Indeed, the metaphor is explicitly mechanical, implying a linear set of cogs, where communication between persons (and machines) may be better described as non-linear—as an embodied, complex, adaptive, dynamic system (see Chap. 15).

This is not to say that medical students should not formally learn how to communicate effectively with patients—the professional context offers challenges that everyday communication does not (e.g. limits of intimacy) and some students will be strongly invested in a disease-centred model of medicine from the outset of their studies. Rather, given the deep ambiguities inherent to communication and the *absences* that are referred to throughout this chapter (such as unconscious dynamics, indirections, and purposefully ambiguous, 'open-ended' communications that allow for 'face saving'), perhaps communication may be better learned as a post hoc exercise. Research indicates that this is best achieved through structured, well-facilitated, small group reflection on actual experiences with patients (Branch, 2001; Quirk, 2006).

These reflective experiences can be offered in various ways—within the work placement as uniprofessional settings or multiprofessional groups or as a regular 'mop up' of what has been experienced in clinical settings, with uniprofessional or multiprofessional facilitation. This has possible consequences for protecting patients from potential harm through miscommunications by students, but the advantages far outweigh these possible disadvantages, where, ideally, students learn to communicate in a formative, supportive setting (Benbassat & Baumal, 2009) that mirrors supervisory and mentorial networks familiar to counsellors, psychotherapists, psychiatrists, and clinical psychologists.

This means placing less emphasis on preparation for practice through the currently dominant, largely instrumental, methods of communication skills training (CST) in simulated settings. The dangers of the instrumental approach are that (1) 'communication' is reduced to a list or tick box, (2) the simulated patient offers an out-of-context 'standardized' experience, and (3) the unexpected is controlled or introduced as a purely theatrical device by an actor-patient (Benbassat & Baumal, 2009; Bligh & Bleakley, 2006).

A 1998 survey of communication skills provision in the UK schools of medicine (Hargie, Dickson, Boohan, & Hughes, 1998, p. 25) showed 'considerable variability in such areas as course content, timing, duration and assessment'. The survey notes 'lack of adequate physical resources and suitably trained staff' with lack of forward planning in terms of curriculum development in this area. A follow-up survey in 2010, following a General Medical Council (GMC) curriculum mandate that required all UK medical schools to provide communication skills 'training' and to identify a lead within the core academic staff, showed far greater consistency across schools' provision, leading to what the authors term a 'modal' model of CST

(Hargie, Boohan, McCoy, & Murphy, 2010, p. 385). The authors note, however, that 'wide variations remain in CST pedagogy'.

It is likely that the next decade will see such variations in pedagogy smoothed out, as CST becomes packaged, involving standard exercises for so-called skills such as empathic listening. Standardization, however, can soon devolve to homogenization. Central to standardization is location—purpose-built clinical skills 'laboratories' and dedicated 'communication suites' with video feedback facilities. Foucault's (1975) work on subtle institutional forms of the uses of power for regulation is readily applicable to the standardized communication suite. Here, the central 'all-seeing eye', or panopticon, is explicitly at work—as the regulatory gaze of the video camera, of the assessor sitting in another room watching (being) the 'monitor', and of the actor-patient who cannot slip fully into role because he or she is also assessing the student and must maintain the assessor's gaze or scrutiny.

Under the guise of a 'safe' environment, in which communication can be tested on actor-patients with videotaped feedback from experts, we then see an explicit form of surveillance and control, which comes to shape a docile identity. Here, we see the more sinister purposes for which such suites are built—not so much educational, in promoting the creative production of knowledge, but regulatory, in promoting the reproduction of docile behaviour. The symptom is evident in the index of Roter and Hall's (2006) primary text, where there are six entries on 'nodding' (the key surface text for empathic listening, but so readily open to dissimulation by the student), but nothing on messy and complex psychodynamics such as transference or resistance. Emotionally charged words such as 'desire' and 'repulsion' are noticeably absent, as are commonly met responses such as lukewarm 'boredom' and icy 'disinterest'.

Just as rigid prescribing to patients by doctors without establishing dialogue and understanding leads to forms of resistance, from 'noncompliance' to 'reduced adherence', so prescribing communication skills to students can lead to a range of resistant behaviours such as simulation (pretending to do what one cannot do) and dissimulation (pretending to do the appropriate thing when one normally does something different). This can be seen as an iatrogenic effect of training, as a 'compulsory miseducation' (Goodman, 1964). These symptoms then infect the assessment process, where students can readily fake performances (Hodges, 2010).

Reinders, Blankenstein, and van Marwijk (2011) show that the reliability of consultation skills assessments in family practitioner training settings is better for real than standardized patients. Benbassat and Baumal (2009) suggest that typical OSCE-based assessment of communication within a clinical skills setting (using standardized patients) is both invalid and unreliable. The assessment may not measure student learning, but rather reflects a 'one-off' teacher judgment that goes against the spirit of the occasion—that students can and should learn communication as a product of reflecting on quality of *dialogue*. Benbassat and Baumal suggest a series of post-consultation debriefs in which students formatively learn about the strengths and weaknesses of their communication capabilities in conversation with expert tutors as a dialogue. This conversation should, of course, include the patient's feedback.

Summative feedback can naturally develop from a cycle of patient encounters and linked formative conversations with tutors and (actor) patients.

For all of its power in reporting and making sense of the research evidence in doctor–patient communication, Roter and Hall's (2006) seminal book-length review of the evidence base does not formally discuss competing theoretical frameworks that may inform such communication, although these are widely debated in psychiatry, psychotherapy, and clinical psychology education. One wonders just what influence psychiatry as a specialty has on medicine and medical education generally. Helpful frameworks developed within psychiatry include broad approaches such as psychodynamic, family therapy, cognitive behavioural, and humanistic existential. There are historical fluctuations in the fortunes of these approaches—for example, psychodynamic approaches were popular in the 1950s and 1960s, only to be eclipsed by humanistic, and then cognitive behavioural, approaches. This is partly based upon available evidence of the effectiveness of approaches, but is more open to political/economic/instrumental influences.

For example, a limited number of sessions of cognitive behavioural therapy (CBT) may show immediate, measurable results in patients, but this approach has been criticized for dealing with symptom rather than cause. Also, CBT is cheaper than longer term therapies, but does this treat the patient merely as a consumer in an economic transaction, putting 'retail' before 'therapy'? The lengthier 'educative' psychodynamic approaches set out to address cause rather than simply treat symptoms. CBT also deals just with the individual, rather than an individual in the context of a system, such as a family group, which systems therapies—such as family systems approaches—address.

Accounts of 'communication skills' training in medical education rarely refer to theoretical basis (or bias), which means that either theory has not been addressed at all, is assumed, or is subsumed within 'practical' concerns. It is difficult to know then how to judge outcomes research in this area because the overall 'outcomes' of major theoretical positions in communication education differ so widely. For example, a medical student in an assessed 'integrated' OSCE station takes a history from a patient and in another station, examines a patient. It is right that we should assess how well students communicate and how well they integrate the technical aspects with the nontechnical (e.g. palpating a patient while explaining clearly what is being done; taking—or, rather, receiving—a history asking an appropriate mix of open-ended and closed questions, rather than mainly closed questions).

However, a psychodynamically oriented approach would not just reduce the encounter to technical skills. There would be discussion about *style* and *demeanour*. Importantly, assessors would look for subtleties in the student's approach that included cognizance of the meaning of non-verbal cues and affect generally in the encounter; the meaning of what was unspoken or remained unresolved; and the *dynamics* of the encounter in terms of transference/countertransference and resistance/counter-resistance (did this patient remind me of someone I know well or someone I dislike; did an inappropriate degree of intimacy or distance emerge in the encounter; did I stop myself from listening fully to what the patient said because he reminded me of someone I do not like, or I was repulsed by the patient; or did I listen closely because I was physically attracted to the patient, although I was perfectly aware of the dangers of this?).

Why do we suggest that a psychodynamic (or a broadly 'depth'-psychological) approach offers a potentially 'deeper' insight? For example, Roter and Hall (2006, pp. 73–74) summarize studies on how 'liking' and 'attractiveness' affect the doctor–patient relationship. These are intriguing—for example, doctors are both less likely to interrupt and more likely to ask open-ended questions that facilitate dialogue from a patient who was rated high on 'good' appearance. But this is left at the level of description or mild exploration and does not shift to the level of possible explanation. Such studies do not say why doctors have preferences in the first place. What is the 'good' appearance of the patient mobilizing in the doctor's psyche or the cultural psyche in which that doctor is embedded? Psychodynamics at least aims for explanation and provides a model of analysis of behaviour, as a basis to supervision. Depth psychologically oriented supervision is currently notable by its absence from the educational supervision/professional development agenda for doctors and related health professionals such as clinical psychologists.

Again, most medical students are not choosing to enter psychiatry as a specialty, but these communication issues within a psychodynamic model would not necessarily be addressed, or thought important, within either a cognitive behavioural or a humanistic model. However, without a theory of unconscious motive, how might we read a student's clever dissimulation in an OSCE with an actor-patient, where she or he does everything right 'for the camera', but has already achieved a reputation on ward attachments of being cynical and callous towards patients? More importantly, how can we now intervene positively to support and help this student?

We have already introduced the idea that poor, or instrumental, teaching of communication skills can have iatrogenic effects. Again, iatrogenesis is medicine-induced illness (Illich, 1975), where the intervention brings unwanted or unpredicted negative consequences. In the realm of the physical, these include medical/surgical errors, the side effects of pharmaceuticals and hospital-acquired infections. In the realm of the psychological, paternalism in medicine can, for example, produce either the passive, unquestioning response of patient dependency or the active response of resistance to, and noncompliance with, the doctor's wishes or prescriptions.

There are more subtle possible iatrogenic effects in medical education. Just as Illich (1975) points out how reliance on medical professionals can 'deskill' a community in losing confidence (and then skills) for self-help and self-medication, so as instrumental or functional training in communication skills, such as empathy, may deskill medical students who already have effective communication skills. This can happen where students become *self-conscious* (rather than *self-reflective*) about what was previously transferred from life experience to patient encounters.

All About Empathy

To move on to the primary focus of this chapter—empathy—we have, first, a fundamental epistemological concern: how can we 'teach' or 'learn' what has not yet been properly conceptualized or at least is open to contestation? For example, Marshall and Bleakley (2009) argue that 'empathy' is a modern, instrumental (mis) reading of what Homer referred to as 'pity'. The complex affective state that is pity for another has been reduced through successive mutations of the everyday usage of 'pity' and through the rise of instrumental descriptors, such as 'empathy', that have filled the gap that the degradation of 'pity', its gradual withdrawal to backstage, has generated.

Further, Arno Kumagai (2008, p. 657) suggests that it may be 'inappropriate— and perhaps presumptuous—for medical schools to "teach" students empathy'. Rather, medical educators have a 'responsibility to engage the students in learning activities which allow them to shape the empathy and idealism that they bring into the educational environment into powerful tools for healing'. But what are the optimum 'learning activities', and where might they best be located? As we have said, an increasingly popular learning activity is teaching empathy in 'safe' contexts such as the clinical skills laboratory setting, rather than focusing upon what Arthur Kleinman (1988, p. 206) describes as 'the messy, confusing, always special context of lived experience'—which could be a description of the medical student's everyday world and/or the clinical setting during work-based learning experiences.

If the undergraduate medicine curriculum is not limited to what happens in the context of the medical school, but has a symbiotic relationship with the lifeworld of the student (as a preparation for being a recognized professional in society), then encouraging students to reflect on their everyday communication is valid, for this lifeworld involves sickness, emotional turmoil, intensity of relationship, and death.

What is different about the professional relationship of doctor and patient to the lifeworld experience is a mixture of three elements: the necessary emotional insulation and management of the countertransference and counter-resistance dynamics, to set up and maintain appropriate distance between patient and practitioner; the employment of a moral imagination and responsibility as a person in a unique power relationship with another; and the ethical responsibility for confidentiality. These three requirements may make the qualitative nature of the *professional* relationship quite different from that of *personal* relationships in the lifeworld, as hinted at earlier. But we should also recognize that where doctors hold responsible positions as citizens, it is sometimes difficult to draw a strong line between private and public worlds and not only a moral responsibility, but also a moral imagination, permeates both.

For Kumagai (2008) and Kumagai, Murphy, and Ross (2009), where reflection is mobilized to educate empathy, this requires students to develop narrative capabilities— understanding patients' stories and retelling these stories to colleagues for further understanding. He describes a program developed at the University of Michigan Medical School in 2003 called 'the Family Centered Experience'. This is a real-time, structured learning experience, involving home visits to create dialogue between new medical students and volunteer patients and their families. The project aims to educate for a humane approach to medicine.

The approach purposefully challenges students' preconceptions (there is, e.g. a healthy 'culture clash'), and they have the opportunity to process what they learn in the field in reflective, small group settings that are expertly facilitated. I did not include 'family centredness' in the list of patient-centred models in the previous chapter. My concern is that the nuclear family is compromised, or made complex, as it extends to more than one family group. In the Metropolitan West, half of marriages end in divorce or separation so that children may be caught between two settings, producing divided loyalties. It is not clear whether students, in the program that Kumagai describes, learn, for example, basic family systems therapy to give them a theoretical frame to better appreciate and understand 'family', 'extended family', 'dysfunctional family', and 'dual family' dynamics. Talk of the 'extended family' is also less common nowadays. Further, North Americans are used to calling 'community doctors' 'family physicians' without the need to articulate critically the meanings of both 'community' and 'family', where the terms are also metaphorical.

It is also not clear how these new students may gain a narrative intelligence, or a sensibility for stories, given that Kumagai stresses that one of the ways in which meaning is learned for doctors is through stories. Does a narrative intelligence simply emerge through repeated exposure to patients, or should it be cultivated through educational framing? For example, in parallel to these important contacts with community members, do medical students study the basics of rhetoric, genre, plot, and characterization? Do they learn ethics through narrative? In what sense does story educate for tolerance of ambiguity?

Kumagai (2008, p. 653–654) claims that education for empathy—defined as 'identification with another individual's suffering'—is at the centre of this narrative-based approach. This is 'fundamentally different' from approaches to learning biomedical sciences, where it is *transformative*: 'a shift in non-verbalized, habitual, taken-for-granted frames of reference towards a perspective that is more open, reflective, and capable of change'. 'Perspective taking' is, again, a descriptor that is increasingly gaining use as an alternative to 'empathy' (Stern, 2006a, 2006b).

If, as Kumagai suggests, empathy is grounded in sensitivity to stories, should medical educators then get to know the bigger stories that lead to 'empathy'—the historical trails? Can history teach us anything about teaching and learning 'communication skills', such as 'empathy', in medical education? Communication skills are usually considered ahistorically, as given (transparent and unproblematic) activities. In fact, we need only return to the first two great books in the Western canon—Homer's *Iliad* and *Odyssey*—to find rich, informing, premodern texts about what modernity calls 'communication skills' (Bleakley & Marshall, 2012; Marshall & Bleakley, 2009, 2011, 2013). In an exercise that reminds us of the value of the medical humanities to medical education (Bleakley, Marshall, & Brömer, 2006), we will ground the story of empathy in the bigger story of the origins of Western storytelling, in Homer's epics.

First, however, let us engage in some contemporary conceptual housekeeping—again, 'empathy' is a problematic term. As Veloski and Hojat (2006, pp. 119–120) warn, 'the theoretical investigation of physician empathy has been hampered by ambiguity in its conceptualization and definition', where 'there is no agreed-upon definition of the term'. Worse, empathy may be an operational term for a psychological state that 'may not even exist'. In other words, empathy could be treated as a metaphor. Indeed, a key text on empathy in medicine—*Empathy and the Practice of Medicine: Beyond Pills and the Scalpel* (Spiro, McCrea Curnen, Peschel, & St James, 1993)—is paradoxically replete with the authors' uses of *metaphors* to describe empathy in a collection that is otherwise characterized by the desire to represent empathy as an empirical phenomenon.

Metaphors of transportation, site, and resonance are common and commonly occur together, describing placing oneself in the lived experience of the patient's illness and entering the perceptual world of the other, as cognitive events of understanding and insight, rather than compassion. In a book-length (empathic) treatment of 'sympathy', Lauren Wispé (1991) discloses the core metaphor for empathy as that of travel or crossing over. This raises questions concerning the motives for that travel gleaned from anthropological study concerning the morbid curiosity of the tourist to the desire for conquest and control of the imperialist or colonist.

Such conceptual ambiguity places us in the same position as the circular operational definitions of ambiguous psychological notions such as 'intelligence'—that 'intelligence is what intelligence tests measure'. Empathy may be what empathy scales measure, or is a *construct*, a useful heuristic, rather than a tangible state of being. Yet, we undeniably feel moved in the presence of suffering, as witness to that suffering. And we can argue that 'witness to suffering' is a core identity construction of the doctor. As introduced earlier, a suitable descriptor for this feeling is 'pity', as described by Homer. Substituting pity for empathy is not merely a semantic sleight of hand.

The dictionary definitions of 'empathy' and 'pity' reinforce the argument that empathy is a modern, operational term, grounded in technical–rational thinking, whereas pity is an ancient term grounded in aesthetics. *The Shorter Oxford English Dictionary* defines empathy as: 'The power of projecting one's personality into, and so fully understanding, the object of contemplation'. In contrast, pity is defined as 'A feeling of tenderness aroused by the suffering or misfortune of another and prompting a desire for its relief'. The first definition implies mastery, the second, a contemplation and appropriate action, importantly qualified by the descriptor 'tenderness'. This is stereotypically a more 'feminine' response of *discrimination*—grounded in aesthetic, rather than instrumental, values.

You would think that the dictionary definition of pity is hard to beat, but the word has been corrupted in modern usage, as a kind of sneering. The novelist Graham Greene (1993) starkly captures this view: 'Pity is cruel. Pity destroys. Love isn't safe when pity's prowling round'. And Michael LaCombe (1993, p. 60), writing in the persona of a senior devil to a junior colleague, recommends using pity to pervert empathy: 'permit them to see their patients as simpering fools, helpless wrecks of humanity with whom they could never identify. Let this pity grow, spread like a cancer within them, and you need not worry'. Such understanding of pity is idiosyncratic. It requires a distancing from the object and a feeling of superiority that most would not think was implicit in the term. We have indeed tipped over into instrumental empathy. Definitions matter. Or perhaps this is a matter of understanding and experience rather than definition.

The roots of empathy and compassion appear superficially similar: -pathy and -passion derive, one Greek, the other Latin, from words to do with suffering. Their difference lies in their prefixes—suffering 'in' ('em') or 'with' ('com'). In fact, the Latin word *patior*, from which 'passion' derives, had a meaning largely confined to suffering or tolerating unpleasant experiences, whereas *pathos* was a much more neutral word meaning experiences both good and bad. *Chambers Dictionary* subconsciously reflects this ambiguity by translating the '-pathy' of empathy as 'feeling' and of sympathy as 'suffering'. The word 'sympathy' existed in classical Greek times with a meaning very similar to today's usage, while empathy had different meanings, either a physical affliction (e.g. in Galen), or to mean a state of emotional engagement (the opposite of apathy). 'Pity' derives from the same word as 'piety', the Latin *pietas*. In Old and Middle English, the two senses were intermingled, only separating in the sixteenth century, when both words took on negative meanings— as a kind of knowing superiority.

Paradoxically, when empathy entered modernist thinking, it was wholly grounded in aesthetics, but has since lost this foothold. Although Jodi Halpern (2001) finds echoes of the term in Hippocrates, it is a twentieth-century invention, formally coined by the German psychologist Titchener in 1909 as a translation of the German *einfühlung*—literally meaning 'aesthetic sympathy'. Indeed, Titchener's description only provides further ambiguity, where he says of empathizing with another's expressions or qualities, such as pride, that he 'feels them in the mind's muscle' (in Wispé, 1991, p. 78). The metaphor is again one of movement, of crossing over, of a paradoxical 'at-a-distance' proprioception, but now we are in the body of the mind, an unfamiliar territory for contemporary cognitive models of empathy.

The German philosopher Theodor Lipps (1851–1914), who had a formative influence on Freud's model of the unconscious, used *einfühlung* as early as 1903, originally in aesthetics, to describe a process of the observer 'entering into' a work of art, and it is only later that such language was used by him to describe entering into the mind of a person. Importantly, in these early formulations, the passions are clearly engaged, and this differs greatly from contemporary definitions of empathy as the *cognitive* or knowing partner to affective 'compassion'. In conclusion, there is not only conceptual confusion concerning 'empathy', but the word carries an inherent paucity.

Communication, Virtue, and Virtuosity

Policy documents typically prescribe how doctors should behave and communicate as professionals and list the virtues that inform these behaviours. For example, the UK GMC's regularly updated *Good Medical Practice* (2006, p. 27) includes 'probity' (being honest and trustworthy) amongst its recommendations, suggesting that 'probity' and 'acting with integrity' are 'at the heart of medical professionalism'.

We should begin, then, as did the ancient Greeks, with such virtues. Discussions of virtue thread through Plato, particularly *Meno, Protagoras, Republic,* and *Laws. Meno* (Plato, 1956, p. 115), a dialogue between Socrates and a young aristocrat (Meno), opens with Meno's question to Socrates: 'is virtue something that can be taught? Or does it come by practice? Or is it neither teaching nor practice that gives it to a man but natural aptitude or something else?' Socrates' rhetorical strategy is to not answer the question, but to direct attention to the key prior question: what is virtue? In answer to this, Socrates says: 'The fact is that far from knowing whether it can be taught, I have no idea what virtue itself is'.

Over 2,400 years later, Louise Arnold and David Stern (2006, pp. 19–21) graphically model medical 'professionalism' as a classical Greek temple, where the supporting base (as three steps) is composed of 'clinical competence' (knowledge of medicine), 'communication skills', and 'ethical and legal understanding'. The roof is 'professionalism', and the pillars supporting the roof are four virtues: 'excellence', 'humanism', 'accountability', and 'altruism'. The authors explicitly equate professionalism with 'virtue'. 'Excellence', currently a buzzword in medical education policy documents, is characterized by 'a commitment to exceed ordinary standards'. Here, a return to classical Greece will help us to further define 'excellence' and also sharpen our understanding of 'virtue'. This, in turn, will lead to a better understanding and appreciation of 'empathy'.

In describing the relationship between rhetoric and athletics in ancient Greece, Debra Hawhee (2004, p. 17) describes a tradition of naming specific virtues, such as courage, but also of describing an overall 'virtuosity' (*aretē*). Hawhee describes Greek athletic competition as a form of 'rhetorical practice and pedagogy' in which competitors persuaded, or won over, the audience through their bodily prowess or virtuosity. In early Greek athletics, winners were judged by their ability to enter the field of play (*agōn*) as a warrior enters the battle, showing the virtues of courage, honourable engagement, and physical prowess. However, as athletic contests matured, virtuosity was judged as excellent where it explicitly avoided moralizing or piety. This subtle shift framed virtuosity as a highly focused or concentrated activity combining physical prowess (skill) with wisdom of the body (*mētis*) that is best translated as 'adaptability', expressing an art of timing or exploiting opportunity (*kairos*). This combination goes well beyond mere competence, turning sport into performance art. In the field of play that is the *agōn* of communication in medical practice, excellence might better be termed virtuosity, where virtuosity is a combination of skill (in reading, and responding to, cues), adaptability, and the art of timing.

Let us explore this a little further with emphasis upon empathy. While technical virtuosity—for example, as surgeon, diagnostician, or psychiatrist—is easy to grasp, how might we frame virtuosity in the nontechnical realms, such as communication and its subset of empathy? Arnold and Stern (2006, pp. 21–24) describe empathy as a subset of 'humanism'—one of their four pillars of virtue—along with respect, compassion, honour, and integrity. Further, these virtues must be enacted (or performed) for them to have any meaning, and this enactment is embodied in communication that is clinically informed and ethical. These authors distinguish empathy from compassion, where empathy is defined as a cognitive 'ability to understand another person's perspectives, inner experiences, and feelings without intensive emotional involvement', plus 'the capacity to communicate that understanding'. Compassion, in contrast, refers to the affective dimension of being 'moved by the suffering or distress of another and by the desire to relieve it'. Where Homer describes what we might now call the skilful employment of empathy, he uses the term 'pity', which artfully collapses the modern technical (and arbitrary) distinction between cognitive and affective components.

The shift from the virtue of the communicator to virtuosity in communication serves an important function—it links us back to classical thought in two senses. First, in Homeric Greek language (and then thinking), there is no sense of personal agency as intention. Medical students come with the modernist cultural baggage of 'introspection', 'autonomy', and 'self-regulation'—descriptors that would have had no meaning in Homeric Greek. Modern 'empathy' is considered as something that comes from within oneself and is projected onto another, as the dictionary definition suggests. However, in Homeric Greek, there is no 'I' who is 'empathic'. Rather, pity is embodied in an action or is a verb. Ruth Padel (1992, 1995), in discussing images of suffering in ancient Greek literature, does what medical educators now encourage—she shows that a value or a virtue can only be understood in terms of a performance. It is not what the medical student thinks that matters, but how he or she acts.

In Homeric Greek, many verbs, often those describing what we would now say as what goes on in the 'head' (cognition) or 'heart' (feeling), do not exist in the active form. Rather, the closest to this is a 'middle voice' verb, which is 'very close to passive, what is done to you by an outside agent'. Not 'I am disappointed', but 'disappointment is upon me', and this is known in the form of the resultant activity— disappointment as consequent, or subsequent, performance. 'Wishing' and 'fearing', for example, do not exist in the active form. If empathy, recast as pity, is considered as a verb rather than a personality trait, it is enlightening to consider it in this middle voice because we can now see that the *origin of pity is in that which inspires pity.*

In other words, we can shift emphasis from describing empathy as a personal character trait to placing the importance in its source. In the context of patient-centredness, *the source of empathy is in patients we treat.* This unhooks us from 'character training' in medicine and undue reliance upon role modelling. Rather, we are now interested in how medical students act with patients. Returning to Homer makes us think of 'patient-centredness' as a *verb*. Patients educate us into empathy as a response to their conditions and self-presentations.

While we have warned against cultivation of personality type in favour of consistently observable activities of patient-centredness, a return to classical thought also helps us to reframe the virtuous personality in terms of professional identity. Let us return to the conceptual model of professionalism proposed by Arnold and Stern (2006, p. 22). As described above, a supporting pillar, or virtue, central to professional behaviour is humanism, which includes empathy and compassion. Humanism is defined as 'a sincere concern for and interest in humanity', without which how could doctors treat a variety of patients with concern? We will not pursue here the difficulties presented by that weasel word 'sincere', connected as it is with probity or honesty. Rather, we are interested in the implications of 'humanism' and its relationship to identity.

Empathy has been both literalized and canonized particularly by Carl Rogers (1957) in the fields of humanistic psychology and person-centred psychotherapy. With little critical attention, Rogers' holy trinity of therapeutic skills—empathy, congruence (genuineness or probity), and unconditional positive regard—have been drummed into aspiring counsellors for over half a century. Training workshops focus on acquiring skills of attentive listening, discriminating between empathy, underplayed empathy, or sympathy ('would a cup of tea help?') and overplayed empathy, identification, or 'compathy' ('you know, I had the same thing happen to me a couple of years ago and ...'). 'Compathy' is a neologism of the person-centred school. The end product of such training can be a caricature of the 'engaged professional', sitting attentively, nodding deliberately, and reflecting ('tell me more ...'). A symptom of this approach, noted earlier in another context, is the index in Roter and Hall (2006) having six entries for 'nodding', but none for 'pity'. (There are 13 for 'empathy'.)

Now, as long as humanistic person-centredness is neither pious nor the exercise of political correctness, surely it offers a good model for patient-centred practice. Well, there are varieties of humanism and one can be humane without subscribing to modern humanism or personalism. Person-centredness readily aligns with narcissism—so characteristic of our age of celebrity status—that is a symptom to be cured and not a mode of curing. It is a short step from the inappropriate role modelling on celebrities, whether associated with eating disorders, body image, or being in recovery from multiple addictions, to the general health choices of impressionable adolescents. Cultivating the self is not necessarily a positive health choice—we have become extraordinarily sensitive to our inner psychological states, yet wholly insensitive to the quality of our environment (Hillman & Ventura, 1993). Egology has replaced ecology.

In an effort to provide an alternative to the humanistic tradition's way of thinking about 'selfhood' and identity, Michel Foucault (2005a, 2005b) made a close study of late Greek and early Roman texts that describe a 'care of the self'. These texts do not address a core self that must then realize its potential (the view of Carl Rogers and other humanistic psychologists), but show how an ethical self can be developed, constructed, or produced within a setting. In the same way that athletes can attain virtuosity through practice and artful engagement, so persons can shape themselves aesthetically, or 'form' character, *in contexts*. Such a background provides a new reading of medical education—not just as a technical training, but also as an aesthetic self-forming, to shape a professional identity. Hawhee (2004, p. 93) equates this process with *phusiopoiesis*. First described by the pre-Socratic philosopher Democritus, *phusiopoiesis* is the '*creation* of a person's nature' (our emphasis) grounded in poetics or aesthetics, not in instrumental 'skill'.

Groopman (2007), Stern (2006a, 2006b), and Ginsburg and Lingard (2006) offer comment on professionalism that critiques the current technical–rational discourse constructing notions of 'empathy', while none of these authors mention *phusiopoiesis*, refer to Foucault's ground-breaking work on classical accounts of care of the self, or engage with the topic historically. As we have seen in a previous chapter, the seasoned American physician and practiced communicator (a staff writer at *The New Yorker*), Groopman (2007, p. 17) suggests that how a doctor thinks (clinical reasoning and diagnosis) 'can first be discerned by how he (*sic*) speaks and how he listens'. Communication and diagnostic acumen are closely related—better doctors discover from the patient through close attention and build a therapeutic relationship.

Groopman's elegant observation could be taken directly from one of the primers on self-fashioning that Foucault interrogates. Foucault (2005a, 2005b, pp. 98–99) discusses texts by Philo of Alexandria (20 BCE–50 CE) and Epictetus (c.55–135) that suggest those interested in care of the soul, as well as care of the body, could form a 'clinic' where you learn collectively how to do philosophy. We can readily translate this into contemporary medical education, where aspiring doctors learn both how to treat the body and how to set up the circumstances that will offer a healing or therapeutic *relationship* with patients. Importantly, at the same time, the medical student is doing work on identity or forming a style of life.

In Foucault's reading, Epictetus (Foucault, 2005a, 2005b, pp. 339–340) provides far more sophisticated advice on speaking and listening than most contemporary texts on the medical encounter. For example, Epictetus warns about being captivated by the speaker and not listening through to what is underneath the surface talk. This recognizes that talk is acting rhetorically and certain persuasive elements must be recognized and challenged. Listening is also charged rhetorically. We can listen in various ways—hearing what we want to hear (rhetorical listening), missing the point (not listening well), or listening well (offering benefit both to speaker and listener), including knowing when to be silent. Speaking and listening are not instrumental but an art, requiring discrimination and diligent practice.

This links us to Stern's (2006, p. 7) suggestion that communicating well can be seen in terms of 'connoisseurship' (a term borrowed from the educationalist Eliot Eisner), as 'the ability to make fine-grained discriminations amongst complex and subtle qualities' and to Ginsburg and Lingard's (2006) warning that communication within professionalism is not about what is a 'right' approach but what is *appropriate for context*. Again, judgment, or discrimination—an aesthetic quality—precedes the functional aspect of communicating (Bleakley, Marshall, & Brömer, 2006). Ginsburg and Lingard switch emphasis from the teaching and learning of communication skills, or a body of knowledge concerning professionalism, to what people actually do in practice, emphasizing prior appreciation of rhetoric (how communication is used deliberately or unconsciously to persuade) and reflection (how do I justify my actions in retrospect, and how will this prepare me for future activity?).

The latter resonates with Stern's (2006, p. 7) suggestion that while connoisseurship is the 'input' for professional relationship with patients, there must be an output, and this is 'critique' or 'public report'—a reflexive form of educational assessment and accountability. This can also be read as a form of monitory democracy (Keane, 2009)—a meta-democracy, appraisal, and quality assurance.

This leads us to suggest that structured reflection on real clinical encounters is a better way of learning communication than artificial (simulated) encounters in the skills laboratory or communication suite.

Finally, to reinforce the point about the difficulties of modern humanism's association with personalism and the cult of the individual, Fred Hafferty (2006, pp. 294–296) notes that 'altruism' is a term that seems to be disappearing as the new lexicon of 'professionalism' takes hold. This also returns us to virtues closely associated with pity—but, explicitly, not with piety (Bleakley, 1992)! Altruism is the opposite of egoism. Modern empathy does not require altruism—indeed, psychological introspection as a basis to cognitive empathy would seem to resist altruism by definition. However, pity and altruism are bedfellows.

In summary, 'empathy' has become part of the unexamined fabric of communication skills teaching, taken as transparent. Through a 'return to Homer', we have problematized the modern notion of 'empathy'—now a pervasive term in medical communication. By questioning what can be seen as a false division between the cognitive act of empathy and the affective state of compassion and by recovering a more poignant, ancient use of the now abused (and sometimes abusive) term 'pity', we have attempted to show how the Classics can enrich contemporary medicine, thus adding weight to the argument presented in Chap. 2 for the value of the medical humanities as core and integrated provision within medicine and surgery curricula. In this grounding in Classics, we follow Michel Foucault's impulse in his later work to map the future through classical, historical reference, articulating a history of the present.

In problematizing 'empathy', we have necessarily demanded complexity and ambiguity in an era where many medical educationists concerned with 'professionalism' have demanded simplification, clarity, instrumentalism, empiricism, and measure. We have called for a return of empathy to its aesthetic ground as a challenge to the reductionist approaches characterized by instrumentalism, where empathy can be read metaphorically rather than literally, and we applaud moves to characterize empathy as a form of connoisseurship.

Finally, we have argued for a reading of empathy as a verb rather than a noun, so that empathy is context-specific, as act or performance, rather than personality condition. However, doctors who distinguish themselves through the quality of their communication and 'fellow feeling' (Adler & Brett, 2009/1938) may be seen as cultivating a style of life or work, as an aesthetic self-forming, a shaping of identity. If the communication dimension to medicine—patient-centredness—is a kind of performance art, then it is better nourished by the deeper structure of pity than the surface operations of empathy. Scripts are also better learned in the real field of play (the *agōn*) than in rehearsal in the artificial communication suite. Empathy may be framed as an overall virtuosity (*aretē*), rather than a specific virtue or character trait, realized as a rhetorical activity.

'Empathy', returned to an aesthetic ground in 'pity', does and should defy definition. However, socialized within an empirical, scientific tradition, most medical students, educators, and researchers prefer clear concepts and well-defined boundaries. They will rejoice at the work of Hojat, Gonnella, and Mangione et al. (2002);

Hojat, Gonnella, and Nasca et al. (2002); and Hojat, Mangione, and Nasca et al. (2004) in utilizing a scale to measure empathy, which assumes that one first knows what is being measured. This reflects a modern mindset that tells us we understand by anatomizing, rationalizing, and articulating. It is an instrumental mindset that may, paradoxically, be the opposite of the empathic mindset that it both examines and teaches. Even if empathy could be taught, would it be fair to our students? Would not classes in narcissism and self-interest be of greater benefit? What if there has been no evolution, no progress in our moral sensitivity? That is why the stories of Greece and Rome resonate with us and can inform our ethical practice, while pity, sympathy, empathy, and compassion have been examined formally in medical education for only half a century (Wilmer, 1968).

Perhaps more complex than empathy is the issue of gender as a framework for discussing communication in medicine. I have already suggested that one of the structural, historical burdens for contemporary medicine to address is its (male) gender bias. Yet this bias is now colliding with an increasing majority of women entering medicine over men. It is this thorny issue that the following chapter addresses.

Chapter 9
Gender Matters in Medical Education

Introduction: The Gender Shift in Medicine

A front-page article in the *International Herald Tribune* by Carvajal (March 8, 2011) entitled 'The changing face of Western medicine' details how 'Across the Western world' a generation of young women 'is transforming the once-male bastion of medicine, swelling medical schools and flocking to the front lines of primary care'. The rhetoric is carefully chosen—'swelling' equating with the flush of pregnancy enjoyed by medical schools, with its expectant, women-heavy cohorts promising new life for medicine, 'flocking' signifying emergence of a new family, perhaps around a new idea or practice.

The article goes on to quote the latest figures: women now constitute 54 % of physicians below the age of 35 in Britain, while the figures in France and Spain are even higher, respectively, 58 and 64 %. Women already constitute the majority of students in medical schools worldwide, with a 56 % intake in the UK in 2010 and over 60 % in other European countries. By 2017 in the UK, women will constitute the majority of all doctors. In contrast to men, however, they will tend to pursue part-time careers in medicine as they choose to have children and raise families. They will continue, as part-timers, to be overrepresented worldwide in primary care and paediatrics but underrepresented in other specialties, especially surgery and anaesthetics, and particularly surgery at higher grades (Jefferson Demographics, 2005; Taylor, Lambert, & Goldacre, 2009).

The chapter discusses a 'feminization of medicine'. But quite what does 'feminization' mean? I argue that 'feminizing' medicine goes beyond the numbers and the literal gender reading. The fact that women are entering medicine in greater numbers may or may not affect the quality of medicine practiced. Further, it may be that 'feminizing' medicine depends on qualities that male doctors can cultivate also, such as collaboration ('flocking') and more sensitive patterns of communication. While we should avoid literalizing 'feminizing' by associating this values complex only with women, how can we discuss 'feminizing' without referring back to women? The arena is highly complex and sensitive.

A. Bleakley, *Patient-Centred Medicine in Transition: The Heart of the Matter*,
Advances in Medical Education 3, DOI 10.1007/978-3-319-02487-5_9,
© Springer International Publishing Switzerland 2014

As a man, should I be discussing the feminizing of medicine at all? My response is 'yes', as long as I am reflexive about stereotypes and archetypes. In the key article referred to above—key because it is in an international newspaper on the front-page and informing a wide public readership—Carvajal (*International Herald Tribune* Tuesday March 8, 2011:1) asks: 'Are female doctors offering lessons in more effective care-giving?' Does this question offer a stereotype or a mother archetype? Well, what we know from a decade of research in the area (Roter & Hall, 2006) is that gender is a significant factor in doctor–patient communication, where:

- Women doctors spend 10 % longer than male doctors with patients.
- Women patients spend 10 % longer than male patients with all doctors.
- Women doctors talk 40 % more than male doctors.
- Patients of women doctors talk 58 % more than patients of male doctors.
- Women patients ask more questions and give more information than male patients.
- Women patients check and paraphrase, forcing the doctor into clearer explanations.
- Women patients, more so than male patients, want a 'feelings-oriented' rather than a 'thoughts-oriented' consultation style.

Does this constitute more effective care-giving? Looking at the issue from another perspective, in a 2010 report by the UK National Clinical Assessment Service, tracking and analysing patient complaints, figures are released for suspensions of general practitioners between 2001 and 2010. When the figures are adjusted to reflect the gender composition of the medical workforce, men attracted more complaints than women, and men were shown as five times more likely to be suspended than women as a result of investigations into complaints. There are two main explanations for these figures. First, women community doctors may take less risk than their male colleagues. Second, women community doctors may engage support and early warning networks much better than their male counterparts. Women will be in a majority in the field of general practice in the UK by 2013 (Carvajal, 2011).

Does Gender Matter?

Imagine: a young woman of Asian origin living in the UK is constantly tired, especially after menstruation, which is unusually heavy. She is told by her family to eat 'hot' foods at the time of her periods and that heavy bleeding indicates that she is purifying her body. She is, of course, anaemic and needs iron supplements. She is registered with a male family practitioner, but will not go to see him because she is embarrassed to talk about her periods with a man.

A 60-year-old man is suffering from benign prostatic hyperplasia and feels that his medication is no longer working. The male urologist he has seen for the past 2 years has moved to another area and the man has been referred to a newly appointed urologist. When he discovers that she is a woman, he cancels the appointment, fearing that she will not be able to empathize with his condition and afraid that she might want to examine him rectally.

A woman in a hospital refuses physical contact from a male nurse on the basis that it is an invasion of her privacy. A male surgeon makes an inappropriate sexist remark about a female scrub nurse within earshot of her and other members of the surgical team, but she is afraid to challenge him. An adolescent man feels drawn to have sex with another man and wants to discuss this with someone in confidence, but is cautious about raising the issue with his general practitioner who he sees as an 'alpha male' likely to judge him and put down his feelings as misguided.

These stories show that not just feminizing, but gender issues in general, are central to medicine, yet they are poorly represented in the medical education literature. Is this because discussion of gender issues so readily invites stereotyping? For example, where medicine is so intimately concerned with the body, should we follow feminists such as Bordo (1993, p. 5), who argues that because of the menstrual and ovulatory cycles and the potential to give birth, the body is 'the province of the female', where men, in contrast, want 'to stand clear of the flesh, to maintain perspective on it'? Bordo is rehearsing a familiar argument concerning the pervasive and invasive 'male' gaze that objectifies, in contrast to the subjective interests of the feminine. But can her remarks be read as a further layer of stereotyping?

Robert Romanyshyn (1989) offers an interesting genealogy of the male gaze, grounding it in the 'discovery' (or articulation) of the rules of perspective by the Renaissance architect Brunelleschi and then adopted by painters. Application of the rules of perspective meant that painting could now represent depth vision. Romanyshyn, however, suggests that the widespread cultural adoption of the rules of perspective literally changed the way that people saw the world. The model preceded and formed vision or ways of seeing. Importantly, as painters were male and their models were women, a male 'gaze' developed that objectified or distanced the world, as it objectified the women models posing for paintings, who became objects of lust or desire within the male gaze, as well as objects of curiosity—both held at arms' length (gaining a literal and moral perspective) and embraced (collapsing literal and moral perspectives into impulse or compulsion) at the same time. Primarily, where 'nature' was archetypally associated with the feminine, so nature was held at arm's length, to be studied objectively, dissected and analyzed, or objectified. This is the historical ground for the development of scientific 'objectivity', again associated with a masculine gaze (Daston & Galison, 2007).

In a recent chapter in this story of the development of 'perspective' (objectifying, distancing, and judging as part of the same complex), Foucault (Bleakley & Bligh, 2009) famously describes the medical or clinical 'gaze' as at once objectifying and penetrating—metaphorically looking into the depths of the body in a diagnostic glance, reflecting the actual opening of the body achieved through dissection and autopsy (which literally means 'see for yourself'). Medicine is then *stereotypically* a profession that is gendered male. The penetrating eye is associated with the penetrating phallus, which in turn is associated with the outlook of 'logic'. The metonymic chain of the penetrating eye-phallus-cold logic extends to the scalpel, as a peculiarly masculine extension of the conducting hand and the pointing or probing finger (Sennett, 2008). Paradoxically, Foucault is conducting this analysis as a gay man in a generally homophobic era and (in)famously sought his liberation in the sexually liberated bathhouses of Californian cities. Foucault's autobiography, however, never entered his cultural–historical analyses. This work was carried out after his death by his biographers. The queering of medicine is as yet an embryonic project.

Institutionally, modern medicine can then be seen to be gendered male and is perhaps still institutionally homophobic, both examples of what the doctor and psychoanalyst Adler (2009/1927) described, nearly a century ago, as the 'masculine protest'. The well-rehearsed argument is that doctors see so much suffering that they must protect themselves, through objectification and distancing, from carrying this suffering. Psychoanalytically, they tend to use the stronger ego defence mechanisms of denial and repression. However, this 'masculine protest' ultimately has a counterproductive effect. First, as medical students and then junior doctors, they learn to 'harden', so they come to objectify patients, concentrating on cure rather than care (which is left to nurses). This is well documented, as we have seen, in terms of the phenomenon of 'empathy decline'.

Second, repressed affect is released in classic, often socially sanctioned, ways such as alcohol and drug (ab)use. I have already noted the high rates of burnout, depression, suicidal ideation, and suicide in the medical profession—in relation to rates found both in the general population and in other professions—from medical students (Dyrbye et al., 2008) through to experienced physicians (Schernhammer, 2005; Serry, Bloch, Ball, & Anderson, 1994). Again, the reader is guided to Abraham Verghese's (1998) account of such personal trials in the social-realist novel *The Tennis Partner.*

The masculine protest characteristically runs through all of medicine's procedures. Thus, the bioethicist Tod Chambers (1999) suggests that even the medical case is written in a way that has, perhaps unintentionally, privileged a male worldview. For Chambers, the same cultural logic that produces the male gaze and the medical gaze are at work in the 'case', where the 'person' is objectified first as 'patient' and then as 'case'. Further, the case is often analyzed in classical bioethics through a generalized 'principles' approach that is widely recognized as insensitive to the particular and the contextual.

A Feminist Medical Education

What would such 'cases' look like, or how would they be written up, if medicine were guided by the outlook of *écriture feminine*—feminine practices of writing, such as those modelled elegantly by Hélène Cixous (1991, 2004) who asks, metaphorically, what is it like to write with 'mother's milk?' This can be read as (re)*inscribing* your writing—in our example of a patient 'case'—with maternalism rather than paternalism, where 'care' precedes control and authority. Cixous's use of 'mother's milk' can be read at several levels—as writing that is nourishing; as writing that is expressive, 'expressed' as breast milk that stains as it sustains; and as writing that can only be performed by women.

Cixous further describes how to get a singular, feminine 'voice' into writing by resisting the conventions of a dominant masculine style. She shows how not to be flattened by the stylistic demands of intellectual writing—the scientific report or, again, the 'case'. How would we, in writing a case report, 'make the text gasp or form it out of suspenses and silences' as Cixous (Cixous & Clement, 1986, p. 92) suggests, describing a feminine style? Could such an approach to writing capture the contours and feelings of the patient, as person embedded in a lifeworld, rather than symptom isolated from that lifeworld?

Annemarie Mol (2008), in discussing treatment for, and of, persons who are diabetic, argues against the stereotypical 'patient-centred' view of 'patient choice' (that she calls a 'logic of choice') and for the 'logic of care', which she explicitly sees as a feminist project. The logic of choice, suggests Mol, is apparently founded for patients and seems supportive, but offers a paradoxical imperative based on consumerism. It frames the patient as consumer in a market and discloses both a masculinist and capitalist view, imposed on patients. The logic of *care*, however, reframes health-care as collaboration between experts (in disease) and patients (as experts in their own illnesses), with a focus upon the quality of relationship. This shifts the ground towards a 'care' rather than 'cure' outlook but cleverly retains the sense that there is logic to care: a framework, knowledge, and a set of values, also subverting the masculine logos in the process as it is juxtaposed with feminine 'care'.

Language matters. For example, it is not political correctness that prevents use of disparaging terms for minority groups, but recognition of the cumulative hurt that use of such language has had on those groups. Paradoxically, one 'minority' group that attracts disparaging language is not a minority at all. This group is women, handicapped, and marginalized in otherwise sophisticated cultures by continued use of (male) gendered language and practices. Such male-gendered language—for example, 'houseman' and medicine framed through martial and militaristic metaphors (the war on disease)—has been commonly employed in medicine and medical education and is only now approaching exhaustion.

Wagner and colleagues (2007, p. 288) suggest that 'Medical education is not only about the acquisition of new knowledge and skills; it is also about the acquisition of a new identity in life—an identity as a doctor, a medical professional, with all the rights and responsibilities that entails'. Such talk of identity construction is now commonplace in medical education, especially in the field of professionalism (Bleakley, Bligh, & Browne, 2011). While there is much talk of identity development as a professional in medicine, far too little of this discusses gender and identity.

Kenneth Ludmerer's (1999, p. 334) classic history of American medical education points to the contemporary 'disappearance of heroes from medicine', where 'academic medicine' in particular 'has grown too large and fragmented for "heroes" to emerge'. This may seem like good news to feminists in medical education. However, while medicine now attracts more women entrants than men, as we have noted, academic medicine is still a male domain. Sandhu, Margerison, and Holdcroft (2007) report that in the UK only one in ten clinical professors is a woman. Paradoxically, the authors suggest that this creates a lack of female role models in academic medicine, where 'role modelling' is read by many feminists as a typically male, heroic strategy and, as reported below, women medical students are less interested in learning through role modelling than by other means.

Not so long ago, few doctors would have bothered to question the meaning of the descriptor of the ward team as a 'firm' or the first year junior doctor (intern progressing to junior resident), a house officer, as a 'houseman'. In the UK, the notion of the 'firm' has now largely disappeared, as clinical teams are increasingly constituted on an ad hoc basis, dissolving the metaphor of quasi-family units (with industrial overtones), and in the UK, 'house officer' has been replaced by 'foundation doctor'. The phallic 'firm' is now flaccid or, rather, flexible and 'liquid'—a metaphor used frequently by French poststructuralist, feminist thinkers such as Luce Irigaray (1993).

How will the new female majority of junior doctors establish their household and is the household not, stereotypically, the woman's domain? Will they, for example, see domestic 'care' values as more important than business values (where the 'firm' typically describes a commercial venture or a legal set up), working against a current discourse of managerialism that frames care as a business and patients as customers? 'Firm', as noted above, also means solid, stiff, unyielding, and steadfast and is readily linked with the penetrating gaze. Will such archetypally masculine values, characterized by contemporary feminist theory as 'phallocentric', be replaced by a different set of values where women doctors are in the ascendant, at least in terms of numbers?

Women Doctors in the Workforce

Let us look more closely at the numbers with which I opened this chapter. Referring back to the *International Herald Tribune* article by Carvajal (March 8, 2011), this is supplemented by some interesting statistics. In terms of the percentage of all practicing doctors in 2008, women constituted 47.5 % in Spain, 41.5 % in Britain, 40.6 % in Germany, 39.6 % in France, 36.0 % in Italy, and 30.8 % in the USA. So, women doctors in America have constituted less than a third of the working body of physicians. However, the longitudinal demographics are telling. The change from 2000 to 2008 in terms of female doctors as a percentage of all working doctors is 9.4 % for Spain, 6.4 % for the UK, 5.8 % for both the USA and Italy, 4.7 % for Germany, and 3.3 % for France.

A quite different picture emerges when we look at female doctors under the age of 35 as a percentage of all doctors working in any one country under the age of 35. This has risen between 2000 and 2008 from 60 to 63.8 % in Spain, 50 to 63 % in Italy, 56 to 58 % in France, 48 to 55 % in Germany, 48 to 53.8 % in the UK, and 40 to 46.5 % in the USA. Statistics are, stereotypically, comforting to the male psyche;

but these will bring tears to the eyes of those who are still under the spell of institutional sexism in medicine. The future of medicine is undoubtedly female.

There is also a well-documented gender-based demographic shift occurring in the pattern of recruitment to medical undergraduate programmes across North America, Australia, Russia, and Europe (Kilminster, Downes, Gough, Murdoch-Eaton, & Roberts, 2007; McMurray et al., 2002). In 2008 in the UK, the proportion of women entering medical school since 1965 had risen from 20 to 55 % and continues to rise (McManus, 1997). This trend is predicted to plateau at 60–65 %, rising to 70 % in some medical schools (Carvel, 2002). On the basis of current demographic data, showing that women doctors work shorter hours overall than male doctors, and that women doctors are likely to choose career paths that accommodate having children, there is a predicted shortfall in filling medicine's future labour demands. This demographic trend raises a number of structural problems. There will be a dramatic shortfall in working time, as women doctors currently work 85 % equivalent of their male counterparts. This has been termed 'the medical time bomb' (Laurance, 2004).

On the basis of current patterns in gender-based choices for careers, there will be a shortfall in certain specialties. For example, a survey of 300 first year students from Guys Kings and St Thomas School of Medicine (UK) shows that 'Women still opt for general practice and paediatrics', and while men constituted only 38 % of the total intake, they nevertheless constituted two-thirds of the population of students hoping to pursue a career in surgery (Fysh, Thomas, & Ellis, 2007).

Those who read this demographic shift as likely to produce a shortfall in supply of doctor hours are concerned with the increasing absence of men from the profession. Are men reluctant to enter medicine because they are no longer attracted to the profession, or are they more interested in other careers? Are male school-leavers simply not good enough academically to enter medicine in comparison with their female peers? Are women applicants getting chosen over men because they fulfil a profile of a new kind of medical student and future doctor fit for practice for a new era of interprofessional health-care? Is this profile acting as a disguised form of discrimination? Also, perhaps the men who now enter medicine cannot be judged against previous generations' values, attitudes, and behaviours.

Another view highlights the benefits that a female-dominated profession may bring as it challenges the current dominant discourse of a male-gendered medicine. As introduced at the beginning of this chapter, will this critical gender shift bring a sea change in values and practices to what has traditionally been a male domain? Whatever view we take of the long-term consequences of this gender shift, the shorter-term reality raises a critical issue for medical education. Where, to help us better understand the gendering of practices, contemporary gender studies and feminist thinking are widely employed in academic study (including critique of practices already naturalized as 'masculine'), such frameworks are not commonly mobilized in medical education.

The current literature in medical education addressing the emergence of a female-dominated medicine focuses upon structural issues such as inequalities and is largely descriptive or prescriptive, but rarely adventurous theoretically.

For example, the literature notes current gender-based structural inequalities that continue to hinder the professional development of women doctors. For example, proportionately: less women doctors than men gain senior positions, women doctors constitute the minority of medical teachers, women are less often employed in hospitals, and, on average, as noted above, women doctors work an equivalent of 85 % of the workload of male doctors (Laurance, 2004; Sanfey, Saalwachter-Schulman, Nyhof-Young, Eidelson, & Mann, 2006). Importantly, in comparison with their male colleagues, women doctors are more acutely aware of such gender inequalities, now explicitly framed in terms of institutionalized discrimination (Laurance, 2004).

Career routes leading to consultant posts have traditionally been harder to pursue for women who wish to have children (Denekens, 2002; Derese, Kerremans, & Deveugele, 2002). This is particularly the case in surgery, where 94 % of consultant surgeons in the UK are men. While more women than men—52 % of all Year 1 junior doctors (interns)—show a career interest in surgery, by post-registration Year 2 (residents), this figure halves to 25 % and drops again to 15 % of surgical specialist registrars, culminating in women constituting only 6 % of the body of consultant surgeons. Women tend to be successful on the career ladder in surgery only if certain structural issues are overcome, such as provision of flexible hours, child minding services, and supportive mentors (Washburn, 2000). Women may lose interest in surgery as they progressively encounter a strong competitive element, where in general women doctors prefer more collaborative clinical contexts (McKinstry, Colthart, Elliott, & Hunter, 2006).

There is not only a structural equality of opportunity problem in medicine with regard to gender, but also an equity problem. Women in medicine get poorer rewards for doing the same job as men (Fysh et al., 2007), and where women are underrepresented in key positions in the senior ranks, institutionally medicine continues to fail women with career aspirations through failing to provide the necessary resources and infrastructure to help them achieve their goals (Boerma & van den Brink-Muinen, 2000). Women doctors earn less than men in academic medicine, go slower through the ranks, and do not readily attain leadership roles (Buddeberg-Fischer, Klaghofer, Abel, & Buddeberg, 2003). Again, this is not due to quality of productivity nor to commitment, but rather to structural constraints.

Such constraints are then realized at an individual level of aspiration—when asked in surveys what their potential earning power may be, women doctors report a ceiling that is around a quarter less than that reported by male doctors (Boulis & Long, 2004). Overall, women doctors consistently rate themselves as less capable than male doctors (Wolosin & Gesell, 2006). Such data are poorly theorized and pervasive institutional gender bias in the professions (Pinar, Reynolds, Slattery, & Taubman, 1995) may be a necessary but not sufficient explanation or may simply offer description rather than explanation. For example, where it is reported that women doctors rate themselves as less capable than male doctors, is this a reflection of reality or a rhetorical effect of an already powerfully patriarchal medicine? Another view is that male doctors overestimate their abilities, where women doctors are realistic and note room for development.

Women doctors in general display different professional interaction styles to their male colleagues, informed by a characteristic set of values concerned with intimacy in patient care. Quality of communication with patients is better than male colleagues (Roter & Hall, 2006), and women doctors are generally more egalitarian, patient-centred, and involved with patients' psychosocial problems than their male colleagues (Chambers, 1999).

A study of role modelling by junior doctors on respected senior doctors notes that women junior doctors report 'communication' as the key element they wish to emulate, where communication was reported as much less important by male junior doctors (Wolosin & Gesell, 2006). There is a wider nexus that reflects the valuing of intimacy in professional care, where women doctors rate having a supportive environment, such as close friends, as more important to work satisfaction than their male colleagues (Verlander, 2004). Further, in the balance between intrinsic and extrinsic motives influencing work satisfaction, where women doctors report intrinsic satisfaction as primary, male doctors show more interest in extrinsic monetary and status rewards.

Drawing on Women's Studies to Enrich Medical Education: Gendered Ways of Thinking

These structural issues are important, but only tell half of the gender story in medicine. The other half is to do with gendered mindsets—thinking and valuing in gendered terms—and this is, paradoxically, not necessarily dependent on whether one is biologically male or female. As mentioned earlier, for example, there is little work in medical education drawing on queer studies. While we think it is vital to study ethnicity in medicine (as doctors will work in multiethnic societies), we do not openly and positively discuss the sexual orientation of doctors, medical students, or doctors working with gay and lesbian patients or conceive of sexual orientation as a resource. We should note that educational theory has a strong queer studies element, promoted by activists such as William Pinar (2004, 2006). If we think of a gender mindset and a study of gendered language, rather than literal gender issues as discussed in the first half of this chapter, men can be feminist and women can be anti-feminist, whatever their sexual orientations.

There are two broad streams of contemporary feminist thinking: Anglo-American and Continental, the latter often referred to as French poststructuralism, where most of the recognized key thinkers are French nationals. The 'Anglo-American' stream is grounded in analysis of structural inequalities—including pay differentials or opportunities for promotion—that can be addressed through economic or political strategies. The 'Continental' stream moves the ground for analysis to language and thought, arguing that redressing structural social issues can be cosmetic, where fundamental ways of *thinking and valuing*, that come to shape activity, remain unaddressed. These ways of thinking, suggest poststructuralist feminists, are grounded in language use and the semiotics of a culture or the meanings that cultures ascribe to human experiences and the symbols that represent these meanings. This school of thought suggests that only by addressing language use and culturally negotiated meanings will social practices change.

For example, the widespread, mute, acceptance of andragogy ('adult learning theory') in medical education, periodically critiqued in the education literature (Bleakley, Bligh, & Browne, 2011), reveals not only a lack of critical attention but also the explicit acceptance of a gender bias grounded in language and thought. The root of andragogy (Greek *andr-*) means 'man' or 'male'. How, then, might a medical education look if it were a 'gynagogy'? Learning theories privileging autonomy also serve to mirror medicine's traditionally heroic, masculine stance, reflected again in the use of martial metaphors such as 'waging war' on disease, 'fighting' illness, and the 'battle' against cancer.

Medical education research may be embedded in such martial metaphors, with its emphasis upon competition for resources rather than collaboration in research. A 'centre' for research is still the most popular descriptor, rather than the more democratic structure of a network, where collaborative models can be seen to be more feminine in tone. For Martha Nussbaum (1999), there is an overarching male privileging of issues of 'justice' in health-care (such as distribution of resources) over a female concern with issues of quality of 'care', and this is echoed by Mol's work on diabetes care (Mol, 2008). Of course, both orientations are important, but Nussbaum argues that an ethic of justice is persistently privileged over an ethic of care, and this can be read as a gender bias leading to inequalities.

Networks will only operate well if they align themselves ontologically as well as epistemologically (Mol, 2002). In other words, researchers who collaborate must know how to communicate, particularly how to manage necessary and predictable tensions. These are issues of affect rather than cognition, and I cited evidence earlier that women doctors and women patients in general work more comfortably with affective issues than their male counterparts. In this case the evidence base confirms what could be read as a stereotype.

Such approaches challenge an unbroken, dominant tradition in the Western psyche, from the warring heroes of Homer's *Iliad* and the lone hero's journey embodied in the *Odyssey*, of the self-sufficient warrior who must get by on his own resources or he will perish, to the heroic individualism endemic to medicine. Contemporary, poststructuralist feminisms challenge the dominance of such traditions. As the face of medicine changes with an influx of women practitioners, perhaps medical education will in time shift its explanatory models of learning from the individualistic models of 'adult learning theory' to the collaborative models of social learning theories such as communities of practice, activity theory, and actor–network theory, the latter two discussed at length in Chaps. 11 and 13.

It is in the space of difference between doctors and patients that a new medicine can be realized—one of the genuine collaboration based on respect for difference. This model argues against essentialism, where doctors realize an identity only in identification with their professional group. In the same vein, I argue that identification with a gendered position of practicing medicine should not be essentialist—I am not arguing that women doctors constitute the future of patient-centred medicine because they are women, but rather that women are more likely to adopt certain, more productive, ways of communicating and working. Again, this does not mean that it is only male doctors who can be boorish and paternalistic and it is not just women doctors who can be caring and tender.

Challenging Binary Thinking

Gender studies are plagued by a tendency to utilize binary thinking (such as male versus female), reducing complex gender issues to essentialism, or referring gender to purely biological differences. Poststructuralist feminisms challenge such rhetoric, first in a critique of oppositional thinking and second in a focus upon language use prior to biological difference. Binary thinking is the fundamental rhetorical device of structuralist thinking. It offers what at first sight appears to be a useful heuristic, and its terms are so familiar as to be naturalized, such as the body/mind opposition, stemming from Descartes, that is a root metaphor for dualism. Such oppositions conceal more than they reveal, failing to describe the complexity of the world. Oppositional thinking can be seen as a basic rhetorical strategy to control complexity by reduction to simplistic descriptive categories. Such mastery becomes institutionalized as the proper way to engage with life.

In oppositionalist thinking and its subsequent practices, one term becomes the positive and comes to dominate the other in an asymmetrical opposition, such as man/woman, human/animal, adult/child, and white/black. The subjugated term is not only governed, or ruled, but is easily belittled, stereotyped, and demonized. In *Sorties,* first published in 1975, Hélène Cixous points out that 'wherever discourse is organized' it is 'always the same metaphor', that of oppositionalism or duality, *leading to hierarchy* (Cixous, 1991, pp. 63–65). Western (North European/North American) 'thought has always worked through opposition', such as activity/passivity and culture/nature, where 'woman is always associated with passivity in philosophy'.

I have argued in earlier chapters that hierarchies in medicine need to be countered if we are to democratize the profession, in light of evidence that 'horizonal' forms of teamworking create patient safety cultures and benefit patient health outcomes. Feminist writers such as Cixous suggest that first, however, we must challenge the habit of oppositionalist thinking that has historically also informed—and attempted to naturalize—imperialism and colonialism (an 'us and them' mentality). Thus, Cixous (Cixous & Clement, 1986, p. 92) offers a challenge to the 'stability of the masculine structure that passed itself off as eternal-natural', a challenge to what she calls the 'Empire of the Selfsame', which is to turn back to oneself as the model for the world and for others, rather than to see oneself as 'different' from others and to respect this difference rather than force others into the mould that is yourself.

Particularly associated with Jacques Derrida, the philosophical school of deconstruction offers the most stringent critique of oppositionalist thinking.

Deconstructive critique exposes the contradictions inherent to the language of ratio-nalist texts, exposing the fragility of claims that such texts offer an encompassing truth or totality. Oppositionalism is a key rhetorical tactic for supposed reasoned argument. For Derrida, there is also always a 'surplus' that texts can never encom-pass and hence their project of mastery ('truth' claims) is doomed to failure. Where language itself is ambiguous, attempts to rationally encompass experience through strategies such as oppositional thinking are inherently flawed. Telling examples of paradoxical language that disrupt oppositional thinking include the Latin *altus*, which simultaneously means both 'high' and 'low' and the Greek *pharmakon*, which means both a 'healing agent' and a 'poison'. Importantly, deconstruction challenges the assumed logic of texts by exposing contradictions and so opens the reader to (an)other reading. This close noticing of and respect for 'otherness' is a characteristic of radical feminist thinking.

Feminist poststructuralists point out that oppositional thinking is actually illogi-cal, where oppositions contain the seed of their own dissolution. Paradoxically, the dominant term cannot exist without the presence of the inferior term. As Hegel pointed out, 'master' is meaningless without 'slave'. I have already noted that there is no 'doctor' without 'patient', and this could act as a more subversive definition of 'patient-centredness' than 'learning with, from, and about patients' that is our stan-dard definition.

I have described the particular feminist view, based in interest in language use, which suggests that the masculine way is invested in the 'selfsame'—where identity is 'in' the person, not in the difference from, or relationship to, an Other. The post-structuralist feminist way, in contrast, is grounded in 'difference', where one's iden-tity is formed in the 'mirror' of the 'other'. Is there any empirical evidence for what seems like an abstract, theoretical view and might we legitimately ask 'so what?' for medical education? How will the focus of this part of our chapter help us with prac-tice? Is it not just a piece of theoretical self-indulgence?

Male junior doctors show a greater degree of direct role modelling on mentors than their women colleagues and these mentors tend to be male. This reproduction of selfsame may be of less interest to women doctors who value difference, a per-spective that also affirms understanding for the other, such as patients and col-leagues. Can we then not learn from women doctors to orient to the other rather than to the self, which would offer a ground for a collaborative patient-centredness, realizing our preferred model of mutuality within a relationship-centred mindset? Research evidence also shows gender differences in medical students' 'hardening' to patients, where male students harden more quickly than female students and retain these attitudes into their medical careers.

Julia Kristeva's (1982) work suggests that oppositional thinking promotes a slippery slope to prejudice. Typically, an opposition takes the form of subject/object. Whatever I oppose is potentially dehumanized and depersonalized. The relegated 'other' can quickly become demonized, moving beyond the status of 'object' to take on the status of the 'abject'—that is considered intolerable. The abject is not only excluded, but pathologized and actively discriminated against, for example, in scapegoating. Discrimination now becomes prejudice. Paradoxically, doctors tend to treat their less-ill patients more favourably than the more ill (Roter & Hall, 2006).

Medical education favouring individualistic learning theories generally approaches communication through the maxim 'know thyself'. This is institutionalized in traditions of reflective practice (Bleakley, 1999; Bleakley, 2006c). Kristeva (1982), in the psychoanalytic tradition, critiques such illusory aspects of 'mastery', where we are always 'strangers to ourselves' or have abject aspects that remain repressed yet actively shape behaviour. In comparison with their female colleagues who are more uncertain about practice, self-image, and career goals, male doctors show assertive confidence in their practice congruent with strong self-image, aligned with focused career ambitions. This difference can be read psychoanalytically, where overconfidence can offer defence against recognition of uncertainty.

Kristeva suggests that it is through 'unknowing', or the recognition of basic instability of self-image, that we paradoxically come to 'know' ourselves. But this is not 'mastery' (another exclusive, masculine term). 'Unknowing' accepts a basic uncertainty in character that has consequences for idealistic models of the education of professionalism in medicine and is reflected in the current shift in interest in medical ethics from an idealistic approach based on consistent application of universal principles, to a more realistic and pragmatic approach that takes account of context or situation. Sensitivity to contexts and their meanings then precedes introspection. Further, we should not strive for ideals, as lists of virtues to be 'achieved', but rather educate medical students to be flexible and tolerant of ambiguity and uncertainty, so that their moral medicine is based on appropriate response to a fluid context, rather than unbending application of principles. At the risk of introducing another oppositional category, this requires 'liquid' rather than 'crystallized' thinking.

'Liquid' Thinking and the Use of Metaphor

Luce Irigaray (1993) and Hélène Cixous (1991, 2004), in particular, suggest that feminism must claim its own language and not be drawn to work through the medium of a patriarchal language. Irigaray describes a fluid or liquid language that is highly metaphorical to capture ways of thinking and knowing marginalized by dominant patriarchal language. Medicine, like any complex praxis, is intimately bound with metaphor. Thinking in medicine works in two ways: literally, as social-realist narrative and figuratively or metaphorically, as expressive narrative. To employ a metaphor to make the point—while medicine treats the literal body, if it does not do this with 'heart', then it is a merely a technical or instrumental practice, showing perhaps a hardening of the heart and not advertising a sensitive practice also of relationship and support.

Sensibility, or deliberate use of the senses, is central to diagnosis and is enhanced by a vocabulary of metaphors. For example, pattern recognition in experts is grounded in an internalized vocabulary of resemblances, especially in the visual specialties of dermatology ('lichen planus'), radiology ('eggshell calcification'), and pathology ('strawberry gallbladder') (Bleakley, Farrow, Gould, & Marshall, 2003a, 2003b).

By turning the literal into an image, metaphors can help us to get closer to the experience of the patient. For example, Vincent Lam's (2006) vivid, contemporary account of the lives of doctors, *Bloodletting & Miraculous Cures,* describes his grandfather's developing tumour, where 'His left flank bulged as if a balloon was being inflated under the skin. ... I pressed the tumour gently with the tips of my fingers. It was firm, hard like cold plasticine'. Metaphors and analogies throughout— *'like* cold plasticine', *'as if* a balloon was being inflated'—employed in expert clinical judgment through pattern recognition. Lam (a male physician) further describes his grandfather's 'bloody pee' as having 'clots like coarse sand'. This close noticing and literal contact clearly illustrates Irigaray's call for tactility, to counter the objectifying and abstracting diagnostic gaze that is characteristically male and also serves to place the patient in a passive role.

We can argue that the metaphorical landscape of conservative, male-gendered medicine both reflects and constructs a heroic, controlling practitioner-centred practice that resists dialogical models of patient-centredness described earlier. This readily aligns with Susan Sontag's (1978) account of how, following the precursor of tuberculosis, contemporary descriptions of cancer and AIDS can move beyond the literal illness to offer accusatory metaphors. These metaphors bring about shame and guilt in those suffering from illness and may prevent them from seeking appropriate treatment. This resonates with cultures of shaming and scapegoating, rather than support and understanding. Medicine may not help patients to deal with illness where it typically employs martial metaphors to describe its work, such as 'fighting cancer'. The already exhausted patient may feel that he or she is not up for the 'fight' or does not characteristically frame illness through such metaphors of direct enemy engagement.

As medicine's literal gender balance changes, will medicine's metaphorical landscape also shift gender bias from its present dominant masculine form to a feminine form? Recall that in the UK an inclusive gender-neutral language ('Foundation Years') has already replaced the masculine, business-like language of 'housemen' and 'firms'.

Importantly, how will this come to affect patients? Perhaps a feminized narrative sensibility is more likely to read the patient as unpredictable person, rather than predictable machine and may, again, grasp the complexity of the patient through a fluid, dynamic sensibility rather than a formal mechanics. Liquid thinking is, as noted earlier, described by Cixous as *écriture feminine*—to metaphorically inscribe the world with 'mother's milk' as a form of expression. Just as milk is expressed from the breast, so Cixous argues, through a literary sensibility rather than a rational argument, that a female way of being can be expressed, where mother's milk acts as the ink that writes out a way of being. This is an elegant metaphor for inscribing the world with nourishing, unconditional care—neither a disguised form of control nor a demand for reciprocity, where the ink makes no mark—it is 'invisible' yet inscribes.

As Medicine Is Feminized, Will Medical Education Follow?

A paradox in the current culture of medical education is, crudely, that women may be better at the job, but are less likely to enter the field (Guelich, Singer, Castro, & Rosenberg, 2002). For example, women medical students tend to make more effective facilitators than their male counterparts (Kassab, Abu-Hijleh, Al-Shboul, & Hamdy, 2005), yet, proportionately, as noted earlier, less women than men go into medical education and academic medicine. Women medical students, in comparison with their male colleagues, tend to be less interested in areas such as research (Guelich et al., 2002). Where gender issues are introduced into the medicine undergraduate curriculum, it is women faculty who tend to initiate this move (Westerstahl et al., 2003). While medicine undergoes a gender-inflected transformation, will medical education also change?

I have argued that medical education could benefit from an influx of feminist ideas, such as 'liquid' thinking, tolerance of the 'abject', and challenges to oppositionalist thinking. This summarizes a sea change and needs to be carried out by influential women in medical education for credible change. There are two main issues at work in the relationship between gender and medical education. First, as indicated above, is the gender of educators themselves, where women doctors, even proportionately, have tended not to be drawn to medical education. This leads to their voices not being represented or being misrepresented. Second is the issue of the lack of discussion of gender within medical education from perspectives other than structural issues of equality and equity.

There is no established, interdisciplinary medical education culture that can draw with ease upon contemporary gender studies and feminist thinking. This may be a symptom of a wider malaise, where medical education traditionally refuses contemporary interdisciplinary theory (Bleakley & Bligh, 2009; Bleakley et al., 2011) and, paradoxically, the depth of theory available from within its parent discipline of education (Bleakley, 2006a, 2006b, 2006c).

Feminists who draw from poststructuralist thinking, interested in relationships between language, the body, identity, and activity, will then generally not be familiar to medical educators with a clinical background. Oriented to life sciences, clinicians are likely to read gender literally, as sex (biology), rather than as a historical, cultural, or linguistic issue. Social scientists who work in medical education, however, may typically read gender as a complex discourse challenging reduction to the biological (Hamberg, 2003; Norstedt & Davies, 2003). Feminists drawing on poststructuralism do not reject the importance of the body. Indeed, they begin with the body as the basic point of identity, but remind us that the body is not to be taken literally, but is inscribed culturally and linguistically. This also applies, importantly, to the suffering bodies of patients. The body must be understood metaphorically. This is fundamental to medicine, where even the contested distinction between the 'normal' and the 'pathological' is seen to be grounded in language use (Canguilhem, 1991).

With reference to a future woman-dominated general practice, Denekens (2002) asks three questions: (1) are women changing the face of care, (2) do women have different interaction styles, and (3) do women have an impact on the way medical practices (such as surgeries) are organized? I have focused on the first of these questions, drawing on poststructuralist feminism as an explanatory framework that is congruent with the research question. I have further signalled the dangers of essentialism in suggesting that male doctors and male medical educators can subscribe to feminist readings and practices. My main concern has been to note that a future world of medicine dominated by women will not be best informed by the conventions of a patriarchal educational framework, but by a medical education familiar with the fields of contemporary gender studies and critical feminisms.

Although women will predominate numerically, it is not clear whether a feminizing of medicine will constitute a significant culture change. The gender shift is also made more complex by a generation shift, where future male doctors may value more flexible lifestyles and working patterns that echo those of previous generations of women doctors (Sanfey et al., 2006; Washburn, 2000). The future of medicine's workforce is then centred not just on gender questions such as 'where have the men gone?', but also on whether gender may be transcended by generational lifestyle issues. Paradoxically, just as traditionally male-gendered specialties such as surgery have been attempting to attract more women surgery is now likely to suffer from a dwindling interest from a new generation of men whose lifestyle preferences will lead them to other specialties. Significant factors, such as dramatic changes in working patterns and salaries favouring general (family) practitioners in the UK, will undoubtedly affect specialty choices for a new generation of doctors.

The most important question is, whatever the gender-related outcomes, what quality of care are patients likely to receive? Pertinent to this question is the level of morale of the workforce as well as its level of expertise. Returning to the question of how patients may be affected by the current demographic shift, it is widely acknowledged that women predominating in medicine may produce positive patient-centred changes in health-care. We have seen that there is evidence that women treat patients with more overt compassion and intimacy than their male colleagues and are more concerned with the psychosocial and communicative sides of medicine (Boerma & van den Brink-Muinen, 2000; Boulis & Long, 2004; Buddeberg-Fischer et al., 2003), although it is strongly debated as to whether patients are, currently and generally, ultimately concerned about the gender of their doctor (Wolosin & Gesell, 2006). It may be that women are now perceiving medicine more favourably than men as a career choice on the basis that they see medicine's culture changing towards a more patient-centred, team-based, collaborative profession. It is this emergent pattern of clinical teamwork that is the focus of the following seven chapters.

Part II
Deep Theorizing in Communication in Medicine: Relationships Between Team Process and Practitioner Identity

Chapter 10
Working and Learning in 'Teams' in a New Era of Health-Care

From Jigsaws to Systems

In 1998, the Chief Medical Officer (CMO) in the UK announced in a speech that health-care had entered 'a new era of partnership where teamwork will be the route to success' (in Arthur, Wall, & Halligan, 2003, p.86). Later, a large, national UK study, The Effectiveness of Health-Care Teams in the National Health Service (Borrill et al., 2000), provided empirical evidence to back up the CMO's rhetoric, showing that where teamwork was of good quality, both effective delivery of health-care and high work satisfaction followed. The CMO's speech went on to suggest how better care might be achieved: 'we must specifically address the rough edges which stop organizations joining together to form genuine partnerships'. Both the focus and the metaphor are interesting. The focus is on cross-team and cross-organization, rather than intra-team, activity. The metaphor suggests that if we smooth out the edges, teams will join together seamlessly, like a jigsaw. This, unfortunately, configures health-care as a puzzle to be solved.

I have placed 'teams' in inverted commas because I see this as a problematic term—as this and subsequent chapters will explore. However, 'team' is a descriptor that is so embedded in health-care language that it is difficult to reinterpret or re-inscribe and harder to abandon. In the following chapter, I argue that 'team' is better thought of as process—as a verb rather than a noun. In this chapter, I warn against simplistic thinking that sees teams as jigsaws, with component parts that can be readily slotted together. 'Team' is a descriptor that lends itself to Jacques Derrida's (1967) process of putting something 'under erasure' (~~team~~) where the term is suspended. This of course does not mean that medical and health-care professionals do not engage in meaningful collaborative activities, it means rather that 'team' may not yet be the best adequate summative descriptor for such activities. Therefore, I do not abandon the term, but signal to the reader that it is inadequate to describe the complexity of such meaningful collaborative activities (as well as many meaningless non-collaborative exchanges). 'Team' will then remain a suspended term or one with a severe health warning.

A. Bleakley, *Patient-Centred Medicine in Transition: The Heart of the Matter*, 129
Advances in Medical Education 3, DOI 10.1007/978-3-319-02487-5_10,
© Springer International Publishing Switzerland 2014

In the period since the CMO's observations, the terrain of clinical teamwork has changed dramatically. For example, Iedema and Scheeres (2003, p.332) describe a 'new work order' in hospitals, where medical work has become 'more inter-dependent, more dynamic, and less certain' as practitioners 'renegotiate their knowing, their doing, and their worker identity'. Such a work order is more about adaptation to permanent revolution than attempting to stabilize the object, or smooth out the surfaces so that the parts of the jigsaw fit. Where health-care planning is determined by management policy that sees 'change' as a necessity rather than an option, the jigsaw metaphor is redundant, not only because health-care is not a puzzle to be solved, but because the jigsaw would never be completed. Importantly, how will practitioners bed in new practices if such practices are constantly changed, or reconfigured (Sennett, 2008)?

There is a rapidly changing landscape in contemporary community health practice, particularly reflecting the needs of patients with multiple chronic illnesses who require both inter-team and inter-agency attention and move frequently between community and hospital care. In 1 year, a person with multiple illnesses may need 20 or more visits to different providers, demanding high levels of collaboration between teams and agencies (Engeström, 2008; Kerosuo, 2007; Kerosuo & Engeström, 2003). Key difficulties prevent successful collaboration between health-care teams and agencies. For example, a standard instrument for management of care—the 'critical pathway'—is flawed, where the implementation of the pathway is based upon a single diagnosis, so that patients with multiple diagnoses are not readily accommodated by the protocol (Engeström, 2000). A key lesson from research studies is that a global, linear, and instrumental solution to cross-team collaboration is doomed to fail because it does not address the dynamic and complex nature of the local systems involved.

The changing terrain of health-care practice, characterized by clinical team practices based on patient pathways, offers a fundamental challenge to traditional hierarchical ways of working. Collaborative care systems do not fit together like a jigsaw, as hierarchical structures might. Rather, the care pathway system around any one patient, or patients grouped by illness category or needs, is an inherently unstable, dynamic set of activity systems. Some areas will achieve relative stability, held together by strong protocols and characterized by habitual patterns. These can be characterized as effective 'networks' or 'meshworks'.

However, habitual patterns may crystallize and the network may become outmoded, ready to crack or dissolve. Other areas will be highly labile or fluid, with fragile protocols, high levels of uncertainty and powerful emergent properties. These are not necessarily negatively decaying pockets of work activity, but often healthy examples of what Engeström and colleagues refer to as 'negotiated knotworking' (Engeström, 2004, 2008; Kerosuo & Engeström, 2003), where effective team process involves high levels of adaptation, tolerance of ambiguity, calculated risk, and collaborative creativity.

The complexity of cross-organizational team collaboration affords a resource and need not be configured as a problem to be solved. Kerosuo (2007, p.138) suggests that beyond the complexities inherent to a person's illness and that person's immediate clinical care is the organization of a health-care service that 'requires new organizational forms linking multiple providers'. However, 'many institutions, particularly those in health-care, are still trapped inside organizational models and practices that derive from conventional management thinking'. By 'conventional', Kerosuo means thinking that attempts to optimize production by rationally and instrumentally atomizing work—breaking activity down into particulars. In contrast, the new era of complex, collaborative work activity requires whole systems thinking, explored later in Chap. 15, such as a shift from multiprofessional to interprofessional activity (Barr, 2007).

This broadly aligns with Giddings and Williamson's (2007, p.10) distinction between 'groups' and 'teams' in surgical education, where 'group working involves individuals coming together to perform a task or achieve a target', whereas teamwork 'involves a broader vision' that includes collaborative activity and full appreciation and understanding of each other's roles.

This distinction between groups and teams may conceal more than it reveals. Below are two short accounts of work from the operating theatre. In the first example, surgical practitioners looking inward act together as a 'team', but when facing outward seem to act as a 'group', failing to communicate with an adjacent team— the unit that sterilises and packs surgical instruments. Also, groups may graduate to teams that are constituted in a negative sense, in adversity, working against the grain and against each other—heroically surviving work rather than gaining fulfilment, putting patients at risk in the process.

In a close call (near miss) incident report taken from a longitudinal study of teamwork in operating theatres (Bleakley, Boyden, Hobbs, Walsh, & Allard, 2006), a scrub nurse describes a day from an orthopaedic operating theatre team involving a busy and complicated list with first choice equipment unavailable: 'the surgeon had to improvise at times with what equipment was available. The whole day caused major stress to staff … not to mention the patient. No one thought that quality care had taken place'.

While the team was resourceful, the scrub nurse summed up the day's work as 'skating by the seat of our pants'. This team had worked together many times before. However, had they become habitual and inward-looking, to some extent crystallized as far as inter-team collaboration is concerned, sacrificing adaptability for stability? Perhaps better communication with the surgical sterilization department may have relieved the increasing tension they carried through the working day, as they turned inward to their own, limited, resources, paradoxically stretching their primary resource of stability.

From the same study, but with a different surgical team, a scrub nurse reports that:

> power kept tripping out in the Surgical Sterilisation Department (SSD) negating the sterility of sets needed for a major case. Due to excellent communication between SSD and operating theatres, the whole team had time to review existing disposable instruments and plan in a controlled discussion whether the case should go ahead or be cancelled. This team included theatre manager, surgeon, scrub team and circulating nurse. The whole procedure was discussed and where an instrument of choice was missing, the whole team could contribute to thinking of alternatives. Because of good communication, stress levels remained low.

Unlike the first team, while again working under difficult, unpredictable conditions, inter-team collaboration (between theatre and SSD) was established, resulting in 'whole team' work. This alleviated stress and potential harm to patients. This team was temporary, constituted on an ad hoc basis from a pool of individual, expert practitioners, where the surgeon may meet a new group on the next list. What this team did, however, was to brief, indeed to establish a running brief (briefing not just at the beginning of the list but also between patients), establishing understanding of each other's roles, and establishing a common mental map of the day's list, or situation awareness (Bleakley, Allard, & Hobbs, 2013).

What Is a 'Team'?

Before we can address issues about both intra- and inter-team dynamics raised above, there is conceptual work to be done. For example, in spite of a large standing literature on group dynamics in health-care, medical education is only now seriously asking 'what do we mean by a team?' Bleakley (2006c) points out that heroic individualism is a given in medical culture, where collectivity is a condition to be achieved. Further, medical culture and medical education are notoriously pragmatic and atheoretical, so that interest in teamwork tends to follow a reductive, instrumental approach.

In a key text on teamwork in multiprofessional care, Payne (2000) quotes 15 definitions of 'team' from the relevant literature, ranging from 1975 to 1997. As early as 1975, in the context of social work, Kane (1975, p.5) was already talking about 'interprofessional' teams, succinctly defining a team as: having 'a common objective, differential professional contributions, and a system of communication'. The common factor across the definitions gathered by Payne is that teams are characterized by what may be termed a will-to-stability. There is no reference to teams as complex systems viewing inherent instability as a resource, where emergent properties may move the team to new levels of activity, particularly in the context of inter-team collaborations.

Payne (2000) does address cross-team collaboration in developing a model of 'open' teamwork, where several teams work in a coordinated fashion around a service user's needs. However, this model, based on conventional networking theory, privileges stability of teams over adaptability.

In contrast to the will-to-stability, Bauman (2000, 2007, p.1) describes the contemporary post-industrial social condition as 'liquid life', defined as a 'society in which the conditions under which its members act change faster than it takes the ways of acting to consolidate into habits and routines'. This mirrors Anthony Giddens' (2002) description of the 'runaway world', impossible to nail down. The new era of clinical teamwork can be seen as a prime example of liquid life in a runaway world, where teams are increasingly constituted on an ad hoc basis and cross-team activities become more complex and accrue fragile protocols. Here, a will-to-adaptability is required. Contemporary clinical teamwork inhabits a place between established 'habits and routines' and improvisation under conditions of uncertainty or ambiguity. The danger in such a model is that new knowledge and skills may not be given enough time to bed in.

Paradoxically, in many medical teams, technical work is becoming safer and routine, where inadvertently putting patients at risk now rests largely with non-technical, systems-based, team communication practices (Vincent, 2005), as I have evidenced earlier. This parallels a shift in emphasis in work practices from doing work to talking work (Iedema & Scheeres, 2003; Iedema, 2007), where an opportunity for negotiation of roles and rules is possible and this has a knock-on effect on construction of identity.

Traditionalists may characterize such a negotiating possibility as an aspect of a new climate of political correctness. However, this misses the point that Iedema and Scheeres make—that new forms of work arise because they are characterized as much by talk as by action. In routine teamwork, things simply get done without the need for verbal exchange. In more complex work, the need for communication exchange arises and this invites verbal negotiation.

This shift is an effect of power—the transition from sovereign power (power over, power as reproductive of social structures) to capillary power (power runs through the system and can be mobilized as forms of resistance, power as productive of new social structures). This shift is a natural consequence of the breakdown of hierarchy for more democratic, collaborative and participatory forms of teamwork. It may be thought of as a revolution of the 'multitude' against the old 'sovereignty' of imperialist conquering and autocratic rule by the consultant culture, to draw on the capital of 'common wealth' in the affective domain of work (Hardt & Negri, 2009). This operates in concert with the drift of clinical teams away from the notion that the surgeon 'leads' the team towards the notion that the needs of the patient 'lead' the team and leadership is distributed according to context.

In capillary power, cognitive (thinking), psychomotor (doing), and affective (feeling and valuing) labor are interlinked and mobilized in the construction of identities. An example of this, discussed in Chap. 12, is how 'moral courage', or 'speaking up'/'speaking out', can be exercised in a clinical team by a member traditionally lower on the hierarchy to legitimately challenge the sovereign power of a member of the team higher on the hierarchy. In this challenge, productive work is done, through talk, in transforming identity.

The other side of this coin is that talk can be used unproductively, to maintain a hierarchy. For example, Bleakley, Allard, and Hobbs (2013), in a local study of the communication patterns of orthopaedic surgeons, show that such communication patterns are characteristically monological (statements and closed questions) rather than dialogical (stimulating exchange). This can be seen as a rhetorical strategy aimed at stemming the possibility of being challenged—that can arise if dialogue is initiated—and of confirming identity as autocratic figurehead. Surgeons may make statements rather than ask questions as a defensive strategy to maintain the status quo, where inviting somebody else into the conversation risks opening a debate, or hints at democracy. The colonized (the rest of the team) must remain silent.

In capillary power terms, this means that resistance is generated unwittingly as power flows through the system of the team, or democratic patterns are established. Such resistance is typically expressed in three ways: as moral courage in speaking out; as delayed and indirect hostility expressed through a secondary medium such as close call (near miss) incident reporting; and as a variety of subtle, indirect tactics of resistance such as 'sly civility' (discussed in the following chapter).

Traditional hierarchies in medicine are grounded in profession-specific knowledge and skills, so that emphasis upon the value of shared communication practices demands renegotiation of identities. Shared communication increasingly involves distributed decision-making, including ethical decisions, where a negotiated and situated ethics of practice, sensitive to emergent context, replaces a traditional principles-based or authority-led decision-making climate (Bleakley, 2006b). Potential communication and ethical practice problems are increased through multiple team involvement. Close call incident reports reveal that communication issues potentially putting patients at risk are three times more likely to be grounded in inter-team issues than intra-team issues (Bleakley 2011a). Such inter-team issues, for the operating theatre, are dominated by ward-to-theatre communications (or, rather, miscommunications).

To better understand teams, we could draw on older, established models of group life from social psychology and sociology, including theories of conformity, risky shift, leadership roles, and group development (Brill, 1976). Central to this body of theory is developmental thinking describing stages of group life: how a group matures through invariant phases such as 'forming', 'storming', 'norming', 'performing', and 'mourning'. Here, ideal group development starts with a tentative getting to know each other, passes through a stage of sorting out differences, and matures as maximum 'adult' performance in first establishing norms and then performing beyond such norms in innovative practices. In some cases, the group life expires and is mourned. Such models, besides suffering from developmentalism (the fantasy that history equates to progress) and idealism (a model of the perfect team performance), are not meaningful when applied to expert clinical teams that are established on an ad hoc basis, as if already developmentally mature. The expectation for such groups is that they will automatically be at the 'performing' stage—now not 'teams', but aggregates of expert 'team players', where stability is wrongly assumed.

Further, as we have already seen, theoretical models should allow us to explore cross-interprofessional activity—learning with, from, and about other health-care teams and their cultures within complex, multiple team and inter-agency care. This challenge of authentic cross-team collaboration has been characterized, within a cultural-historical activity theory approach, as one of 'boundary crossing', where several activity systems meaningfully interact (Engeström, 2000; Kerosuo & Engeström, 2003). Boundary crossing is facilitated particularly by 'negotiated knotworking', described in detail below.

For Iedema and Scheeres (2003, p.317), the new complex work order demands that professionals 'engage in discourse about their work, with others with whom they would not normally negotiate the details of their work'. This means crossing previously strongly held 'hierarchical, occupational, professional, or organizational boundaries'. Negotiated knotworking is an activity-led response to these challenges (Varpio, Hall, Lingard, & Schryer, 2008).

'Nets' and 'Knots' in Team-Based Learning

How has the research community risen to the challenge of theorizing clinical inter-team collaboration? There is a significant gap between traditional social-psychological models of groups applied to contemporary clinical teams and current interdisciplinary research drawing on more complex models such as cultural-historical activity theory (Engeström, 1987; Bleakley 2006c). The former focuses largely on discrete teams, tending in the psychological literature to gravitate back to the experience of the individual team member through an emphasis upon personality styles, roles, and leadership. This atomizes teams. Where such literature describes inter-team, rather than intra-team, activity, it tends to draw on conservative network theory, rather than the more innovative activity theory (Payne, 2000). Activity theory has influenced and updated network theory, largely through alignment with actor-network-theory (Miettinen, 1999; Bleakley 2011a) (discussed at length in Chap. 13). Here, we focus upon the tensions between traditional network theory (derived from Gestalt psychology and borrowing basic concepts from mathematics and topography) and activity theory.

Traditional literature on teams in health-care also privileges tropes—metaphors and images—of place and space, so that groups, teams, and networks are described using terms such as 'points' and 'lines' drawn from the mathematics of networking and 'field', 'boundary', and 'bridge' drawn from graph theory and popularized in social psychology (e.g. Moreno's sociometry with its network 'sociograms' and field theory in Gestalt psychology) (Payne, 2000). These metaphors collectively describe a 'network' and act rhetorically to persuade us into the importance of 'settlement', or stability through reduction of complexity, working against uncertainty. In contrast to conservative or traditional network theory, activity theory privileges metaphors of time over space and place, describing teams as dynamic systems that are inherently unstable and complex and constantly working with horizons of possibility and temporary stabilities. Complex, adaptive systems typically show emergent properties—factors that cannot be predicted and which require improvisational response (see Chap. 15 and Bleakley, 2010). Working with a greater or lesser degree of uncertainty is a characteristic of contemporary 'liquid life' teamwork and inter-team collaboration.

The primary unit of analysis in the work of Engeström and colleagues in Helsinki has been cross-organizational, rather than the discrete team (Engeström, Engeström, & Vähääho, 1999; Kangasoja, 2002). This research group has progressed Victor and Boynton's notion of 'co-configuration' (Engeström, 2004, 2008) to describe a form of work organization that they term 'negotiated knotworking', defined as 'rapidly pulsating, distributed, and partially improvised orchestration of collaborative performance between otherwise loosely connected actors and activity systems' (Engeström, 2000, p.972). It is a valuable descriptor partly because of its pun (in English) on addressing what is 'not working'. Potentially, knotworking can be hit-and-miss, fragile, clumsy, and subject to quick decay, as well as beautifully improvised, timed well, and creatively developed. In the context of this chapter, which discusses intentional rather than serendipitous, or accidental, collaboration between practitioners, the term 'negotiated' in 'negotiated knotworking' is considered superfluous, as 'knotworking' in its own right refers to intentionally democratic or collaborative practices.

In production of goods and services, co-configuration refers to how interaction with consumers comes to shape or tailor provision. Producers do not dictate to consumers or shape their choices, but rather gather intelligence from consumers on how to provide services and what resources (goods) are required. An example of co-configuration is authentic patient-centred health-care, defined and discussed in previous chapters. Engeström and colleagues' work considers how the principle of co-configuration may be realized in the new era of complex inter-agency health-care. This work recognizes that complex care provision may be mapped as a rational exercise but actually entails a good deal of improvisation under conditions of uncertainty and is then better treated as a dynamic system inviting knotworking.

Knotworking is grounded in recognition of complexity and uncertainty: teams that knotwork effectively produce new knowledge and innovative practice strategies because they tolerate high levels of ambiguity and work at maximum complexity without falling into chaos. Knotworking advertises the need for this new mindset in its description of the absence of a 'centre' to the 'knot' of activity (Engeström, Engeström, & Vähääho, 1999). Where several, apparently separate, threads of activity between teams need to be tied, untied, or re-tied to achieve better patient care, this is not reducible to an agent or an organization as a point of control—hence the challenge to traditional—hierarchical and personality-bound—models of 'leadership'. Again, we can have patient-centred care without a centre.

Knotworking can be seen as an emergent property of the system of several clinical and care teams working around a patient, mediated by a complex of artifacts, such as a patient's medications, records, and charts. Knotworking resists reductive analysis—where it is more than the sum of its parts—and resists universal definition, where, as an emergent property, it is subject to local context. Knotworking is created across and between a range of activities, including conversation and related artifacts that Engeström (2000) describes as a 'strategic alliance'.

Knotworking offers an important refinement of co-configuration. It is a 'muscular' term, conjuring up strong literal images of activity. Along with other neologisms of the Engeström research group such as 'teeming' (the dynamic act of teamwork) and 'cognitive trailblazing' (radicalizing thinking in practice)—a progression of Cussins' (1992) notion of 'cognitive trails'—knotworking awaits future critical review and further pragmatic application. It is still a 'raw' idea.

Knotworking can be progressed as follows:

1. Through collapsing distinctions between knotworking as an idea, concept, theory, or model, and knotworking as a practice, where knotworking can be seen as an activity offering theory in practice.
2. Through comparing and contrasting knotworking and networking (the focus of the following chapter).
3. Through applying knotworking to discrete, intra-team activity, as well as cross-team collaboration (a factor increasingly recognized in the work of Engeström and colleagues that has previously focused on larger cross-organizational communication) (Engeström, 1999).
4. Through empirical work cataloguing kinds of 'knots' appropriate for context—this can draw on analogies with literal catalogues of knots from boating (the classic work being Ashley's Book of Knots).
5. Through drawing on related work—for example, 'knots' is used as a metaphor to describe the workings of the individual psyche in Jacques Lacan's (1998) later topographical work (Miller, 2005) and to poetically describe dysfunctional family (and then team intimacy) relationships in Ronald Laing's (1972) work *Knots*.
6. Through reconsidering visual representations of how activity systems work. Current models (triangles with double-headed arrows to indicate interconnections and zigzags to indicate perturbations and disruptions) offer an internal contradiction. Such graphics tend to atomize the whole system (reducing the system to the sum of its parts) and fail to capture the dynamism of the system. This graphic failure becomes more acute where systems are shown interacting with one another, again privileging space over time. While such graphic representations may be seen as conveniences and then may be forgiven their flaws, they do not follow the spirit of Vygotsky's imperative—that the artifact mediates learning. Given the power of new technologies to represent in time as well as in space, there is work to be done in authentic graphical representation of the interaction of several activity systems.

A further rich area for theory and research is the alignment of cultural–historical activity theory with contemporary actor-network-theory, the latter discussed at length in Chap. 13. This has been pursued in particular by Reijo Miettinen (1999) at the University of Helsinki and Lara Varpio (personal communication 2007, Varpio et al., 2008) at the University of Ottawa and by Alan Bleakley (2011a).

Engeström (1999) describes three generations of activity theory. First, Vygotsky's original work pointed out how learning is mediated by both artifacts (tools, instruments, languages and now, particularly, computers) and culture and is then paradigmatically human and social, rather than animal and individual. Vygotsky's work, however, focused on child development. A second generation, from the 1970s, applied activity theory to other contexts, primarily how people learn in work-based settings in differing cultural contexts. The new, third generation, focuses on how activity systems interact with one another in what are variously termed networks, meshworks, flows, aggregates, plateaux, and assemblages.

Both activity theory and actor-network-theory describe how learning and work practices, mediated by artifacts, languages, and symbols, are becoming increasingly complex and expand as new forms of collaborative practices emerge between teams, organizations, and institutions. This work can now be progressed to include empirical studies of knotworking and more sophisticated modelling of the dynamics and complexity of knotworking.

In the next section, reviewing networking, it will become clear that traditional networking theory and contemporary knotworking describe two qualitatively different ways in which people and teams may interact. Further, networking and knotworking are grounded in different epistemological frames. This is not only in terms of tensions between spatial and temporal and analytic and synthetic approaches, as described above, but also reflects distinctions between metonymy and metaphor, described later. Knotworking is a more appropriate description of the day-to-day complexities and uncertainties of teamwork as it aims to become explicitly interprofessional and collaborative and is interested in the local context and proximal issues that Engeström (1999) describes as 'radical localism'. Networking is about the horizon of organizational work and is interested in general principles and distal issues.

The proximal focus of knotworking is captured most powerfully in improvised communication activities that can be described as tying, untying, and re-tying, which can also be configured as deliberate learning and 'unlearning' (Rushmer & Davies, 2004). Unlearning can be described both as undoing 'overlearning' (habit), but also as inoculation against unproductive habitual practice, offering a resistance. Positive networking seeks to consolidate 'habitus' (Bourdieu & Passeron, 1977), as the collective honing of necessary practices, where knotworking seeks improvisation and renewal. Finally, Engeström (2000) suggests that knotworking is related to the ebb and flow of temporary groups. In the following chapter, I expand these ideas through knotworking and networking primers.

Chapter 11
Theorizing Team Process Through Cultural–Historical Activity Theory (CHAT): Networking and Knotworking

A Networking Primer

As described in the previous chapter, classical networking theory draws on metaphors of space and place. Knotworking typically places activity in time. Networks describe topographies, fields, locations, and distances between points. Distances between points are given 'weighting', where, for example, medicine and health-care 'actors' in a network of roles show relative distance from a patient and from each other and show relative density of weighting in terms of the strength of connection to other actors in a network field. If actors in a field of activity are closely aligned, this is termed a 'bridge' and is graphically displayed as a heavy print, double-headed arrow. Paradoxically, the graphic tropes that activity theory uses such as varieties of arrows (double-headed, light or heavy type, lightning bolt as disjunction) are also stock vocabulary for network theory. This is typified in sociograms, where social distance and power of relationship are reduced to shorter or longer, heavier or lighter, and double-headed (reciprocal communication) or single-headed (unreciprocated communication) arrows.

Payne (2000) suggests that there are three key paradoxes facing teamwork in traditional multiprofessional care: First, the historical concerns with 'group' and 'group dynamics' that force teams inward, avoiding issues of inter-team and organizational dynamics. Second, what management wants from teams may not conform to the desires of professionals who work in those teams. Third, teams may exclude patients or service users from their activities, yet the purpose of clinical teams is to provide care for those patients or users. Payne suggests moving from thinking 'teamwork' to thinking 'open teamwork', where traditional social psychology team thinking is combined with networking, providing an outward looking team ready to work closely with service users, while sorting through its own dynamics and goals in relationship to management's strategic concerns.

In traditional network theory, there is an assumption that networks will conform to certain implicit rules or rule structures. As suggested above, a network is a set of lines and points plotted out to reduce complexity. Networking thus has sympathy with structuralism, which seeks fundamental structures, guiding rules, or generative simple categories behind complex phenomena. For example, Lévi-Strauss contends that myth generation follows a small number of universal patterns based on binary oppositions such as the 'raw' and the 'cooked'. Chomsky contends that language generation (grammar) follows a small number of generative, inherited rules. Piaget and Kohlberg contend that development of cognition and moral reasoning follow invariant, rule-bound stages.

Networks are thus surface imitations of inherited and invariant 'deep structures', seeking to embed or acquire permanence. In contrast, knotworking follows the post-structuralist critique of structuralism—that the world is not an effect of oppositional thinking and that there is no universal 'deep structure'. Rather, multiple and competing discourses are historically and culturally determined and show local variety or differ-ence, even at the level of multiple ontologies for everyday material phenomena (Mol 2002). For example, a material object of concern for health-care such as 'blood' will be appreciated differently by differing practitioners and by patients—where the cardiologist sees an arterial system as pipework, blood is conceived as the fluid flowing through those pipes under differing conditions of pressure and density or fluidity (blood is an object of fluid dynamics), whereas the nurse sees blood as something to be contained through pressure and clotting and the laboratory technician sees blood as a configuration of cells under the microscope with normal and abnormal presentations.

Knotworking does not seek to stabilize in terms of a 'best' way of working, a universal solution, or a distant 'cool' consideration. Rather, knotworking seeks 'hot', local, and contextualized ways of doing things that may not be transferable or universal. Knotworking is infinitely adaptable as it seeks to do, undo, and redo according to context, serendipity, and moment. Knotworking is especially sensitive to complexity and dynamic, working in time with unpredictable contexts. In this sense, knotworking is inherently risky.

A Knotworking Primer

Knotworking describes expert work taking place in rapidly shifting contexts, where a number of 'loose ends' of activity are constantly being tied together or untied, to create the conditions for collaborative production of knowledge or new work prac-tices. In two earlier illustrative examples, we saw how one surgical team knotworked internally, to improvise where the correct equipment was not available, but at the expense of knotworking effectively with the surgical sterilization unit. Here, although the team was able to continue working, both patient safety and team morale were compromised. In a similar, unpredictable context, the second illustra-tion showed knotworking across teams (boundary crossing between the surgical team and sterilization unit) where improvised communication led to an effective climate for patient safety.

Knotworking is frustrated where teams pursue habitual, rhetorical patterns of practice in which boundary crossing is weak and patient information is sequestered (and then duplicated). Adhesion may be profession-based (e.g. surgery, anaesthetics, nursing) or team-based (e.g. ward team, surgical team, physiotherapy team), either way spelling out multiprofessional rather than interprofessional activity, where teams do not internally reconfigure activities or externally co-configure new ways of working together.

Where activities are reconfigured as both inter-team and interprofessional, teams of professionals and experts learn with, from, and about each other to become expert teams with a common object—the shared patient. This has four main components in clinical teamwork:

- Information reproduction (shared across teams)
- Unlearning (undoing habitual practices that no longer serve the needs of collaborative care)
- Knowledge capital (collaborative creation of new knowledge)
- Social capital (collaborative creation of new work practices and related identities, changing climates, and even cultures of work and patterns of relationship)

'Capital' is used here to describe team-based common ownership of the means of production of knowledge and work practices.

Where information reproduction is high, but unlearning and collaborative creation of knowledge and social capital are low, reconfiguration of work will be limited—with focus on stabilization and habitus—and we can characterize this as a networking opportunity. Where information reproduction is low, but unlearning and collaborative creation of knowledge and social capital are high, reconfiguration is replaced by co-configuration, and this characterizes knotworking. Importantly, knotworking is used to describe concentrated, task-based collaborative activity between people or groups who may not have worked with each other before and need to quickly establish ways of working. Working at high tempo and often with risk, creation of new patterns of work is common. New practices emerge and knowledge is produced rather than reproduced.

Nets, of course, are made using knots, but these are explicitly tied to be permanent. A net is then a stabilized system of knots focusing on the distal—the long view. Knots that can be tied and untied offer a further dimension beyond a stable net—that of dynamic complexity. Knots have powerful symbolic presence. As Gschwandtner (2006, p.40) suggests, 'string ... has delivered language' and has been used to 'embody ideas'. She is referring particularly to the Inca use of quipus, 'bundles of twisted and knotted colored threads each feature of which—length, color of string, number of knots, and type of knots, for example—is thought to convey information'. Importantly, quipus were used for temporary information and communication, where unknotting was as important as knotting.

In the literal world of knots (3,700 are described in the encyclopaedic sourcebook The Ashley Book of Knots), they take on more than their function of tying one thing to another. In the various modes of tying—for example, a slipknot as compared with a hitch knot—there is a narrative that helps us to progress Engeström's notion of 'knotworking'. Knotworking cannot be used as a blanket term. We must discriminate between kinds and functions of knotworking. Empirical work such as observation and video recording of clinical teams at work would readily produce a typology of knotworking. What kinds of encounters produce what kinds of tying and untying of threads? What purposes do particular 'knots' serve? This would translate 'knotworking' from an abstract to a concrete heuristic and provide models of collaborative practice. Is knotworking merely descriptive or does it have explanatory power? Is it a heuristic or rule of thumb? Or is it used metaphorically? Can knotworking be taken literally?

Two Ways of Coming Together: Metaphor and Metonymy

As two differing approaches to work activity, networking and knotworking are grounded in different epistemological frames. In rhetoric, a crucial distinction is made between metonymy and metaphor. Metonymy describes contiguity or association, where one entity stands for another (ruler—king—crown). Metaphor describes similarity and transfer, where one entity is viewed as another ('crown of creation'). For Roman Jakobson (1992) metonymy and metaphor describe different and pervasive form of organizing language. While serving different purposes, they are not to be placed in opposition. Metonymy describes the typical structure of prose—sentences in contiguity or narrative, often instrumental or descriptive—where metaphor describes the typical structure of poetry, where transfer of meaning in word and phrase is paramount.

In terms of how threads of work practices or activities meet and come together or come apart, metonymy and metaphor offer quite different approaches that can be seen, respectively, as networking and knotworking. The difference is evident in the conventional images of nets and knots. Where nets are made to last from particular kinds of knots, other kinds of knots are temporary, made to hold but also to easily untie and retie. Traditional network theory describes the stabilization of a previously unstable system. Cultural–historical activity theory describes the inherent instability of work activities as dynamic systems. Where a net works because it is inherently stable, a knot works because it is inherently flexible and where a network is an object, knotworking is a process.

Metonymy is the organizing principle of networks (which is why nets work), where metaphor is the organizing/disorganizing principle of knotworking. Knots then serve different purposes as components of nets in striving for permanence. A key difference between networking and knotworking, where 'threads' come together in different ways, is that networking strives for 'settlement' and follows the paradigm of the tree, where knotworking strives for 'nomadism' and follows the paradigm of the rhizome (Deleuze & Guattari, 2004a, 2004b), or mycorrhizal structure (Engeström, 2008).

Three illustrative examples may help to clarify the distinction pursued here. Cultural–historical activity theory is fond of neologisms, especially describing objects as verbs, thus translating potentially static identity into dynamic activity. An example is Yrjo Engeström's notion of 'teeming' to describe the activity of teamworking. 'Teeming' best captures the dynamic and unstable element of team life as a metaphor, offering a perspectival shift through transferring a source domain to a target domain. Teeming widens our horizons of meaning to make us think of teamwork as a running river, a herd of animals, and an army of ants. The more familiar 'teamworking' is metonymic or employs contiguity. Where policy documents exhort us to establish 'teamworking' in clinical teams, are they implicitly inviting a move to stability or establishment of the 'network'? Is this an invitation to 'habitus' or familiar patterns? Imagine a policy document supporting 'teeming'!

A second example involves Adrian Cussins' (1992) notion of a 'cognitive trail' that suggests an unconscious or tacit dimension to work practices. A cognitive trail is the tacit thinking dimension to repeated activity. As an activity is worked over and over and becomes practiced (expertise), what came to inform the novice now becomes tacit as a 'cognitive script' or an informing metaphor (Eva, 2005). For example, the doctor, as expert, makes a diagnosis based on pattern recognition, no longer needing to draw explicitly on the informing biomedical science. This is now an established network. An equivalent cultural phenomenon is the Australian aboriginal 'songline' (Chatwin, 2005). Different cognitive trails intersect—for example, the surgeon has an 'anatomy knowledge' trail, a 'physiology knowledge' trail, and an 'eye–hand coordination' skill trail, all working together throughout a familiar procedure. Where these cognitive trails intersect is a permanent marker—a node, or a secure knot. This is the pattern recognition 'button', organized as a visual or linguistic shortcut.

Now imagine that the whole procedure shifts to mediation through new technology, such as keyhole surgery using transmitted televisual images. A whole new network has to be established for stability. Old intersecting nets of cognitive trails are abandoned, undone, and erased—to be replaced by new nets. This is 'trailblazing' in one sense—that of establishing new habits of practice (and the habitus of new communities of practices). In a period of new learning and more importantly, unlearning of the old, a surgeon lays down new cognitive trails, now knotworking for a period, before new networks are established.

A third example addresses knotworking as a co-configuration of activities where the centre does not hold. The meeting of threads as a knot—tying, untying, and retying—describes movement between intentional learning and unlearning. But there is no identifiable agent or object that 'makes' or 'holds' the knot. Rather, the 'knot' is the metaphor for the coming together or collaborative process through which work activities are reconfigured, raised to new levels, allowed to transform, and so forth. We can reconfigure the 'knot' itself, not as a literal tie but as a metaphorical 'attraction'. Central, knotty metaphors characterize periods of work activity. Recall the scrub nurse who described the working day as 'on the edge' and 'skating by the seat of our pants', where the surgeon improvised with available equipment. Other days 'run smoothly'. Active, dynamic topographical and tactile metaphors are commonly employed to describe such work. This returns to the starting point of the previous chapter—the jigsaw requiring smoothing out of the edges for a better fit as a (problematic) metaphor for co-configuration. While an appropriate description of networking, the metaphor is wholly inappropriate for knotworking.

In its infancy as a concept, knotworking is open to progression and refinement. For example, knotworking is seductive and may promise more than it delivers conceptually and practically. Where knotworking conjures strong visual images, the notion is poorly modelled visually through traditional activity system graphics and such graphics need to be revised to better capture the temporal bias in knotworking. However, knotworking is a radically important idea for exploring the new era of complex teamwork in health-care, where traditional networking has limited explanatory power to address these new unstable contexts.

Decolonizing Teamwork to Open Up New Horizons

In Chap. 17, I discuss the tension between medical education academics who research clinicians and the clinical community itself that is the object of research—and how this tension may be resolved. Mathieu Albert (2004) describes the tension between 'production for producers' (academic researchers) and 'production for non-producers' (non-academic practitioners) in medical education research, while Albert, Hodges, and Regehr (2007) describe the difficulties in balancing service and science in such research.

There is another way of reading this tension, within a model of postcolonial studies. Academic communities may attempt to colonize clinical communities with their disciplinary ideas (and ideals), sometimes in a heavy-handed manner. Most famously, critical and often confrontational, medical sociology has been characterized as 'doctor bashing' by members of the medical community, where, for example, it critiques paternalism (Friedson, 1970) or engages in emancipatory work on behalf of patient autonomy (Coulter, 2002). Similarly, medical communities may be seen as attempting to colonize academic communities by exerting the traditional authority they enjoy in clinical culture as they transfer interest to academic settings. Just as the world has moved beyond colonialism into an era of globalization and post-colonialism (Hobsbawm, 2008), so medical education can constitute its own mixed research teams based on the hybridities that characterize the global moment.

The world of medicine can be seen to be still in a colonialist phase with the postcolonial imminent. As medicine changes historically, for example, reconsidering its traditional professional autonomy and paternalism after the Bristol, Alder Hey, and Shipman scandals in the UK, so it will enter a phase equivalent to globalization, where hybridities emerge as standard. The key hybridity in this chapter is the doctor taking on an identity of the 'interprofessional', where he or she engages in genuine collaboration and dialogue to work with other professionals and to learn with, from, and about them. This is the basis to shifting teamwork from multiprofessionalism to interprofessionalism and depends upon collapse of traditional hierarchies to allow emergence of new working practices.

Hardt and Negri (2001, 2006, 2009) suggest that the transition from the imperialist (colonialism) era to the post-colonial (that they call 'Empire', referring to globalization as a new form of imperialism) is a phase in progress towards 'multitude' or a global democracy, characterized by the realization of 'commonwealth' or potential as shared capital. This overview may help us to understand difficulties in transitions in clinical teamwork. We would predict from Hardt and Negri's model that the initial phase of transition from traditional hierarchical structures to more fluid and collaborative structures would be difficult. Indeed, the post-colonial stage of Empire or globalization is characterized by conflict, as differences (between identity-led groups) remain unresolved. We have local ethnic conflict in the wake of withdrawal of the colonizers and larger conflicts of interest in the global setting. Here, 'difference' is a source of disquiet, not of celebration. The parallels with 'silos' in clinical teams can readily be drawn.

Hobsbawm (2008: 18) reminds us that 5 % of all casualties in WWI were civilians. This rises to 66 % in WWII and, by 2000, a staggering 80–90 % across wars globally. In other words, wars are fought at the expense of the peaceful 'multitude'. The analogy with clinical teamwork is clear. The 'turf wars' of professional discipline interests lead to an inability to form cohesive, collaborative teams. Poor teamwork is a systemic issue in health-care, and as previously noted, systems mistakes lead to an estimated 70 % of medical error (Xyrichis & Ream, 2008). While team members fight their wars of 'difference', patients are the main casualties, as their safety is compromised.

In the multitude or democratic future and commonwealth, difference will be a cause for celebration and 'boundary crossing' will be a 'core competency'. This shift from multiprofessional to interprofessionalism (and from pluridisciplinarity to interdisciplinarity and transdisciplinarity) will offer new identities. This can be described as 'epistemological alignment' (agreement on why we are doing team work) and 'ontological alignment' (agreement on who we are as team members), underpinned by 'axiological alignment' (agreement on informing and shared values).

Rachael Finn (Finn & Waring, 2006; Finn, 2008) suggests that there is disjunction between writing and talking about teams (as in research) and doing teamwork. She describes the first as the discourse of 'teamwork' (this also includes policy statements such as the one that opened this chapter) and 'team work' as a practice. She distinguishes between the two by eliding team and work to describe the discourse of 'teamwork' and separating them to describe on the ground practices of 'team work'. This is an interesting distinction, but becomes untenable as we see the evolutionary development of clinical team practices from imperialist and colonizing practices to hybridities in the post-colonial phase, to democratic practices in the phase of 'multitude' and realization of a commonwealth. We are confident about such evolution, because, without it, teamwork practices would become extinct as they failed to adapt. The future of teamwork is full collaboration and mutuality. There is an emerging evidence base for this claim. The patient's needs, as the heart of the matter, will shape such collaborative endeavour in teamwork.

Where the clinical community, as an activity system, has patient care and safety as its objects (and outcome), researchers might focus more on work that leads to benefit for patients. This would provide a common outcome, facilitating collaboration and dialogue. I (Bleakley, 2011b) have developed a research interest looking at the relationship between team practices and practitioner identities, in which practitioners learn to research their own practices in collaboration with academics, as an educational process. In this research program, the tensions between academic researchers and clinicians are resolved through identification with a common goal of patient safety and a common philosophy of lifelong learning. This can act as a mode for boundary crossing within clinical teams, who learn to work collaboratively and research their efforts as both team-based appraisals and audits, for patient benefit.

The future literacy of teamwork will probably be based on models such as networking and knotworking, introduced above, within a wider perspective of complex, non-linear, adaptive systems theory. Other informing models will be actor-network-theory, cultural–historical activity theory and the work of Deleuze and Guattari on plateaux (2004a, 2004b), and Manuel DeLanda (1997, 2002, 2006) on assemblage theory. All of these perspectives are discussed at length in subsequent chapters. If the past 3 decades have been dominated in some circles of creative thinking within medical education by the work of Michel Foucault, the emerging era is likely to be based more on the work of Gilles Deleuze and Felix Guattari (Bleakley, 2011a) and students of their work such as Manuel DeLanda.

By way of an introduction and taster to Deleuzian thinking (expanded in Chap. 14), DeLanda (2006) describes an alternative to hierarchies as 'assemblages', a term that can be used to characterize contemporary, ad hoc teams in clinical work. Assemblages are not 'finished' products but in a state of 'becoming' (Bleakley, 2011a). They may retain vestiges of hierarchies such as 'standing' rules, but mainly they are 'moving', not standing, and in this movement power is generated as a potential in the system, as the ideological shift from autocracy to democracy. How this power may be expressed is through 'moral courage' (speaking up and speaking out), discussed at length in the following chapter. Assemblages are not totalities (self-contained units), where they are constantly changing in relation to other assemblages within more complex dynamic systems (such as activity systems moving about each other).

Assemblages have components, both expressive (humans) and material (artifacts). These interact to form 'intensities'. In crisis, this interaction is multiplied. Assemblages do not seek stability, but less intensity suggests greater stability and more intensity suggests instability. Assemblages seek to stabilize through territorialization (imperialism, colonizing) and then will crystallize. Good teamwork attempts to deterritorialize through resisting colonizing impulses, to keep the team fluid, open to ideas, and capable of producing new knowledge, rather than reproducing old information. An assemblage can be thought of as a local ecosystem in fine balance. Evolution works by chance small differences and variation (gene mutations) that form the basis for natural selection. Local ecosystems must maintain a balance between allowing for variation while recognizing competition for resources.

The system, assemblage, or team is therefore constantly self-regulating to maintain stability in the face of change.

Better performing teams establish a 'situation awareness' (Bleakley, Allard, & Hobbs 2013), for example, through briefing, where members have a sense of what others are doing throughout the rhythm of the working day. Hardt and Negri (2006) describe the 'multitude' (our collaborative, interprofessional team) as knowing 'what is to come' through 'circuits of collaboration'. They have transcended a state of conflict in which difference is a barrier to working around patients, to utilize difference as a resource for patient benefit. Such a team becomes an engine for biopolitical production—the production of identities, forms of relationships, and patterns of communication. This is important, because the teams themselves are the producers, and not the discourses of social scientists on how teams best work. Importantly, the patient is the key element in how the team works, as the team shapes itself around the patient's needs. Patient-centredness again appears without a centre, as the purpose of the assemblage configured as a horizon of possibility on a trajectory of work.

In the following chapters, I expand in depth upon key theoretical perspectives that have been previewed in previous chapters. This reminds us that no one theory can comprehensively explore and explain clinical team process at the heart of which is effective communication. Rather, theories are fit for purpose.

Chapter 12
Theorizing Team Process Through a Foucauldian Perspective: Gaining a Voice in Team Activity at the Clinical Coalface

'I Was Unhappy with Him to Carry on': Fearless Speech and Moral Courage in New Team Work Settings

There is a sea change at work in surgical education. While anaesthetists have had a long-standing interest in patient safety, surgical culture now more widely recognizes the importance of improving safety through reform of clinical team practices. For example, Beger and Arbogast (2006, p. 147) describe the importance of a surgeon's capability in the non-technical realm, involving 'the ability to communicate' for 'seamless cooperation within the surgical team'. Giddings and Williamson (2007, p. 4) suggest that 'Patient safety is at the centre of care' and explicitly guide all surgeons to actively improve teamwork in order to enhance safety. They call for structured team briefings and debriefings to create common understanding as a basis to decision-making. Importantly, setting up such collaborative work practices is explicitly couched as a 'moral obligation' for surgeons.

The key report by Giddings and Williamson (2007), in effect a policy statement from the Royal College of Surgeons of England, does not however explore in depth just what the 'moral' dimension to collaborative operating theatre work might look like in practice. It is couched in the technical language of skills and competencies acquisition, rather than the language of values that may inform (and form) practices. Indeed, the use of the term 'moral' obligation, rather than an ethical obligation, is telling. Lorraine Daston and Peter Galison (2007, p. 40) make an important distinction between ethical and moral, where 'ethical refers to normative codes of conduct that are bound up with a way of being in the world, an ethos in the sense of the habitual disposition of an individual or a group, while moral refers to specific normative rules that may be upheld or transgressed and to which one may be held to account'. Examples of an ethical disposition are commitment to the best possible patient care or to evidence-based approaches, where a moral issue may be the transgression of a particular protocol such as a sterility rule (not touching sterilized equipment in the operating theatre, washing hands between seeing patients on the ward).

A. Bleakley, *Patient-Centred Medicine in Transition: The Heart of the Matter*, Advances in Medical Education 3, DOI 10.1007/978-3-319-02487-5_12, © Springer International Publishing Switzerland 2014

In terms of the order of work, there is remarkably little change in operating theatre culture since the account of Strauss, Schatzman, Ehrlich, Bucher, and Sabshin (1963) that focused upon how work is negotiated generally in hospitals in the absence of explicit rules. Indeed, the increasing complexity of work in hospitals has increased the level of ad hoc negotiation that resists formal structure and this, in turn, demands more sophisticated ways of capturing such complexity through work-based research processes (Iedema, 2007; Sorensen & Iedema, 2008a, 2008b). Although operating theatre work is sometimes framed as protocol driven, protocols are often both labile and fragile. Rather, a characteristic local ethos dominates. For example, there is wide variability amongst operating theatre teams in the extent to which they apply practices such as briefing, debriefing, and close call (near miss) reporting, where these are guided by ethos and code rather than the moral obligation of an explicit rule (Allard, Bleakley, Hobbs, & Vinnell, 2007).

Instrumental approaches, which identify patient safety gaps to be filled by protocols, overlook the possibility that such protocols may be followed grudgingly where they do not sit readily with the ethos of the culture, paradoxically creating another layer of risk. In contrast, the ethos approach would see the entire operating theatre culture adopting safety practices because such practices are valued as they follow best evidence. Unidirectional culture change, involving building new practices for patient safety, will be difficult to establish and harder to sustain if it is enforced, offers unwelcome colonization, or attempts to build on a values quicksand. Values and attitudinal change are foundational, where they precede and form behavioural and performance change (Bleakley, Boyden, Hobbs, Walsh, & Allard, 2006; Bleakley, Hobbs, Boyden, & Walsh, 2004; Bleakley, Marshall, & Brömer, 2006).

Further, while surgeons may have a moral obligation to create good patient safety climates through teamwork practices, what of the other practitioners in surgical and anaesthetic teams? What are the ethical obligations of team members traditionally lower on the hierarchy than surgeons? This ethical, or values-laden, dimension to teamwork in the operating theatre is explored here through the notion of parrhēsia—ethical courage.

I (Bleakley, 2006a, 2006b) have explored how operating theatre practitioners voice concerns and represent work through rhetorical strategies. For example, in narrative accounts of close calls ('near misses'), where an issue that might have led to an accident was avoided by intervention or serendipity, a typical rhetorical strategy is to speak on behalf of a professional group, such as nurses, by stereotyping another group, such as surgeons. This is potentially divisive at the level of the team and has a detrimental knock-on effect for quality of patient care. Another strategy is to identify all operating theatre team members as pulling together in the face of adversity (such as lack of equipment) against the common (rhetorical) enemy of 'management'. This is potentially divisive at the level of the organization. The rhetoric here is, typically: 'we', as practitioners, privilege quality of care; 'they', the management, privilege cost-effectiveness and efficiency. Indeed, 'management' is parodied as the 'dark force', and practitioners who become managers or are seduced by management-speak are ribbed about 'going over to the dark side'.

In this chapter, the focus moves from use of rhetorical strategies in critical accounts of work in the operating theatre to issues of parrhēsia, or ethical courage, that is formally the opposite of rhetoric. The terms 'rhetorical' and 'parrhesiastical' do not simply apply to representations of work such as reflective accounts but describe work strategies themselves or constitute two sides of the coin of daily work practice as these strategies serve different communication purposes.

Where rhetorical work explicitly persuades through the flow of convergence upon team needs or divergence of professional interests, parrhēsia explicitly shows, or exposes, ethical tensions and injustices arising from power and legitimacy issues. Parrhēsia is an issue of 'human rights' embedded in 'human rites'—in this case the rituals that formulate the ethos of the collective household that is the anaesthetic room and operating theatre (in the UK these are physically separate domains, where in North America the operating room is also where anaesthesia is carried out) and recovery room. Parrhēsia was first posited by the ancient Greek world as an alternative to rhetoric and now may be thought of, paradoxically, as a kind of rhetoric in its own right, albeit a 'degree zero' rhetoric.

There is a new wave of research in work-based hospital activity that focuses upon the intersection between power and identity as this emerges in explicit acts of resistance to habits, conventions, and associated protocols. Such research, as we have seen, is informed particularly by Michel Foucault's analysis of power as both capillary (running through a system) and productive (of resistance, knowledge, relationships, and identities). The operating theatre practitioner traditionally lower on the hierarchy may resist, indeed collapse, a traditional power structure through a carefully timed intervention showing ethical courage. This, in turn, produces a new identity for that person and sets up a new structure of relationships.

This view may be combined with the work of Giorgio Agamben (1998) who aligns Foucault's model of productive capillary power with traditional models of sovereign power to explore the dividing line between legitimate authority and authoritarianism (Bleakley, 2006b). Agamben's work reminds us that, in the operating theatre in particular, sovereign power is evident—the King is not yet dead!

We have not yet evolved, in Hardt and Negri's (2001, 2006, 2009) model, from imperialism (colonizing, authority-led, hierarchical), to empire (hybrid practices), to multitude (democratic, collaborative practices) and then to expression of a 'commonwealth'. The sovereign power of the surgeon must still be taken into account to temper an analysis of power that privileges the notion of resistance and production of knowledge, relationships, and identities. There may be circumstances, explored later, where the potential for resistance through capillary power is simply overwhelmed by the exercise of sovereign power (as legitimate or illegitimate exercise of authority).

In the new wave of complex, work-based hospital research, Lorelei Lingard and colleagues in Toronto (Whyte et al., 2008) have applied ethical courage to their own program of research in the operating theatre by comprehensively accounting for the paradoxical and unintended negative effects of interprofessional briefings on operating room team performance. Briefings were introduced as a consistent protocol ('checklist') to improve practice, and a body of evidence was accrued for such improvement.

However, in line with comments above about the difficulties of introducing fragile 'moral' protocols into a tough and idiosyncratic local ethos, briefings also produced resistance and either no impact or even negative consequences, including the perpetuation of the very professional divisions briefings set out to overcome.

Rick Iedema (2007) and colleagues in Australia have shown how labile complex work is as they explore everyday practices embedded in and often frustrated by organizational structures. For example, Riley and Manias (in Iedema, 2007, p. 67), using a Foucauldian approach, analyse 'power relationships in communication between nurses and surgeons' in structuring the operating room list—the order of patients. They report that 'nurses are positioned between competing organizational discourses that privilege time and efficiency and the hierarchical dominance of surgeons'. Nurses, however, still 'challenge surgeons' traditional and hierarchical right to determine the order of the operating list'. This act of resistance, read as parrhēsia, challenges the stereotypical identity of the operating theatre nurse as 'handmaiden' to the surgeon. Let us now consider parrhēsia in more detail.

Parrhēsia

Michel Foucault (2001) delivered six lectures at the University of California in Berkeley in 1983 on the topic of 'Discourse and Truth'. These lectures centre on the contemporary relevance of the ancient Greek notion of parrhēsia that Foucault describes as a particular discourse of truth concerned with 'fearless speech' (or 'frankness', 'licence', and 'free speech'). Parrhēsia literally means 'to say everything' and has been translated as 'plain speaking' (Flynn, 1987), 'truth speaking' (Rabinow, 1994), an 'ethical practice of freedom' (Franĕk, 2006), 'all telling', 'truthfulness' and 'probity' (Sharpe, 2007), and 'freedom of speech' or 'candid speech' (McGushin, 2007).

McGushin (2007) describes parrhēsia as central to the practice of askēsis, a conscious shaping of the self as an ethical pursuit, or becoming a parrhesiast (Bleakley, 2001). McGushin delimits the parrhesiastical act as 'one speaks one's mind where the stakes are high'. To speak one's mind plainly in the presence of authority is an act of ethical courage. As Frank (1999) suggests, the parrhesiast does not merely confront, but actively disturbs, established relations of truth and power through ethical intervention. The parrhesiast seeks to alter relations of power. The complex notion of parrhēsia should not be reduced to 'assertiveness', which captures only a technical dimension. 'Assertion' may not be 'truth saying' but purely rhetoric or persuasion.

Parrhēsia first appears in the fifth century BC in the work of Euripides as a counter to rhetoric. In rhetoric, where the speaker may set out to persuade a listener, the speaker does not necessarily identify with what is said. In parrhēsia, identification between what is said and the speaker is total. Further, where parrhēsia is a way of being or a virtue, rhetoric is a craft and a technology of control. Where parrhēsia is concerned with how one is, rhetoric is then concerned with government of others. Further, parrhēsia is not a form of self-examination, either of conscience (reflexivity) or ideas (reflection). These are practices that refuse who we are, or make strange the 'familiar' self (now a stranger). Rather, a parrhesiastical act 'refuses' others, or engages with others critically as an exercise of truth telling.

One who speaks 'the truth' is a foil to the ruler or king, bearing the same relationship that the Fool bears to King Lear. The parrhesiast speaks from a social position of inferiority and therefore exerts ethical courage as risk. This difference in status is critical. The ruler cannot be a parrhesiast because there is no risk in speaking against oneself as ruler. Parrhesiastical behaviour thus constitutes an identity, first as underdog and second as truth teller, pointing out that the emperor is indeed naked. Another quality of the parrhesiast is timing—judging the opportunity or critical moment for intervention. These qualities collectively constitute not only an ethic of existence, but also an aesthetic of existence, forming a style of life or work.

Besides political parrhēsia, or truth telling as Fool in relation to King, there is parrhēsia as Socratic dialogue. This is informed critical debate around the touchstone of an ethical problem. Such ethical problems are common in the operating theatre (Bleakley, 2006b), but again they are often framed as instrumental or technical and open to solution by rules and protocols. Both political and critical parrhēsia offer useful analytical maps to inquire into the nature of relationships between practitioners in the operating theatre. In the political incarnation, the traditional hierarchy of roles sets the frame for parrhesiastical 'games' centred on power and legitimacy issues: medical staff showing authority over nursing staff and anaesthetic assistants; nursing staff showing authority over auxiliary staff such as porters and cleaners; surgeons showing authority over anaesthetists; surgeons showing authority over everybody (except, in the UK, in the anaesthetic room that is the anaesthetist's and anaesthetics assistants' domain). In the ethical incarnation, the touchstone, around which debate ensues, is the patient and the ethical issue is how to create the optimum climate for patient safety.

Under what conditions and for what purposes might members of operating theatre teams need to speak out, or exert ethical courage, to promote patient safety? Giddings and Williamson (2007 p. 13) provide a stark, high profile example. Due to a series of errors, including the consultant viewing the X-rays on the viewing box back to front, a patient had the wrong kidney removed and later died. The consultant had instructed a registrar to carry out the operation. The authors go on to say that 'A medical student observing the operation suggested to the SpR (Specialist Registrar) that he was removing the incorrect kidney but was told by the SpR that she was wrong'. Here, a medical student speaks out against a surgeon. Usually, the need for ethical courage is from a non-medical member of the team, such as a scrub or circulating nurse, speaking out against a surgeon or anaesthetist. However, such speaking out (again, not simply 'assertiveness' but moral courage) may depend upon a prior condition of possibility—a climate in which constructive dialogue between members is possible at all.

In the remainder of this chapter, the notion of parrhēsia is used to explore and illuminate interactions in the operating theatre that serve to either facilitate or frustrate the establishment of a positive communication climate for patient safety. Such interactions are recorded in two levels of data: first, scripts written by operating theatre staff, describing typical (mis)communications, used to produce video vignettes for teaching purposes; second, from close call (near miss) incident reports (Hobbs & Bleakley, 2005).

Speaking Up and Speaking Out

Surgical errors are rarely the mistake of an individual surgeon's technical error but are grounded in systems errors, where the basic system is the clinical team (Gawande, 2009; Gawande, Zinner, Studdert, & Brennan, 2003; Pronovost & Vohr, 2010). Further, operations generally depend on 25 % of manual skill, where 75 % rests with cognitive performance (Beger & Arbogast, 2006), and important elements of cognition are distributed across a team. Team communication involves both collaborative cognitive problem solving and ethical decision-making. For teams to communicate well, they must generate what Pignatelli (1993) calls 'democratic habits'. Parrhēsia is a key democratic habit (although it can be argued that if democracy were working within clinical teams, the need for parrhēsia would be dramatically reduced) and fits with the general argument of this book—to shift medical education in both undergraduate and postgraduate education towards collaborative models based on evidenced patient benefits.

The operating theatre is a high-risk work context, and tension between practitioners is a common, and understandable, occurrence (Lingard, Reznick, DeVito, & Espin, 2002; Lingard, Reznick, Espin, Regehr, & DeVito, 2002). There are many reasons for such tension, including cultural differences in approaches to patients between doctors and other professionals such as nurses and between surgeons and anaesthetists. However, where collaborative teamwork is a critical factor in ensuring patient safety, it is important that tensions arising from issues such as professional differences are addressed productively.

A study by Bleakley, Allard, and Hobbs (2013) of communication in orthopaedic theatre teams showed that miscommunications are a typical symptom of 'monological' rather than 'dialogical' (Bakhtin, 1981) teams, where surgeons usually set these atmospheres or climates. In a monological climate, the surgeon models one-way communication. It may not be authoritarian but is 'authoritative' as opposed to 'facilitative' (Heron, 2001), where the communications are typically statements (mild or confrontational), information giving (the most common), or telling (also common). In contrast, in a dialogical atmosphere or climate, there would be more facilitative exchange—question and answer, open-ended discussion, supportive comments, and tolerance of, indeed encouragement of, emotional expression.

In a deeply monological climate, a surgeon may display authoritarian behaviour that denies the possibility of democratic participation and open communication in the team. Here, for example, briefing and debriefing would not occur and situation awareness would not be established. This creates a poor climate for patient safety. In contrast, where a surgeon holds a brief before the list begins, displays warm and courteous behaviour towards other members of the team, and encourages open dialogue, the patient is at less risk from potential systems-based communication errors, such as a wrong side or site operation (Gawande, 2009; Pronovost & Vohr, 2010).

Below are two typical exchanges from the operating theatre scripted by an operating theatre team minus the surgeon. Actors then used these scripts in preparing videotape scenarios for teaching purposes (www.ttrm.co.uk). The first is a typical miscommunication scenario in a team that clearly never briefs or debriefs. In the second, the surgeon is prepared to brief and is led into this by the staff nurse, who helps to guide the brief to consider 'who is on the team today?' as well as technical issues such as 'do we have the right equipment?'

In this short encounter, there are 12 utterances. Two of those are requests from the surgeon that are close to demands ('Send for the next patient' and 'Ring the

---

General surgery theatre, team around anaesthetized patient with surgeon sewing up and clock showing 16.45:

Surgeon (male) (assertively): 'Send for the next patient'.

Scrub Nurse (female) (gently): 'I'm off at five, we'll need to see if another scrub nurse is available'.

Runner (circulating nurse) (male) (gently): 'So am I. The list is supposed to finish at five; if we do the next case we won't be finished until six thirty at least'.

Surgeon (aggressively): 'No bloody commitment! How am I supposed to reduce my waiting list if theatre lists are always cut short?'

Scrub Nurse (assertively): 'This wasn't cut short, we were ready at 1.30 and you were 20 min late!'

Surgeon (accusingly, glancing at anaesthetist): 'We would still have had enough time if the anaesthetic on the second patient hadn't taken so long'.

Anaesthetist (somewhat defensively): 'Hang on a minute, if you were having a laparotomy you would like to have an epidural for post-op pain relief. The problem is that you don't think about the anaesthetic time when you write the list … and you let the registrar do the anastomosis which took 20 min longer'.

Surgeon (assertively and accusingly): 'Well, who is going to tell the patient they are cancelled?'

… Long pause (heads of the other OT practitioners drop, averting eye contact) …

Surgeon (smugly): 'You see, it's always down to me. Ring the ward and tell them to feed the last patient'.

Silence, everyone studiously avoids everyone else's gaze, especially the surgeon's … fade to black.

---

ward and tell them to feed the last patient'). Eight are statements with varying degrees of emotional overtones (such as 'I'm off at five', 'Hang on a minute', and 'You see, it's always down to me'). Two are hostile rhetorical questions ('How am I supposed to reduce my waiting list … ?' and 'Well, who is going to tell the patient … ?') The emotional atmosphere is tense; the communication climate is surgeon-led and monological. This is a typical ethos, where there is failure to set up constructive dialogue.

Is this a stereotype of surgeons by other members of the team preparing the script, and is it untypical of work? The answer to this is emphatically 'no'. The scripts and the subsequent video scenarios have been used countless times in educating surgical teams, including surgeons, and their veracity is supported.

Further, in videotaping surgical teams live (Bleakley, Allard, and Hobbs, 2013) and analysing encounters, monological interaction initiated by surgeons is the default communication ethos, suppressing dialogical interaction.

To return to the script—while the scrub nurse, runner, and anaesthetist start to challenge the surgeon, importantly, they fail to turn assertiveness into parrhēsia. The surgeon exerts a faux moral authority and the rest of the team capitulate while the surgeon turns the whole event to his advantage by agreeing that they will finish the list but chastising at the same time. In the process, the surgeon takes the wind out of the sails of the team, so that they are dispirited and deflated, and they give up on their challenge. No prior condition of democratic habit or dialogue had been set up, and the team is a pushover for the passive–aggressive style of the surgeon. The potential for resistance through capillary power is simply overwhelmed where the surgeon says: 'You see, it's always down to me'. By this time, there is no stomach for resistance, heads have dropped, and gaze is no longer maintained. No doubt the team, when the surgeon leaves, will engage in a corrosive 'corridor debrief'. Moreover, while the surgeon exerts authority as leader for the team, taking 'responsibility' for the patient, the behaviour, in terms of patient safety, is irresponsible and does not recognize that actually patients 'lead' clinical teams.

In contrast, consider the following exchange, which stimulates a briefing prior to a list, set up by the surgeon but progressed collaboratively:

Venue: general theatre—male anaesthetist checking machine, male anaesthetic assistant fixing suction tubing, a young male scrub nurse and an older female staff nurse counting equipment. Male surgeon walks in.

Surgeon (pleasant and confident demeanour): 'Morning everyone. Nice straightforward list today. First patient on the way?'

Staff Nurse (politely): 'Of course, Mr S...; but I have a couple of queries; can we just run through the list please?'

Anaesthetist (enthusiastically): 'That would be good as I think we might have to change the order'.

Surgeon (taking the list off the wall): 'OK, let's have a brief then'....

Staff gather round, scrub nurse keeps himself sterile (stands to one side and avoids touching anyone).

Surgeon: 'First patient is the bilateral orchidopexy; he's young and fit; no queries there?'

Staff Nurse: 'No, that's fine. Before we go through the rest of the list, can I just introduce my runner, Simon, he's new here, and as the first case is straightforward, he will be scrubbing for you'.

Surgeon: 'Hello Simon. As long as you have all my sutures, I'm sure we will get on very well. .... The next case is the insertion of JJ stents for bilateral ureteric obstruction—that's straightforward too'.

Anaesthetist: 'Well, no. His creatinine was 400 yesterday and the potassium 6.1; we may have to delay him until we get today's blood results back. They hadn't been taken when I was on the ward'.

Surgeon: 'O.K., but he needs to be done, or else he will need nephrostomies. However the third case is a removal of ureteric stone, so we can move that up, if the results aren't back. Is there a problem with this case?'

Staff Nurse: 'That depends if you want the lithoclast or the laser'.

Surgeon: 'I suppose that means the laser isn't back from repair, but the lithoclast will be fine. By the way, have we warned radiology?'

Staff Nurse: 'Of course, but thanks for asking'.

Surgeon: 'And that just leaves the open nephrectomy'.

Scrub Nurse: 'Which side is it? I know we will all check the side again when the patient is here, but it just helps with setting up the trolleys'.

Surgeon: 'It's the left side. If there's enough time I may let the registrar do some of the dissection, O.K.? .... I think the first patient has just arrived, and as we all know what we're doing, let's get on'.

Staff Nurse: 'Now we're all singing from the same song sheet everything should be smoother—but we just need to keep communicating about the second patient; and perhaps at the end we could debrief to see how well we did'.

Recall that the surgeon did not initially see any reason for a brief, but was quickly persuaded by the collective parrhēsia of the team channelled through the nurse, and much good flowed from this. In the encounter there are 28 utterances. Seven of those are questions or requests, all posed in a positive way. While all others are statements, they are supportive, affirming, or clarifying. The tone of the exchanges is positive, the talk inclusive, and the conclusion upbeat. While the difference between the emotional tones in the two scenarios is important, a key difference is that the first scenario is monological where the second is dialogical. In the first, questions are closed or hostile and statements do not invite response. In the second, both questions and statements invite dialogue. Importantly, as dialogue evolves, so a facilitative climate is set for further parrhesiastical intervention.

Narrative accounts of 'close calls' or 'near misses'—issues that arise that did not lead to harm to a patient or a member of staff—are good sources of understanding teamwork, albeit through retrospective accounts. The good news about a close call is that an accident was avoided, and this is often through collaborative resourcefulness of the team, who may have to improvise. The bad news is that many close calls do not escalate to an accident only by luck or chance. Also, accidents are known to arise from the cumulative effect of small incidents, so it is important to respond to close calls. Close call accounts are necessarily remembered and then subject to narrative shaping through rhetoric. We can account for this and suggest what functions such rhetoric may serve (Bleakley, 2006a, 2006b). Nurses usually submit close calls, sometimes on behalf of surgeons or anaesthetists. While anaesthetic culture is familiar with incident reporting and utilizes reports for monitoring purposes, close calls are rarely submitted directly by surgeons, and this is a reflection on their cultural values including a general scepticism towards protocols (Pronovost & Vohr, 2010).

Given these concerns, the narrative close call can still be seen as an important auto-ethnographic method that brings authenticity and strength to the collaborative inquiry. Here, the practitioner writes an account of work as if she or he is an ethnographer describing an Other's culture. This turns the familiar into the strange, as a basis to both reflexive accounting and parrhesiastical account. Narrative close call reports offer a substitute debrief—a way of 'speaking out'—where this may have been stifled by team dynamics. The narrative opportunities for close call reporting are widely exploited by staff members, who will often write reports as stories rather than simply technical accounts. Differing professional groups—nurses, surgeons, anaesthetists, and operating department practitioners—then go beyond merely descriptive recall of the near miss to craft both rhetorical and parrhesiastical statements.

The following examples illustrate a 'first-level' parrhesia—ethical courage operating through close call reporting because the opportunity to speak out at the time was stifled by context. Again, while open to rhetorical devices, the accounts given below seem remarkably free from rhetoric. The first is a report from a nurse:

Close Call Report 1

'The on-call endoscopist organized a patient to be brought to theatre and called in the on-call endoscopy nurse for 9 am without informing the anaesthetic, surgical, or nursing staff. The endoscopist arranged for the endoscopy nurse to come back at 16.00 h for the patient to have an upper GI endoscopy. He did not inform the anaesthetists or the on-call surgical team that he had done this. The on-call surgeons were in the theatres operating all day, and at 16.30 h when the endoscopist brought this patient to theatre to perform an endoscopy, the surgeons were in the middle of performing a procedure on a patient and had several more patients to be operated on. He then demanded that one of the general nurses assist him and also an anaesthetic assistant needed to maintain the patient's airway after he had had some sedation. This left the department with low levels of staffing as 3 theatres were then in use and maternity needed cover. While operating, the endoscopist was rude to the staff. When he couldn't stop the bleeding, he then went into Theatre 7 where the general surgeons were operating and informed them of the situation and asked them to stem the bleeding. He did not communicate with the theatre staff or the anaesthetists and just walked out of the theatre. The patient was moved into the recovery unit where he was cared for until the surgeons and anaesthetists were free. The endoscopist had written on the patient IV chart to have blood transfused; the consent form only had the word "surgery" on it and he still had not spoken to the anaesthetists. When he was phoned and politely told all of this, he said he would get his registrar to sort it out. His registrar duly came up to the recovery unit but had not had any dealings with this patient before and so had no knowledge of the patient's history. He had to sit and read through the patient's notes and talk to the theatre staff before he could "sort out the problem"'.

The second report is by a scrub nurse:

Close Call Report 2

'I was asked to scrub for a case. I was told the patient was sent for so I washed my hands to get ready. She was sent for at 16.40—I waited in theatre having got the set ready for the operation. The patient arrived in the anaesthetic room at 16.57. I was later informed that the operation had been cancelled by the consultant anaesthetist as the surgeon hadn't turned up. I waited around then; I was asked by the junior anaesthetist if I could dress the leg which had been exposed down to the dressing. At 17.25 the surgeon then turned up, and the junior anaesthetist still present told him he had been told he was not allowed to anesthetise the patient by the consultant. The surgeon wanted to look at the leg and started to pull the dressing off. The patient was crying out in pain; I said I was unhappy with him to carry on. The patient was really in a great deal of discomfort and pain. I dressed her leg as quickly and gently as I could. She went back to the ward via the recovery department.

I was very unhappy that the patient had been put through this ordeal—(1) the consultant cancelled because of the time; (2) the surgeon was doing a ward round when he should have been in theatre; (3) the patient was put through unnecessary pain and discomfort'.

The nurse's parrhesiastical intervention 'I said I was unhappy with him to carry on' appears to stop the surgeon in his tracks and cut short the 'ordeal' of the patient. The account draws attention to a web of miscommunications putting the patient at risk. If good teamwork is an ethical obligation, then here a vacuum at the heart of ethical practice is reported.

Dialogical Climates and Hospitality

The emergence of parrhēsia may then require a prior condition of possibility: a 'dialogical', rather than 'monological', climate. As mentioned earlier, these terms are borrowed from the literary theorist Mikhail Bakhtin (1981). Bakhtin challenges the need for finality or closure in talk, suggesting that dialogue requires no finality or identity to achieve shared meanings. The monological is a rhetorical device of the voice of authority, used to close down debate, at worst to prescribe in an authoritarian manner, drowning out the possibility of open or democratic debate. Here, dialogue's creative division of voices is collapsed into a single, overriding voice, and the possibility of collaborative teamwork is frustrated.

A dialogical climate is produced and maintained through facilitative exchange and interventions, whether in consensus or dissension: question and answer, reciprocation, expression and recognition of cathartic or emotional release, ethical recognition of the face of the Other, hospitality, generosity, exchange, mutuality, democratic participation, invitation, call and response, collaboration, and coordination. A monological climate is produced and maintained through prescription, informing without exchange and confrontation without recognition of response. In short, a dialogical climate is about questions and response, a monological climate is about statements and silences.

This crude distinction needs some refinement. Questions of certain kinds—such as rhetorical or closed questions of a negative sort or 'loaded' questions that are cynical or barbed—are not positively dialogical where they do not invite reciprocal engagement. Certain statements such as the confirmatory, self-disclosing, and purely technical do not necessarily produce or add to monological climates. Tone of voice in both question and statement, signalling intent, will often be read as the main cue to invitation to dialogue or closure in monologue.

The primary conditions of possibility for the emergence of a dialogical atmosphere are work-based friendship ('collegiality') and hospitality (Bleakley, 2002, 2006b). Work-based 'friendship' (not an intimate relationship but a collegial one) engages interprofessional aims and collectively orients to the patient's needs. 'Hospitality' follows Emmanuel Levinas's (1969) description of self-recognition as dependent upon recognition first of the face of the Other. Hospitality means, first, not setting conditions for the stranger who arrives in your house, but rather learning from that stranger about your own limits and identity and, second, offering your help as a freely given, or unconditional, 'gift' (Bleakley, 2002). Levinas's approach to hospitality describes one way of framing patient-centredness, now grounded in how practitioners open up their collective house to welcome strangers.

'House' at root means both a dwelling place and place of worship. It therefore brings together, albeit temporarily, domestic and ethical life as shared work or turns work groups under the same roof into quasi-families with a shared ethos or style of life. Ethos is the common genius of a system. The shared deity or spirit of the clinical household of the operating theatre is the 'patient'. As described earlier, also once known as the 'firm', 'house' has a long history in UK acute care or hospital-based medicine, referring to the clinical team. Junior doctors (interns becoming residents)—now 'foundation' doctors in the UK—were once 'house officers', as noted previously. The household, the ancient Greek oikos, may be thought of as the total ecology of care under one roof. The patient is a visitor in the clinical house or household. In the operating theatre house there are (two in North America, three in the UK) rooms with professional groups—the anaesthetic and surgical room(s) and recovery room. The ward offers another, adjacent household. The overarching household is the hospital, literally the place of hospitality.

In the turn towards collaborative practice, teams must be attuned to the ecology of the work context, indwelling their respective households. In establishing a dialogical atmosphere through questions promoting engagement rather than statements promoting disengagement, an atmosphere of trust is established in which parrhēsia can be exercised. Again, in an ethical dilemma, the scrub nurse speaks up and out against the surgeon—reminding him or her of options to the choice he may have voiced. Ethical positions arise from context, especially as an improvised response to value conflicts or situations of uncertainty emerging from the dynamic unfolding of work activity.

Collaborative intentionality produces 'horizon' thinking—the team plans ahead or briefs as it goes along. A central value of this collaboration, whose edge, inventiveness, and dynamism are kept open through the welcome attitude towards parrhēsia, is then unconditional hospitality. Hospitality constitutes the 'centredness' of patient-centred practice, where the patient is a welcome guest in the houses of the operating theatre teams. Sensitivity to patients' needs is necessarily embedded in the ecological attitude that allows education of attention, a close noticing of both the patient (care) and team (safety). It is through close observation of what the patient 'wants', especially when anaesthetised and under the knife or the scope that demonstrates an ecological awareness at work. This witnessing or sensitivity describes how one indwells the household as a gracious host.

As an ecological practice, parrhēsia displaces habitual egological practices of monologue, heroic individualism, self-concern, narcissistic self-examination, and instrumental practices of 'assertiveness' learned as skills in workshops. Heroic individualism is heavily embedded in medical culture and has come to influence all health-care professionals. Again, collectivism is not a given condition but is seen as a condition to be achieved. Parrhesiasts follow Aristotle's definition of the virtuous friend as 'those who wish well to their friends for their sake', replacing Descartes' 'I think, therefore I am' with 'I think of the Other, therefore I become'. Care in the operating theatre is shaped by inclusion rather than exclusion, boundary crossing rather than boundary maintenance. How can a horizon of professional friendship and hospitality be offered to patients if it cannot first be modelled across operating theatre teamwork?

Conclusions

This chapter has described two possible forms of resistance to the traditional and habitual hierarchy of the surgical culture by those lower on that hierarchy (often nurses): rhetorical and parrhesiastical. Each approach serves to construct or reinforce identity and is intimately tied to power and location. I have shown how power operates across both sovereign and capillary dimensions, as surgeons in particular exercise authority and nurses in particular muster forms of resistance. Location is vital as the operating theatre is traditionally the house of the surgeon, but is also a common household for a team, into which a patient is invited as welcome guest. (For an exposition of the Identity–Power–Location triangle as a framework for analysis of both medical work and medical education practices, see Bleakley, Bligh, & Browne, 2011.)

Rhetorical forms of resistance may, paradoxically, be reproductive of existing structures, where parrhesiastical resistance may produce new patterns of relationship and identity. Where resistance is focused on moral obligations such as following protocols, rather than changing the ethos of a practice culture, they may paradoxically exacerbate problems. However, expression as parrhēsia may be frustrated by lack of a communicative climate in which monologue dominates over dialogue. Where patient safety climates are improved by collaborative teamwork, parrhēsia will emerge as a communication option and strength within an open team and should be tolerated for its transformative power, as resource rather than hindrance.

Chapter 13
Theorizing Team Process Through Actor-Network-Theory (ANT): Communication Practice as a Theory in Action

Prologue

Imagine: you are sitting in the bath reading this chapter. Normally, you look forward to this relaxing moment, this mini-holiday, an opportunity for time out in a hectic day when you can also fully concentrate without distraction. However, it is late, you are overtired, the bath is neither hot nor full enough, you cannot settle into a comfortable position to read, and you are now irritated that you have not got the hang of the paragraph you have just read. Nevertheless, from the late evening's ruins, a nascent idea dawns, and you want to get it down before it evaporates—but you do not have a notebook and pen handy! You go back to the paragraph and read it again, but find yourself drifting and nodding with tiredness so that you nearly let the book fall out of your hands and come back to reality with a jolt, the edge of your expensive and once pristine book now stained with bathwater. The book suddenly feels very heavy and awkward to hold.

Your idea, in the absence of notebook and pen, has already dissolved along with your patience, and now your book is close to following the same course as your concentration is shot. This lost learning scenario is ripe for analysis through actor-network-theory (hereafter 'ANT'). There was no Archimedes' 'Eureka!' moment. Rather, the glimmer of an idea dissolved where a network failed to form. The initiation of a network offers a potential transformation, but you are dead in the water. Your body was tired and your concentration poor and this was aggravated by having to hold up what felt like an increasingly heavy book. There was no paper or pen at hand.

And what is the point of this depressing little story? First, context matters where learning is concerned. Second, context centrally involves objects—artifacts such as the contours of your bath, the temperature of the bathwater, and the shape and weight of the book you are reading. These are, in ANT, all significant 'actors' in the drama of learning. I am introducing them early in this chapter so that their significance will not be forgotten. On another day, the context may not have bitten

A. Bleakley, *Patient-Centred Medicine in Transition: The Heart of the Matter*,
Advances in Medical Education 3, DOI 10.1007/978-3-319-02487-5_13,
© Springer International Publishing Switzerland 2014

back, but rather acted to promote learning as a network was formed in a stream of connections between hot bathwater, engaging book, relaxed body, and buzzing brain.

Section I: The Architecture of ANT

Introduction

ANT resists reduction to a concise description. Bruno Latour's (2007) so-called introduction to ANT is a closely argued text of 300 pages. However, Akrich, Callon, and Latour (2002, p. 205) offer a concise account of ANT as a research method where they say that 'Innovation is the art of interesting an increasing number of allies who will make you stronger and stronger'. Where ANT-inspired clinical education research makes claims for promoting innovation, knowledge production and transformation of practices, this can be summarized as *the formation, and subsequent widening and strengthening, of a learning network*. What, however, is a 'network'? And who or what are the 'allies' that must be increased or enrolled to make a network stronger? We have already seen that such 'allies' can include the temperature of your bathwater. I have also previously discussed, in Chap. 11, models of networks and related 'knotworks', as conceived by cultural–historical activity theory (CHAT).

ANT Offers an Apology

ANT has acquired a potentially unhelpful mystique as a left-field approach, offering 'a body of unsettling and rather audacious work' that operates 'around the edges of educational research' and sets out to 'rupture central assumptions' within educational theory (Fenwick & Edwards, 2010, p. viii). The rhetoric is clear and the supporting metaphors powerful: 'unsettling' and 'audacious', 'edges' and 'ruptures'. We expect to find ourselves at our limits, the ground taken from under our feet.

We would feel that we were on reasonably safe ground if someone explained that ANT involved 'actors', 'networks', and 'theory' and, as the hyphens suggest, that these are linked in some way. It was therefore disconcerting when Latour (1999a)— the single most influential voice in ANT—famously announced that there are four things wrong with ANT: 'actor', 'network', 'theory', and the hyphen! Latour's tongue was not in his cheek—rather, he feared that ANT would be reduced to a formulaic approach and misinterpreted in the process, the acronym coming to act as an aphorism or an old saw—a pithy statement supposedly embodying wisdom, but paradoxically disembowelling wisdom. Further, where reduced to an acronym, ANT is capitalized—a rhetorical device that offers declamation and *gravitas*. For this reason, I have reduced ANT to lower case—actor-network-theory—throughout this text, to get closer to its democratic promise as one amongst a number of exploratory, predictive, and explanatory models explored in this book (CHAT suffers the same fate).

In a later overview of ANT, Latour (2007) offers an apology for his earlier rather grumpy decision, recognizing that where use of the acronym is widespread, he may as well turn it into a virtue. 'ANT', suggests Latour (2007, p. 9), is 'so awkward, so confusing, so meaningless that it deserves to be kept', on the basis that it is a good descriptor for a 'myopic, workaholic, trail-sniffing, and collective traveller'. For good measure, Latour added another hyphen (from the convention of 'actor-network theory' to 'actor-network-theory') to further emphasize linkage between the components. In this chapter, I follow Latour's sentiment and prefer to keep my own nose close to the ground, mainly for the rich research detail that this posture affords. Also, to maintain the tone of democratic collaboration, readers will note that I get ants to chat—or, I see valuable connections between the perspectives of ANT and CHAT. I also retain Latour's usage of the double hyphen, to stress that actor-network-theory is a linked whole, a worldview and way of being, exceeding the limitations of an applied technique. Later in the chapter, however, I will point out some key objections to ANT, signifying limitations to its use within clinical education and its research arm.

The second hyphen in actor-network-theory also serves to repair the historical separation of theory and practice. ANT can be taken as an example of what Schatzki, Knorr-Cetina, and von-Savigny (2001) describe as 'the practice turn in contemporary theory', where theory is *performed*. Mind and knowledge are constituted, and social life is organized and transformed through action and interaction or activity. ANT is not an analytical apparatus but 'more like a sensibility, an interruption or intervention, a way to sense and draw nearer to a phenomenon' (Fenwick & Edwards, 2010, p. ix). Medicine is often characterized as an Aristotelian *phronesis*—a 'practical wisdom' (Bleakley, Bligh, & Browne, 2011)—and medical education and its research arm are consequently infected with such pragmatism. With its emphasis upon educating sensibility rather than analytical reasoning, ANT would seem to afford a ready-made pragmatic research approach for medical education, and it is puzzling that its uptake has not been more vigorous within this field of inquiry.

What Are Actors and Networks and How Do They Link?

In ANT, 'actor' refers to any phenomenon—human, material object (artifact), or concept (the imaginary, ideas). Phenomena in self-presentation are irreducible to any other expression—such as higher order categories—so ANT researchers resist drawing, first, on grand theoretical frames (such as Marxism or Psychoanalysis) that shape or prejudge data collection and, second, on the use of themes in data analysis, typically employed to order otherwise disorderly data. Fenwick and Edwards (2010,

p. 146) suggest that 'What ANT brings to its ethnographic methodological approaches is a sensibility for mess and it attempts to suspend a priori assumptions'. The ground rule is to stick with (and to) the mess in closely following the actors.

Because 'actor' is associated with persons in the English language, ANT also uses 'actant'. Throughout this chapter, I will refer to 'actors'. Actors interact in meaningful and nonmeaningful ways. For ANT, a meaningful interaction is where one actor has an effect upon another (e.g. a mobile phone ringtone captures the attention of somebody who is daydreaming) to realize a *transformation*, a change of state, an innovation, or a production of knowledge. This linkage is dynamic, moving through time. ANT calls this a 'translation' because the actors involved are now no longer the same as before.

The actors are mediators of this process of translation or are affected by the movement of translation. For example, the person answers the mobile phone to discover that her best friend has just died in a car accident, at which point a potential, and emotionally painful, network is initiated. If the actors are linked but no translation occurs, then a network fails to form. In the example above, the person may have missed the call. Where actors interact without transformation (such as automatically deleting spam mail), they act as 'intermediaries' rather than 'mediators'. Educational activity for ANT is a mediated network effect—a series of mutual translations between actors leading to transformation such as adoption of a new work practice. ANT is a way of accounting for how persons, material objects, and ideas become linked as fluid networks through tracing effects generated by the 'work' that is the assembling and strengthening of the network. ANT's concerns are inevitably 'work-based'.

Symmetry Between Humans, Material Objects, and Immaterial Languages

ANT's key philosophical contribution is the radical notion of *generalized symmetry*— where all phenomena, whether human, material, or semiotic, are afforded equal ontological status within a network effect (Harman, 2009). This notion separates ANT from other approaches to clinical education, where both objects and concepts are often given secondary ontological status to persons, or only the talk and activities of persons are recorded, as if the world of material objects that these persons interact with is of little consequence. Where the human is figured as having equal ontological status with MRI scanners, libraries, cutlery, and ocean currents, ANT is often referred to as a 'posthuman' outlook (Schatzki et al., 2001).

This radical idea of generalized symmetry has important consequences for clinical education. For example, in studies of practices of 'care', Annemarie Mol (Mol, 2008; Mol, Moser, & Pols, 2010, pp. 7–26) challenges the habitual opposition of 'cold' technologies and 'warm' humans to demonstrate that health 'care' is usually a product of interaction between the warmth of technologies (e.g. giving oxygen)

Fig. 13.1 Generalized
symmetry

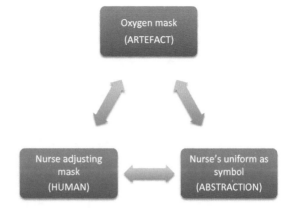

and the warmth of persons (the nurse adjusting the oxygen mask). To this we can add the potential warmth of the symbol, such as the reassurance signified by the nurse's uniform (Fig. 13.1).

Shifting focus away from just persons (as actors) affords the opportunity to appreciate both the complex and multiple appearances and translations of objects, as they interact with persons through codes and languages, as an ontological effect. The notion of multiple ontologies—states of being—is illustrated by the instability of complex objects of research across contexts. In studying the management of alcoholic liver disease, Law and Singleton (2010) report that keeping this object (the 'illness') to a single meaning is impossible as it comes in and out of focus according to the context in which it appears. Rather than seeing this as a methodological failure, the authors suggest that research methods are ill equipped to study messy objects. Mol (1999) offers a multiple ontological reading of anaemia, where the condition is 'performed' in at least three different ways: clinically (through medical diagnosis and treatment), pathophysiologically (through laboratory routines), and statistically (through epidemiological analysis).

In a later extensive study, Mol (2002) tracks the diagnosis and treatment of atherosclerosis by a variety of practitioners in a Dutch University hospital. Her ethnography reveals that what is described to patients in information leaflets as 'the gradual obstruction of the arteries' is conceived differently by doctors, vascular surgeons and nurses, and is further modulated by differing professional and lay languages and through varieties of imaging artifacts such as microscopes, X-rays, and ultrasound. Mol problematizes the study of the illness by, for example, taking the perspective not only of the human but also of the blood as this is configured in contexts such as the haematology laboratory. Here, 'atherosclerosis is enacted as deviance that involves the blood clotting mechanism', and where the patient's blood now flows across a variety of investigative sites, its 'anatomical location is completely lost' (Mol, 2002, p. 109).

ANT is drawn to suspect and problematic research contexts, from failures and fault lines to 'black boxes'—habitual or routine activities that disguise complexities such as multiple ontologies. ANT wrestles with the contents of the black box, typically 'tokens' or 'quasi-objects' that are reifications. Examples in clinical education research, as previous chapters indicate, include terms such as 'teams' (Engeström, 2008) and clinical 'guidelines' (Gabbay & Le May, 2011) used as if they were transparent and had commonly agreed meanings but are actually problematic, concealing more than they reveal.

Without entertaining the radically democratic notion of generalized symmetry, the practices of ANT will never be properly understood. Indeed, as the main philosophical position, generalized symmetry can be taken as the 'theory', conceptual architecture, or organizing framework, shaping, informing, and developing the practices of ANT, bringing actors into significant relationships as network effects. Generalized symmetry can be equated with the hyphens in actor-network-theory, which act not only as links to turn the individual components into a whole, but also as mediators or translators (actors form networks and afford theory) and, finally, as levellers, or signifiers of democracy, where actors (persons, artifacts, and languages), the networks they form, and the theory they produce to explain and further strengthen such networks *potentially* have equal power or potency.

What Are Networks?

As one actor acts upon or mobilizes another as a work of translation (so that the actors are both now transformed, as mediators), a network is initiated. Further translations expand the network through alliances. However, 'network' is neither a tangible structure nor a diagrammatic representation. It is a metaphor through which we give meaning to the series of translations that occur as actors work transformatively on other actors.

Networks involve things but are not things themselves or resist reification. As unpredictable processes, networks cannot be studied like blood samples under the microscope, yet everything *realized by the network effect* can be treated as concrete and sensible—as things that happen present themselves to the senses or mind or can be measured by instrumentation, including floating concepts and intuitive leaps, as well as cold-steel and congealing blood. As a dynamic net effect of a series of actor translations and transformations that the researcher attempts to partially retrace, a network is then a net *working* whose echo we closely observe through fieldwork and remember through research reports.

'Networking' as described in ANT is then different from networking as described by CHAT in Chap. 11. There, networking was described only in terms of stable structures and contrasted with the more labile, temporary processes of knotworking. In ANT, 'networks' are on a continuum from temporary and unstable to long term and stable. Networks may be initiated but never mature or develop through forming more and more allies. Or, networks may be conceived but never actually initiated.

Or, networks may be developed that have a feel of permanent structures, with strong associations formed, always attracting new allies and promoting translations.

'Network', as ANT understands it, is unfortunately overshadowed by the black box of the 'Internet' that does not usually act as a dynamic network. When I visit a website for information, buy from an online catalogue, or send an email, neither I nor the website is necessarily transformed in the process. I am usually an intermediary in a predictable consumer exchange and reproduction of knowledge and values, rather than a mediator effecting change, innovation or knowledge, and values production. What has occurred is transaction rather than translation. For ANT, a network goes beyond transaction, as a traceable 'set of relations defined as so many translations' (Latour, 2007, p. 129).

Latour (2007) now prefers to call the problematic tracing of the translations across phenomena a *work-net* rather than a network. The emphasis turns from a passive network waiting to be used (a telephone, electricity, or sewage system; pipelines; the Internet as a web of computers and exchange sites) to an active web permanently in construction, requiring 'work' both to maintain its momentum (search) and to record its traces (research). Latour (2007, p. 132) then makes a distinction between the work-net as an 'active mediator' and the network as a 'stabilized set of intermediaries'. In ANT research, one must work on and at the fluid net to apprehend the 'trace left behind by some moving agent'. ANT research, as applied to clinical education, is necessarily concerned with 'work'-based learning, where labour can be material (relocating a dislocated shoulder) or immaterial (puzzling out a dislocated sentence uttered by a confused patient).

If a formula for ANT research work were to be proposed, it would be to dramatically increase the relative proportion of mediators to intermediaries, going against the grain of the usual state of affairs where intermediaries will far outweigh mediators. Another way of putting this is that life is mainly a series of *events* (equivalent to 'intermediaries') that fail to promote innovation. Where events turn to *experiences* (equivalent to 'mediators'), something deep happens in the way of learning. Often, a mediator is troublesome or irksome, already getting under the skin, to turn an event into an experience. Here, ANT reformulates Harold Garfinkel's (1967) ethnomethodology, which explicitly sets out to problematize the social contexts it researches. Ethnomethodologists deliberately breach social rules and conventions through planned interventions, such as cheating at board games or acting as a stranger in one's own home to record reactions.

Rather than intervening in terms of the researcher breaching a convention (which may also have ethical implications), ANT researchers seize upon social phenomena that are already inverted, divisive, or calamitous. For example, Latour (1996) studied the conception, but ultimate failure, of a project in Paris for a rapid public transport system—Aramis—showing how a potential network could be initiated but not maintained, so that the project was abandoned as sterile. The frustration of possible translations across actors may cause a potential network to falter. In Aramis' case this was an economical–technological–political hitch—complicated engineered couplings proved too expensive to produce, and there was a parallel failure of coupling in lack of political support for the project despite a public will.

Feasibility

In such a retracing of the work-net—and having decided that its focus will be inclusive—how does an ANT approach make such a study manageable? Surely, any social phenomenon under investigation is always too complex and its manifestations too numerous to offer any kind of comprehensive account. ANT does not seek a comprehensive account but a close description of a slice of activity, getting so close to the ground that an overview is impossible. ANT research prides itself on its radical localism, suggesting that 'generalizability' in research is a convenient fiction, where all research projects are necessarily local and situated. Will an ANT study then either miss the point completely by its self-inflicted myopia or will it get lost, indeed suffocate, in excessive detail?

Fortunately, ANT has addressed such questions of scale. To achieve focus, as mentioned earlier, ANT places two primary restrictions upon the study of the initiation, development, and future of a work-net/network or a series of interacting networks. First, ANT research focuses upon the work of actors as mediators rather than intermediaries. It is interested in transformations promising innovation, rather than the maintenance of the status quo. Second, ANT chooses to research what is already showing symptom, signs of wear and tear, instability, or a fault line. ANT feeds off controversies, even fiascos. ANT is then selective of the slice of activity for study, but this may be the only explicit marker you will find of its research 'design'.

Where ANT research focuses upon the apparently unremarkable or routine, such as Mol's interest in anaemia, it is because a black box has been opened to expose complexities and contradictions. ANT is sceptical of linear, problem-solving approaches and the hunt for final solutions that together constitute a genre of research typified by the hero's journey—where monsters, riddles, and labyrinths are rendered unproblematic and the Grail is revealed or the Minotaur slain.

Section II: Let's Go to Work! ANT as a Research Methodology

Introduction

In this section, I describe how an ongoing collaborative inquiry focused upon improving teamwork across operating theatres in one UK teaching hospital has been informed and shaped by an ANT sensibility (e.g. Allard, Bleakley, Hobbs, & Vinnell, 2007; Bleakley, 2006a, 2006b; Bleakley et al., 2006; Bleakley, Hobbs, Boyden, & Walsh, 2004; Henderson et al., 2007; Hobbs, 2005; Hobbs & Bleakley, 2005). The inquiry—the Theatre Team Resource Management (hereafter 'TTRM') project—was conceived in 2001–2002 and initiated in December 2002 to progressively assemble a patient safety work-net/network through strategic alliances focused on a common object: incremental sophistication of communication between team members within the operating theatre (hereafter 'OT') and across perioperative environments. This analysis from an ANT perspective adds to the work already reported in previous chapters, such as the accounts of moral courage in the OT by staff positioned lower on the traditional team hierarchy, such as nurses.

TTRM has been gathered as an open access website (www.ttrm.co.uk). The website will be updated to include interactive elements, continuing to strengthen the network through a technological ally, and has been adopted by the hospital trust concerned as a platform for developing a rolling in-house staff development programme. This offers an opportunity to develop stronger strategic alliances, particular with trust management, in supporting practice development and innovation. However, strengthening the work-net/network has inevitably invited resistances threatening ruptures, detailed below along with successful alliances.

Research projects tend to be reported as if they were discrete, ahistorical events. A project of course has a life cycle. There are initial grant applications to be made (including unsuccessful bids, where potential networks remain unrealized), grant obligations to be fulfilled, steering committees to be set up and dissolved, interim and final reports to be submitted, researchers to be appointed to short-term posts, Ph.D. theses to be completed and examined, journal papers, conference presentations, and so forth. All projects are necessarily punctuations in a bigger narrative.

Further, as practice changes are adopted and absorbed by the clinical community involved, they become hybrids, locally adapted, and mutable. For example, while we modelled, early in the study, an ideal pre-list team-building briefing, at least five local hybrids evolved including nurses, leading the brief in the Day Case Unit and one surgeon developing a 'horizon' brief a week before lists, scanning potential issues. These hybrids have now been eclipsed by the introduction of a mandatory briefing protocol—the World Health Organization's Surgical Safety Checklist (Gawande, 2009), which itself is destined to be locally adapted and sometimes resisted despite its 'mandatory' status.

The TTRM project tracks the cumulative impact of a number of collaborative changes in activity on the ethos of the OT as a basis to improving patient safety. The 'interruption' to habitual work practices promises a culture change in communication style, from autocratic and hierarchical patterns to democratic, participatory, and dialogical patterns (Bleakley, Allard, & Hobbs, 2013). While ANT's approach is less interventionist and more about interruption, it readily aligns with the values of collaborative inquiry, to research *with* and not *on* practitioners. Practices researched in this context include collaborative briefing and debriefing, before and after a surgical list.

Problematization

ANT is drawn to conundrums, including practices that are historically crystallized, lacking innovation. CHAT, discussed in detail in previous chapters, is a close companion of ANT. CHAT's major proponent, Yrjö Engeström (1999, p. 5), describes how in activity research:

A new theoretical idea or concept is initially produced in the form of an abstract, simple explanatory relationship, a "germ cell". This initial abstraction is step-by-step enriched and transformed into a concrete system of multiple, constantly developing manifestations. In an expansive learning cycle, the initial simple idea is transformed into a complex object, into a new form of practice. At the same time, the cycle produces new theoretical concepts.

An example of this process in action can be drawn from the TTRM project. The core research team argued that the assumption amongst surgical teams that only the lead surgeon could initiate a team briefing should be challenged on the basis that briefing was centrally about establishing team morale and mutual situational awareness (where each member of the team comes to understand other members' roles in a mini-rehearsal of the day's work ahead). This is Engeström's 'germ cell'. As this abstraction was turned into practice, where, for example, nurses led briefings, this challenged assumptions about autocracy as the default political position for the surgical team, to be replaced by participative democracy. As this was further tested, for example, with nurses progressively leading briefing as the norm in day case surgery, so objections to such a model from surgeons were challenged and dismissed.

The initial idea is now established through expansion of the learning cycle as anaesthetists and surgeons begin to see the value of the nurse leading a briefing, where the nurse is already the centre for information exchange and the first stop for patients in the Day Case Unit's extended team. As the practice is developed, so nurses reformulate identities as team leaders, transforming the initial idea into a complex practice that has the immediate effect of collectively raising morale amongst nurses, but also implies the need for parallel, tailored professional development. Theoretical gain emerges from the process of expansion of the activity of briefing, where surgical teams can now be seen to be experimenting with new forms of work-based democracy, and the identity construction of the nurse is positively and radically reformulated.

The activity cycles of expansive learning in CHAT and the strengthening of networks in ANT act as neither sponges nor cookers—respectively, cleaning up and processing raw data. ANT likes its data rare, challenging research studies that draw on a variety of tactics and rhetorical devices to disguise the mess in research that is, after all, a slice of a messy life. By 'rare' I mean data that are not overly analysed or processed ('cooked' would be an alternative here, but not in the sense of manipulating data unethically, to purposefully mislead). A model for this kind of research account is Mol's account of the relationships between people living with diabetes and those professionals who care for them (Mol, 2008). Mol derives an argument that critically addresses the logic of 'patient choice' by showing how such logic, in the cases of the diabetics she follows, often frustrates rather than facilitates good care practices. The argument is derived elegantly from the fieldwork—that exposes multiple ontologies—without the mediation of an overwrought epistemology, or predisposing framework, that may provide a fog to obscure the objects of the research.

Latour (2007, pp. 146–7) notes that approaching research analytically is premature: 'we are in the business of descriptions. ... we go, we listen, we learn ... it's called inquiries. Good inquiries always produce a lot of new descriptions', where 'if your description needs an explanation, it's not a good description'. Conventional research texts often deliberately bracket out context, such as the political, historical, and organizational. ANT texts lean towards thick descriptions and baroque detail.

The design of the TTRM project has its origin in an ethical dilemma that is the central concern of this book. While sometimes high-risk, surgery has an unacceptably high rate of error, and this is grounded not in technical mistakes but in poor communication. Again, an estimated 70 % of medical errors result from miscommunications within and between teams, and 50 % of this is thought to be remediable through improving communication (Kohn, Corrigan, & Donaldson, 1999; Pronovost & Vohr, 2010). Better clinical teamwork in hospitals correlates with lower morbidity and mortality rates and high levels of work morale (West & Borrill, 2002). Improving communication and teamwork in the OT should ultimately benefit patient safety and challenges work practices that jeopardize patient safety. Engeström (2009, p. 5) suggests that:

> The expansive cycle begins with individual subjects questioning the accepted practice, and it gradually expands into a collective movement or institution. The theory of expansive learning is related to Latour's actor-network theory in that both regard innovations as stepwise construction of new forms of collaborative practice, or technoeconomic networks.

On a first round of surveys of 300+ OT staff in 2003 as part of the wider TTRM research that included elements of inquiry other than ANT, we found that perceptions concerning quality of communication differed across professional groups. For example, where 90 % of consultant surgeons said that they have good communication with their surgical colleagues, only 50 % of consultant anaesthetists, 40 % of nurses, and 25 % of trainee anaesthetists reported that they had good communication with consultant surgeons. When asked how often a pre-list briefing occurs, 10 % of surgeons said 'never', 50 % 'occasionally', and 40 % 'always'. When anaesthetists were asked, however, 70 % said 'never', 20 % 'occasionally', and 10 % 'always'. So what model of 'briefing' did those surgeons hold and with whom did they imagine they were briefing? We meticulously followed this fault line.

When we carried out an intensive audit on briefing practices soon after this survey, we found no OT teams who held a properly structured whole team brief, where 'briefing' was often configured as, literally, a brief conversation between the surgeon and anaesthetist and not a team meeting. Five years after introducing our ANT-inspired 'interruption' with OT allies, an audit showed that 20 % of surgical teams were regularly briefing and 15 % debriefing, but that 50 % of individual practitioners reported having been part of a brief that week and 30 % part of a debrief that week. Given what we know about the pace of practice change in conservative surgical environments, this was relatively good news.

In terms of initiating and strengthening a work-net/network through strategic alliances, we knew how problematic this could be in the face of a surgical culture grounded in hierarchy and meritocracy focused on technical ability and knowledge, rather than in participative democracy focused on shared capabilities in communication. In 2004, we videotaped orthopaedic surgical teams. Analysis revealed a clear and consistent pattern that favoured one-way communication (telling, informing, confronting) over dialogue (asking questions, inviting participation), working against 'assembly' democracy (Keane, 2009).

Coordination of care across clinical teams is greatly enhanced by participative democratic structures (Iedema, 2007), sometimes facilitated by objects (artifacts) such as protocols (Gawande, 2009). However, autocratic structures retain a strong, historically contingent presence in medicine and, particularly, surgery. While there is a solid base of evidence suggesting that expanding out to collaboration and connection, rather than shrinking back to the individual, is fundamental to developing a learning organization (Christakis & Fowler, 2010; Surowiecki, 2005), this again bumps up against a historically contingent ideology in medicine and surgery of heroic individualism—itself grounded in the Protestant ethic of self-help.

Where collaboration is not in the historical grain of surgical practice, it has to be learned. Ikegami's (2005) study of the development of 'aesthetic networks' in feudal Japan shows that horizontal, shared, and democratic practices can develop within historically conditioned autocracies and hierarchies. Mutual interests in art and craft encouraged horizontal social interactions that suspended normal, strict rules of conduct based on vertical social hierarchies. The 'nontechnical' or shared elements of surgical work (Flin, O'Connor, & Crichton, 2008)—communication, teamwork, and aspects of decision-making—can be configured as practice 'artistry' (Bleakley et al., 2011), an aesthetic network of immaterial or emotional labour, binding practices horizontally, while technical practices can be expressed not in terms of autocracies but meritocracies.

Initiation of a Network: Champions Meet Sceptics

In late 2002, we were faced with how we could *initiate* a network through increasing our number of allies, mobilizing actors to affect other actors in translations yielding innovations. Enrolment of allies includes negotiating terms of participation, and this forum initiated a key debate about how the entire range of OT personnel could be centrally involved in the project through shared communication and teamwork practices.

We set up an exploratory dialogue between six champions (four consultant anaesthetists, a consultant surgeon, and an experienced nurse) and six sceptics (two consultant surgeons, two consultant anaesthetists, and two senior nurses) in a 2-day human factors seminar. This initiated a dialogical process, where 'an interventionist research methodology is needed which aims at pushing forward, mediating, recording, and analyzing cycles of expansive learning in local activity systems' (Engeström, 2009, p. 2). Some key sceptics (surgeons), for example, were persuaded to road test briefing. Others were deeply ambivalent, mistaking research for management surveillance and already threatening to rupture a delicate, nascent network.

Some radical ideas emerged—for example, how nurses or operating department assistants traditionally low on the hierarchy could be empowered to speak out (a form of 'moral courage' but also an act of professionalism) if they saw activity that may jeopardize a patient's safety. The more 'moral courage', discussed previously, was slighted by sceptics (including some nurses), so the network paradoxically strengthened, and moral courage became an actor and key ally in its own right (Bleakley, 2006b).

Funding

Funding is patently a key actor in research, allowing for enrolment of allies. Funding can, however, act as an intermediary rather than a mediator, supporting a sterile network with lack of translations and a poor net effect, rather than a dynamic network of fertile associations and translations promising innovation, knowledge production, and practice change. Funding translates across actors, for example, buying in the expertise of clinicians to work as researchers.

Grants allowed us, for example, to collaborate with the author of a North American, validated Safety Attitudes Questionnaire (SAQ) in anglicizing the SAQ for UK practitioners (Sexton et al., 2006); to buy in a full-time researcher and two Ph.D. students; to buy in expertise to develop team self-review (briefing and debriefing) (Henderson et al., 2007); and to install videotape recording facilities in two OTs, where, once ethical clearance was received, we could record routine work to supplement ethnographic observations. Videotaped extracts were played back to teams as a stimulus to a 'hot' debriefing, offering a major innovation in research methodology and a powerful addition to the overall educational 'interruption' (Bleakley et al., 2004).

While no surgical team members were in any way forced to engage with the project, a few did harden opinion against the value of the project, culminating in an act of defiance (or sabotage) through physically dismantling connecting cables in the video setup. After 6 months of sporadic filming—gaining key insights—we abandoned the video ethnography to appease the minority of dissenters. By not engaging in open confrontation but accepting the depth of feeling of the clinicians concerned and their rationale for such feeling (suspicion that the project was ultimately a form of management surveillance, questioning surgeons' autonomy), we gained some respect from those clinicians. We followed the advice of Sun Tzu's *The Art of War* that strategy and not hostility wins allies.

Other grants allowed us to, first, employ an experienced theatre nurse to support and evaluate briefing activities over a period of 6 months (Allard et al., 2007); second, to develop a close call reporting system that later included hiring a recently retired consultant anaesthetist to close the loop locally on reports, where an issue raised by a report is addressed with practitioners in an effort to resolve the issue (e.g. ensuring that protocols are adhered to or that faulty equipment is fixed rapidly) (Hobbs & Bleakley, 2005); and third, to set up a centre of excellence recognized by European Social Funding as a platform for international networking and to develop the open access website (www.ttrm.co.uk).

The website offers a mixed blessing through a design fault. While promising to act as an ally in mediating translations between actors, an interactive component was not built in so that the website paradoxically became an intermediary rather than a mediator—a frozen web and repository of authoritative information, rather than a site for translation and negotiation. One of our aims for the near future is therefore to raise funds to develop interactive elements for the website.

A Multiprofessional Conference

In December 2002, we arranged a 1-day human factors symposium for as many staff as possible to advertise and kick-start the project. OTs closed down apart from emergency provision, and attendees ranged from cleaners and porters to consultant surgeons and key members of management and the public, including the Chair of the trust. The morning offered unique small group discussions, where cleaners and porters discussed issues along with researchers, managers, and clinicians. Many reported that this was the first time that they had experienced such a democratic levelling. The afternoon offered specialist input from an ex-airline-pilot-turned-safety champion and human factors researchers, including data from observation of paediatric heart surgery teams.

Consciousness raising was clearly established and the network effect was powerful and formative. However, the conference also had the paradoxical effect of producing a kind of toxic shock. While bringing home the message concerning the importance of improving teamworking to establish a patient safety culture, the news from the airlines that such a culture change took around 15 years to establish produced a kind of numbing amongst some participants, as if the challenge was actually too great to contemplate.

Hard and Soft Design

Cumulative, unidirectional attitude change creates a climate and lays the foundation for culture change. We saw no point in attempting to change work activities without first changing attitudes towards that work. This would be equivalent to introducing a mandatory protocol without the will of those who would have to follow it.

Our key outcome measure of climate change was cumulative scores on each component of the SAQ—particularly 'teamwork' and 'safety climate'. Significant positive changes in scores from a baseline measure would indicate a climate shift. We were also—serendipitously—able to offer the intervention to one discrete OT complex and then to a second complex of similar size 1 year later to compare both cumulative SAQ scores across complexes and changes from baseline scores within complexes. To gauge culture change, we employed qualitative methods guided by an ANT framework—ethnographic observations, videotaped examples of practice, open-ended interviews, and free-text comments on the SAQ.

In using the SAQ, alliances were made with an international community of researchers, widening the network effect and multiplying the numbers of actors as mediators, again facilitating translations leading to innovations. The author of the SAQ was able to insert our baseline data into an international database, so that we could compare scores from our hospital cohort with those from other OT cohorts internationally. This proved to be an effective leverage data in persuading our senior management to become mediating actors in the widening network where, in comparison with a large number of international hospital cohorts, our SAQ scores indicated a relatively low level of development of an active safety culture as perceived by OT personnel. This one piece of evidence served initially as an effective way to gain senior management allies in strengthening the patient safety work-net/network, although key senior management figures in general have acted as intermediaries rather than mediators in the project.

Team Self-Review

Having confirmed through observation lack of a culture of team self-review, a team of social science researchers and clinicians modelled, initiated, and facilitated briefing and debriefing practices across a sample of OT teams. A comprehensive handbook of techniques was produced and distilled down to bullet points on credit card-sized prompts circulated to all OT staff (Henderson et al., 2007). Suggested practices encouraged team building through communication, reflective practice (debrief), and reflexive accounting (innovation resulting from team self-review) (Bleakley et al., 2011), cumulatively building a safety net for patients. This was further networked through the key artifact (actor) of a regular newsletter circulated amongst all OT staff that kept them up to date on research findings and implications, including the percentage of teams carrying out briefing and/or debriefing and accounts of local styles. Data were also fed back and discussed face to face at audit and education meetings.

Networking with Clinicians and Academics

Networks are expanded and strengthened across the clinical education community through dissemination of research texts by publication and conference presentations. Through invitation, we have taken TTRM on the road to many national hospitals and three Canadian hospitals. Where ANT is still perceived as a radical or even wayward approach within clinical education research and particularly within health services research, where positivistic models dominate, strengthening network effects through creating alliances is an exciting challenge.

Research Texts

Texts, such as this chapter, are naturally and sometimes frustratingly partial—but then so is the slice of life that is researched. The point of an ANT approach is to render interesting objects visible that might otherwise remain black-boxed. Visibility of actors and translations between actors is the focus of the research text, researching issues through tracing the network.

For example, Frode (2010) describes complex interactions between members of a breast cancer care team—cytologists, surgeons, and radiologists—with emphasis upon key objects, such as X-rays, cytology pictures, and a form held by the patient used to record diagnoses and passed between surgeons, cytologists, and radiologists as the patient visited each in turn. Frode followed the breast cancer unit in a Norwegian hospital for 18 months and also conducted interviews, showing how team meetings based around a patient led at best to a 'loosely coupled' system and at worse to disintegration.

In loosely coupled systems, networks might be traced but were faint and did not stabilize from week to week as the forms of connections between the three specialties were more or less reinvented on every occasion in discussing patients. Tightly coupled systems leading to strong networks were never realized. Potential networks were also frustrated or quickly disintegrated. For example, a radiologist within the team used specialist knowledge to frustrate potential collaboration between specialties by insisting that X-rays could only be properly read by radiologists. The form held by the patient came to be utilized sequentially by the three specialties, and then acted as an intermediary between those doctors, rather than being used as a mediator in a common meeting. Frode's account offers a thick description of a potential network that is constantly frustrated, as the inherent potency of objects as mediators (such as the patient's form) is never realized, where such objects, actants, or actors only act as intermediaries.

Law (2004, p. 21) suggests that ANT research is guided by a baroque rather than a Romantic sensibility, where we should 'look down' to get an overall grasp of relations between actors and the messy, sensuous materiality of practice—detail and texture—rather than looking up for some guiding ideal, a framework, or principle. Latour (2007, pp. 133–5) suggests keeping a series of notebooks during fieldwork to record the voices of the actors and the effects of translations, the recruitment of allies, your own responses, your wild ideas, and effects of feeding back data to participants.

Public Engagement Through the Arts

The public has come to see medicine and surgery through the rather distorted lens of UK and North American television soap operas (Bleakley et al., 2011). TTRM has widened and strengthened the research network through alliances with dramatists, actors, and visual artists in particular to develop public engagement and education projects. These have included schoolchildren making films about their experiences in hospital; visual artists tracking the patients' perspectives from diagnosis through surgery to recovery, presented as video, drawing, and painting; and use of actors working with clinicians in scripting and preparation of video vignettes for teaching purposes, also uploaded to the website for open access. The work-net/network effect then also includes the enrolment of web designers. The point of engagement has included gallery exhibitions, public open days, and conferences, and the video resources are widely used in teaching medical students and junior doctors. Through medical humanities and medicine and arts funding bodies, these activities have attracted significant research funding.

In summary, the movement into the public arena initiates new actor-network possibilities, where the innovation resulting from translations across the network between actors is the opening to public gaze of what has, historically, been a closed profession.

Work-Net/Network Effects

Rather than list 'outcomes' of the research, an ANT approach would look at the dynamic work-net that has been created. This goes well beyond the immediate instrumental outcomes of research that may be required by a particular funding body, as the section on public engagement above illustrates. In ANT, since the outcome of a project depends on the alliances created and the translation effects across an unpredictable number of persons, material objects, and ideas, an a priori statement about aims or goals is considered premature. Rather than rational(ized) outcomes, we need to speak of the aggregation of interests determined by the nature of the net effect of the research. Or, what is the quality of impression or trace left by the work-net/network as it is cut at the point of writing up the research work?

What is held primarily as a net effect of the TTRM project so far is a shift in attitudes towards the importance of communication within and across team settings. The cumulative effect of this is the establishment of a safety climate, which we see as the necessary condition of possibility for the emergence of a safety culture—a distinctive change in work practices. Some of this innovation is evident. For example, not only was the ground prepared for the introduction of the WHO surgical safety checklist but also it is already being translated—*mindfully* utilized within a team-building ethos rather than instrumentally, simply as a checklist. We know, for example, from further empirical work that those practitioners who report improvement in safety climate across surgical environments are also those who engage in briefing—in other words, values precede and shape behaviour (Allard, Bleakley, Hobbs, & Coombes, 2011). There is no point in trying to introduce an educational intervention or a protocol without first establishing a fertile ground, a 'climate' or common attitudinal state, that is receptive to the desired practice (Genn, 2001).

Section III: Limitations to ANT-Based Research

ANT Research Demands Specialists

By now, some readers will have decided that ANT is not for them—it is perhaps too cavalier; others will find it theory heavy or simply out of their comfort zone, employing an already idiosyncratic vocabulary idiosyncratically. Others will be attracted to its apparently naïve realism, its refreshing unorthodoxy, its attraction to the problematic, its refusal to offer reductive answers, and its radically democratic agenda of generalized symmetry.

ANT sets out pretty stringent conditions for membership. Special qualities are needed for taking ethnography into the territory that ANT delineates, such as sensibilities of witnessing, close noticing and attention to context that are aesthetic and ethical, and not primarily instrumental. Patience and restraint are needed, as fieldwork is intensive and time consuming. Just how such qualities and related identities are developed and performed is not well articulated in the ANT literature. Paradoxically, while ANT proposes a radical democracy of phenomena, it appears to encourage an elite body of researchers.

Key writers such as Bruno Latour and Annemarie Mol are stylists and use experimental forms that set very high standards. Latour in particular takes delight in baroque sentences. Here is a piece of advice for the novice fieldworker concerning translation from notebooks to research text: 'The unique adequacy one should strive for in deploying complex imbroglios cannot be obtained without continuous sketches and draft' (Latour, 2007, p. 134). Well, 'imbroglio' means entanglement, and surely 'complex' is then redundant. Deployment is a militaristic word meaning to get in place ready for battle, and is this really how ANT researchers must go about their business in both fieldwork and writing up? Indeed, ANT's overall stance may look militaristic. This chapter uses similar rhetorical devices—particularly metaphors of 'strengthening' networks and conversely, nascent and delicate networks open to rupture. Perhaps we should use less militaristic tropes, encouraging an ANT sensibility of 'presence' rather than 'force'. For some, the language of force is already gendered male. Perhaps ANT's genesis in science studies rather than the humanities already affords tough-mindedness rather than tender-mindedness.

Can ANT Demand Both Precision and Ambiguity?

ANT seems to demand precision and ambiguity at the same time and this may infect research practices. While Latour (1993, 2010) is at pains to point out that the curse of modernism is to aim for purity (whether through truth seeking or ethnically and racially), and where reality is hybrid and messy, what do we make of his insistence on a precise definition of the key notion of 'network', where 'The word network is so ambiguous that we should have abandoned it long ago' (Latour, 2007, p. 129)? ANT feeds off uncertainties, unexpected turns in events, upsets, slippage in practices, impressions, and traces. Surely 'network' must retain ambiguity? As ANT researchers are we not expected to readily tolerate such ambiguity? Further, in cultivating ambiguity as a virtue, where does morality rest in a network? ANT is strangely silent on the ethics of research.

Does ANT Support Animism?

ANT's philosophical position (Harman, 2009) raises the spectre of animism. Where 'actors' include material objects, do objects have agency, and how can interaction between material objects produce non-material effects? ANT's answer to this is straightforward—it does not posit agency for objects, but is interested in the potential and actual connections between things and the outcomes of such connections. As an example, here is a close call report from the operating theatre, part of the dataset of our TTRM study:

> The operating table had a new mattress in place. The patient needed to be positioned naked on a gel mat on the mattress in order to prevent slipping off the table when steep head down tilt is applied to the table. The gel mat was positioned on the table. When the patient was moved onto the gel mat, the gel mat slipped across the table mattress. Because the mattress is very smooth, there is no grip to allow friction between the gel mat and table mattress.

The report does not, however, assign agency to the gel mat or the table mattress. Rather, it points out that the *relationship* between the two is translational or has a transformative effect—of putting the patient at risk through slipping and then of effecting practice change. Something now has to be done to prevent a reoccurrence. Somebody and something has to get a grip. I warned that ANT research is drawn to slippage!

Here is a more serious slippage—one of attention. This report also illustrates the logic of generalized symmetry:

> A valve came loose/detached from a disposable laparoscopic port and into a patient's abdominal cavity. It was only by chance it was noticed inside the patient and then removed.

It is because person, material object, and protocol are brought together in translation and mediation in safety-sensitive care that such a scenario would normally never occur. In this case, again, we should suspend thinking about agency for objects and think about connections between things. Indeed connections and disconnections abound, while a main connection was not immediately made—double-checking the patient and the equipment before, during, and after procedures so that there is no 'by chance' and a valve does not 'come loose', to ghost in 'by chance'. It is the connection between laparoscope and person that does the work of 'noticing' and picks up on the loose valve and not the disconnection between person and instrument that is signified in the phrase 'by chance'. But 'chance' is not good enough for optimum patient safety.

Resisting Reduction

Finally, and paradoxically, for ANT itself to recruit allies and strengthen its work-net, it must be able to tolerate reduction to its Wikipedia form of presentation (http://en.wikipedia.org/wiki/Actor-network_theory) where it is readily black-boxed, confirming Latour's (1999a) fear that a complex apprehension is reduced to a rule of thumb centred on a misunderstanding of 'network'. While Wikipedia explicitly invites revision, entries appear authoritative, soaked in the ethos of encyclopaedic knowledge and resisting interventions. ANT's Wikipedia entry—strangely spawning a paper equivalent (anonymous: actor-network theory, 2010) is a good example of a congealed network. The site actually exerts minimum sweat, doing little work where it has settled and crystallized, failing to interact with other actors in a work-net effect of translation. Will ANT's entry over time into clinical education research lead to a similar dilution and congealing of its dynamic concerns or will it stimulate a welcome revolution in research thinking and method?

I believe that ANT's future as both an exploratory and explanatory framework in medical education research is guaranteed because of its power to understand communication at the level of network. This is the level at which we may best improve team-based communication, where cross-team networks with patients as attractors are the norm. These networks are unfortunately called patient 'pathways', which I suppose conjures up an image of progression, but which fails to capture how a 'safety net' can be established for patients as a living network creating allies and translations across its components.

To this picture of dynamic team interaction, resulting in varieties of networks (some of which are planned, but fail to be initiated; others fail to involve translations, where intermediaries outweigh mediators, and they crystallize; where others are vibrant and develop with gusto), we must now add the fact that team members tend to be 'nomadic' or 'fluid'. The days of the stable 'firm' are over. How might we theorize this emergent nomadicity of team members? In the following chapter, I extend ANT to a discussion of 'Deleuzian rhizomatics'. If the twentieth century was the century of Michel Foucault and new understanding of power (as capillary, to form resistances, as well as sovereign), the twenty-first century promises to be the era of Gilles Deleuze. Let us now move to his potential contributions to understanding team-based communication in medicine and medical education, where the focus shifts to identity constructions in the liquid world of medical work.

Chapter 14
Theorizing Team Process Through Deleuzian Rhizomatics: Becoming a Medical Professional in Nomadic Teams

Introduction: From Being to Becoming

We have seen how the so-called 'nontechnical' (communication) in medicine has become as important as the technical aspects of the work. When research first began in earnest in the field of communication in medicine, especially as it shifted from initial interest in the consultation to team-based hospital work, 'work' was relatively stable. In less than 2 decades since the first wave of intensive research in communication in hospital settings, work has become much more fluid and unpredictable, complex and dynamic. I have borrowed terms such as 'fluid' and 'liquid' (also more feminine descriptors) to describe the new regimes of hospital work. Engeström's (2008) key work on managing patients with multiple chronic illnesses in the community shows that similar levels of complexity now inhabit family or community medicine, where family practitioners are less part of a 'team' and more part of a dynamic web of activities.

We need powerful, contemporary theoretical models to understand the changing face of health-care in these new, liquid, and complex settings. Importantly, we also need to grasp how epistemological, ontological, and axiological dimensions to the new work cultures play out—by this, I mean the relationships between theoretical frames for understanding (epistemologies or theories of knowledge), the experience of persons undergoing activities such as medical and health-care work (ontological dimensions or issues of 'being' and 'becoming'), and the values that inform such work and identity constructions and management of plural identities (moral positions). In this chapter, I draw on the work of Gilles Deleuze to illuminate this complex emerging relationship between what we know, who we are, and what we value in communication in medicine and health-care.

This will draw us away from discussing systems at the level of the team and the organization, to the system that is the person, the professional, and practitioner. As work becomes liquid, so identities multiply and have to be managed as fluid forms. Deleuze, drawing on the inspiration of the seventeenth-century philosopher Baruch Spinoza in particular, characterizes this world of fluid identities as one of

A. Bleakley, *Patient-Centred Medicine in Transition: The Heart of the Matter*, Advances in Medical Education 3, DOI 10.1007/978-3-319-02487-5_14, © Springer International Publishing Switzerland 2014

'becoming' rather than 'being'—shifting focus from *who* we are, as if we have essences, to *how* we are, in terms of managing multiple roles and then multiple identities—first and foremost as 'professional' practitioner (technical specialist) and as 'interprofessional' team player (nontechnical or communication generalist).

The instrumental process of becoming a medical professional has followed a similar pattern worldwide for a century (Ludmerer, 1999). This may seem to be a mark of medical education's enduring success, but it can also be read as a failure to adapt to cultural change (Bleakley, Bligh, & Browne, 2011). Since the revolution in undergraduate medical education provision brought about by Abraham Flexner's (1910) report on North American medical schools (Flexner, 1910), prequalifying programmes in medicine have followed a model of a preclinical (classroom knowledge) phase followed by a clinical (applied knowledge) phase. Programmes vary in whether they have direct entry from school (normally 5 years) or graduate entry (normally 4 years). Graduation normally leads into a qualifying junior doctor apprenticeship (internship) ranging across medical specialties and concentrating on hospital medicine. Specialization may then follow a career path to senior clinical grades in a hospital specialty, surgery, or as a community (family or general) practitioner. Adjunct specialties, such as academic medicine and management, may also be pursued. The UK Tooke Report (Tooke, 2008, pp. 203–220) on postgraduate medical education reforms provides an international comparison of provision across seven countries.

An instrumental accounting for career stages tells us little about the identity construction of the doctor—of what it is to become a medical professional. Policy documents such as the UK General Medical Council's *Good Medical Practice* (2006) and *The New Doctor* (2007)—prescribing the basic content of undergraduate and postgraduate medical education curricula—offer instrumental accounts of what medical students and doctors are expected to know and do at various stages of their careers. Where such documentation strays into the territory of identity, it is vague and often pious. Becoming a doctor may be reduced to an ideal of the consummate professional described by a set of traits—such as probity and the ability to maintain one's own health—through which 'professionalism' can be both conceptualized and measured (Stern, 2006a, 2006b).

The flipside of the focus upon virtues of the consummate professional is the interest in students' and doctors' 'professional lapses', and in students' willingness, or reluctance, to report perceived professional lapses of their seniors (Ginsburg & Lingard, 2006). Paradoxically, research evidence, quoted at length throughout the opening chapters of this book, suggests that the profession of medicine as a whole has already lapsed professionally, where there is a continuing, chronic, inability for doctors to communicate well, or 'professionally', as measured against prescriptions of the policy documents noted above. This includes poor communication with patients (Coulter, 2002; Roter & Hall, 2006), between medical specialties (Wadhwa & Lingard, 2006), and with other health-care professionals (Kohn, Corrigan, & Donaldson, 1999).

Gabriel Weston (2009, p. 135), a surgeon who writes about her work, describes how 'It is no longer enough to be technically proficient; nowadays, we need to be nice'. This may be tongue in cheek, or it may just show a typical reluctance to engage with the surgeon's wider role, where 'nice' is a rather strange choice of word for the necessity of clear and supportive communication, now supported by a good evidence base. Another surgeon who writes about his work, Atal Gawande (2002, 2007), is clear about the need for effective communication, reminding us that patients are put at risk not just because of technical errors, but also as a result of miscommunications. As insistently reported many times throughout this book, the Institute of Medicine (Kohn et al., 1999) and The Joint Commission on Accreditation of Health-care Organisation (2001) figures concur—that as much as 70 % of medical errors are grounded in nontechnical issues, as systemic miscommunications (see also Singh, Thomas, Petersen, & Studdart, 2007). Further, half of these may be avoidable through improving communication and collaboration between doctors themselves and between doctors and other health-care professionals. Becoming a medical professional is also becoming an effective communicator and collaborator, helping to restore the professional 'lapse' of an entire culture, rather than simply lapsed individuals (high profile 'bad apple' doctors such as Harold Shipman) or individual lapses.

The instrumental description of how medical students and doctors proceed through, respectively, an undergraduate and postgraduate medical education has typically been fleshed out through longitudinal ethnographic studies of the socialization of medical students, doctors, and surgeons (Atkinson, 1995; Becker, Geer, Hughes, & Strauss, 1980; Cassell, 1991, 2000; Katz, 2000; Millman, 1976). Here, we learn of the 'hidden curriculum' of medical education—rites of passage, role modelling, and uses of symbols in, sometimes brutally, shaping character, style, and identity. But these accounts are already historical curiosities, as we are now entering a radically new era of medical education, reformulating earlier notions of what it is to become a doctor.

This chapter seeks to understand the becoming of medical professionals of the future and utilizes a theoretical approach to identity construction that is future focused. This approach is drawn mainly from the work of the French philosopher Gilles Deleuze, with reference also to Deleuze's extensive collaboration with the French psychiatrist Félix Guattari (Deleuze & Guattari, 2004a, 2004b; Guattari, 1995), offering an exploratory and explanatory framework that responds to the cultural and historical shift from high modernism to an emerging cultural era variously called postmodern and late modern, a 'risk society' and 'runaway world' (Giddens, 2002) and 'liquid modernity' (Bauman, 2000).

The ethnographies studying socialization into medicine and surgery mentioned above describe a chronically conservative legacy, where doctors and surgeons were typed—or more often stereotyped—as heroic and paternalistic individuals. Medical students were seen to emulate these traits as a central part of their education of character, absorbing them through role modelling as the main form of identity construction. Reading these studies through Deleuzian eyes, doctors can be described, historically, as 'becoming autocrats'. In the new era of patient-centred and collaborative medical practices, doctors now enter a process of 'becoming democrats'.

Although systematic and well chronicled, and following in an established philosophical tradition of vitalism (Deleuze, 1991), there is no easy way in to Deleuze's thought, which relies heavily on neologism and idiosyncratic readings of vitalist philosophers such as Spinoza and Nietzsche. A Deleuze 'primer' is an oxymoron, although Stivale's (2005) edited collection of essays promises to present Deleuze's 'key concepts' to the neophyte. More importantly, once inside Deleuze's world, it may seem as if there is no easy way out as one of the characteristics of this world is its fascination. One of Deleuze's central metaphors is the 'fold', borrowed from the German philosopher Leibniz. To be inside a fold is to experience the interiority of a phenomenon through an enfolding, or full immersion, in that phenomenon as a dynamic process. This is perhaps the closest we will get to a complete description of the 'becoming' of the medical professional, the identity construction of the doctor. The doctor's clinical experience, particularly in the early years, is so all-consuming and pervasive—the realization of a vocation—that it can readily be described as an envelopment in the lives of others, primarily patients and secondarily colleagues.

Conventional studies of the identity construction of doctors, such as the ethnographies mentioned earlier, describe how stability is achieved in identity, how a core self is realized and expressed. This is to be expected of a generation of academics writing at the height of interest in existentialism, phenomenology, and the search for 'authenticity'. Academic interests and foci have changed, and in this chapter a different approach is taken to these traditional ethnographies. From a Deleuzian perspective, one would ask how a permanently labile and multiple identity construction is managed, temporarily stabilized, and understood as a process amongst many intersecting processes. The main shift is from stability to dynamism. This is prefigured in the vitalist philosophers who inspired Deleuze, particularly Spinoza and Nietzsche, both interested in 'power' as personal 'potency' or intensity.

The identity of the doctor is then not treated as 'selfsame' (the stabilization of a professional self, identified with similar others in a stable professional community of practice), but as a consequence of 'difference' in a context of instability—difference from the 'other' with whom one works, primarily other professionals (such as nurses), but most importantly the stream of 'others' the doctor meets as patients. It is in the face of the Other that the identity of the doctor is realized, in an inherently unstable space of difference moving through time.

This model of becoming, realized in dynamic difference, is described in three ways—first, as a 'self-forming' in terms of an assemblage of characteristics shaped by a shifting culture; second, as the undoing and distribution of the modernist medical gaze; and third, as an effect of three levels of textual practices—work-based, autoethnographic, and virtual (as representations of doctors in television soap operas). These three faces of 'becoming a medical professional' are centred on the key identity *activity* of the doctor—as diagnostician or symptomatologist—where the bread and butter work of a doctor is to make a diagnosis through reading symptoms and listening to the case history, offering a prognosis, and formulating a treatment plan.

Deleuzian Becoming: Processes and Assemblages

As introduced above, Deleuze and Guattari, most famously in the two-volume work *Capitalism and Schizophrenia* (2004a, 2004b), develop a complex model of 'becoming', situated in the philosophical tradition of vitalism—Spinoza, Bergson, and Nietzsche in particular. This worldview privileges dynamism over the static object. Life is necessarily unformed and forming—in a state of 'becoming' rather than 'being'—where process is privileged over essence.

In early and high modernism, particularly from the Enlightenment period at the end of the eighteenth century, emphasis was placed upon the stabilizing of identity—the expression of a core self. Indeed, forms of 'madness' have been described mainly as the loss of a sense of core self (alienation, neurosis) or multiplication of selves (psychosis). Psychology became the dominant discipline for exploring identity, which became associated with personality and character rather than as a product of cultural forces. As Louis Sass (1994) suggests in *Madness and Modernism*, late modernism of the early twentieth century had already signalled radically new approaches to the self—through the avant-garde of art and literature—that challenged the notion of stability equating to health. The self was recognized as split, fractured, and multiple in its 'ordinary' states, where a fixed, frozen, or congealed self was now described as potentially authoritarian, rigid, and neurotic.

Postmodernism challenges the notion of self as constitutive or given, reading identity as constituted or constructed socially, and 'situated' (Bleakley, 2000a, 2000b). A constituted identity is not a subject (an expression of a coherent interior 'self'), but 'subject to'—a product or construct of cultural, historical, and social circumstance. In this view, a work-based 'professional' self is not seen as a 'given', a personality expression, but as situated, an effect of a variety of unstable and dynamic historical, cultural, and social forces that are temporarily stabilized through processes of learning, examination, and practices—most importantly in medicine as cumulative patient contact leading to gaining expertise as a diagnostician.

In his last published work on late Greek and early Roman forms of aesthetic and ethical self-forming, or 'care of self', Michel Foucault (1990, 2005) draws attention to the paradox of a contemporary Western culture in which we celebrate the supposed 'freedoms' of self-hood (especially in sexuality) but are actually constrained by a variety of forms of regulatory structures, forming an overall 'governmentality' within a surveillance society. These include new forms of what the Classical world saw as 'self-forming', a making of character, through self-help techniques. Self-forming or 'self-fashioning' (Greenblatt, 1980) was revived in Renaissance Europe as an educational process. This shaping of character is a form of positioning identity within a web of regulatory devices, where identity can be described as 'assemblage' (DeLanda, 1997, 2006) and potential, always in process. In the professional identity formation of the doctor, often expressed as 'lifelong learning', there is not just an accumulation or sedimentation of knowledge, skills, and attitudes, but a process of 'becoming doctor' as assemblage—a dynamic identity construction shaped within a web of regulatory devices.

Foucault's work draws attention to the interplay between a governed identity and processes of resistance to particular forms of identity construction, where Deleuze's work emphasizes interplay between, and intensities within, assemblages that shape professional identity, such as 'becoming doctor'. From Deleuze's (1993) analysis of 'the fold', 'becoming' involves an (en)folding into (and unfolding out of) an assemblage that, read through Spinoza, affords a certain potency. This view is in sharp contrast to the idea of an unfolding of a given self as the realization of innate potential, where the dimension of potency is weakly expressed as 'potential'. An assemblage affording potency may be any point in the career trajectory of the doctor, such as graduation as a medical student, passage through junior doctor (intern) education and training, and beyond, through specialty grades (resident) and membership examinations, to the achievement of consultant (attending) status.

Where new thinking about professional identity construction—as becoming rather than being—stresses process, dynamism, lability, and fluidity, this mirrors a wider 'runaway' and 'liquid' culture, as noted above. In such thinking, models of stabilizing identity are given less credibility than dynamicist views of 'managing' an inherently unstable identity in which 'becoming' is not something to be mastered, but is always in production and carries an unpredictable surplus.

Where identity is not given, but is *made as a work*, the identity of the doctor is a work achieved in the workplace, in clinical contact with patients and primarily in acts of diagnosis. Where subjectivity is read not from the inside out (as expression of self) but from the outside in (as subjectivation or positionings of identity in relation to sets of dynamic forces), then becoming a doctor can be seen to be a *series* of identity positions held in network or assemblage—a set of constructions of identity. As Bruno Latour (2007, p. 217) suggests, within actor-network-theory: 'attachments are first, actors are second'. The actor is networked, or engaged by the system, as a product of the potency of attachment. Medical students and junior doctors characteristically learn their work incrementally through a series of clinical 'attachments'. Such attachments offer a series of assemblages that are identity positions held temporarily in place, also invoking emotional attachments of various intensities, producing varieties of affective capital.

It is not just knowledge and skill that sediments to produce a 'doctor' or drives the doctor to specialize in a certain field. Rather, values entrenched in certain specialties entangle doctors or enfold them, in ways that permanently stain the psyche and leave lasting impressions. These gather to provide an axiological dimension to becoming a doctor—the acquisition of values—that informs both ontological development (identity construction) and epistemological development (knowing).

Félix Guattari (2008, pp. 24–25) does not speak of the subject, but of 'components of subjectification'. The becoming of identity (rather than its being, say as an 'authentic self') is a continuous making—the product of the meeting of a number of vectors or forces in a life. These are larger historical and cultural forces (such as the changing position of women in medicine or the reorganization of junior doctor training) and local forces (such as this particular hospital unit's methods or the idiosyncratic style of this supervising consultant). What has been called 'interiority' of the self—available through introspection—is, for Guattari, again a product of a meeting of forces, so that 'Interiority establishes itself at the crossroads of multiple components', vectors, or 'force fields' (Massumi, 1992).

A significant vector is the presence of the 'other', such as a patient or colleague. Guattari focuses us back on how difference comes to act as an engine for identity construction in a process of 'doubling'. Not only is self realized in difference from another (recognition) but also is the other realized as the inside of thought in oneself that is speculative about thought inside the other. Thus, as a diagnostician, the doctor comes to be *inside the somatic 'thought' of the patient*. This is more than 'empathy', a rather weak contemporary construction, as previously argued in Chap. 8, where it is a stark realization of 'difference'.

Persons are subject to various forces in time and space that crisscross and, at points, form assemblages, temporary stabilizations. A language is needed to describe this model that goes beyond psychology's tradition of 'subject', 'personality', 'character', and 'traits'. For Deleuze and Guattari, borrowing from the vitalist tradition, a 'becoming' is best described in terms of nonlinear powers, vectors, intensities, and lines of flight. Professional development, as becoming rather than being, is neither a singular nor a coherent process, but involves several processes at once, operating at different speeds.

Three Planes of Becoming

Deleuze and Guattari do not dismiss traditional ways of accounting for identity construction, as a process of being, or character expression characteristically learned through role modelling (Deleuze & Parnett, 2007, pp. 124–5). Rather, they offer staged challenges and alternatives to this view in a spectrum of possible ways of describing identity. At one end of the spectrum is segmentation.

A segmented identity is defined, bounded, bordered, and patrolled. This is the traditional professional structure and the official story of identity construction. Its core elements are personality or character, role, and role modelling. It is a process necessarily subject to transcendent organization or rule. Segmentarity in medicine and medical professionalism is represented in policy regulation and prescription of role, as the official story of how professionalism may be achieved. As indicated earlier, in this view professionalism is a set of ideal performances grounded in character traits, such as 'honesty' and 'trustworthiness', further grounded in good personal 'health'. While professionalism has a developmental dimension, including a proto-professionalism, 'professional lapses' are subject to censure. The segmented identity suggests a strong character with an internal backbone (a sense of morality) developing like a tree (aspiration), where growth is a product of strong governance internalized as self-governance.

A second level of identity construction challenges this strong model of agency and puts more emphasis upon the context in which the tree develops. Segmentation is replaced by suppleness. Deleuze and Parnett (2007) pun on the idea of a (supple) ment (an added extra to the strong model of agency), where they describe a supple(mentarity). Here, there is some loosening of structures in identity formation to account for the potential of the system(s) within which identity develops, containing unknown qualities. The sense of a strong core (a consistent 'self') is replaced by ideas of nodes, attractors, and flash points as places where critical changes may occur in identity construction. Here, the idea of a linear development in career is disrupted, taking into account a range of realities such as maternity breaks, career shifts, structural employment problems, burnout, illness, and serendipity. There is now a shift from 'being' to 'becoming', and the idea of connections is introduced as key to understanding a shift from content to process explanations. Development of identity is no longer a 'straight-down-the-line' affair but involves modifications and detours.

The idea of an identity influx is introduced, with the notion of thresholds of change. As an illustration, if we take the identity of the undergraduate medicine curriculum itself, this has a formal and informal face. The informal face is the hidden curriculum. This is necessarily unstable, unpredictable, and unplanned. It is by definition neurotic, anxious. The identity construction of the doctor will necessarily have a hidden curriculum. The tapestry that is the official, orderly, story of the policy document (segmentation) is now turned over to reveal greater uncertainty—in a tangle of threads—as the vulnerable human encounters the ideal segmented structure. The model of the tree must now include its context for development, its environmental surround that is in flux, both seen and unseen.

Focus drifts from the trunk to the hidden roots that feed the trunk and the supportive structures that engage symbiotically with the far reaches of the root structure. Here, we find rhizomatic and mycorrhizal structures (Engeström, 2008). The rhizome tangles with other rhizomes to form an underground structure that may look messy to the above ground view, but is perfectly adapted as a network or meshwork. Mycorrhizae (fungal structures) live symbiotically with plant roots and can form huge underground structures from which an occasional mushroom emerges above ground as the reproductive structure. In this shift from segmentarity to supplementarity, we recognize that becoming a doctor—even as a career trajectory—has an unconscious life and an absent story. The doctor's identity construction is necessarily *enmeshed*.

A radical break with segmentarity, and even with (supple)mentarity, occurs with lines of flight. Here, we are in the world of Spinoza's potencies and potentials—forces and possibilities. In terms of development of identity, 'lines of flight' operate as a rhetorical device, a trope, persuading us out of fixed ideas of identity as interior and stable. We are now prepared for radical shifts, transversality, sudden irruptions and reversals, chance and fate. Lines of flight cut across previously segmented organizations and structures with unpredictable force. Now, identity is a product of assemblages, has greater ambiguity and uncertainty, and is always labile. Lines of flight are not abstract potencies but products of the real. Ironically, policy makers act as if they bring stability, but are obsessed by change—new ways of organizing clinical work, new management structures, and new patient charters. This places doctors in contexts of nomadism and deterritorialization, where they can no longer put down roots in practices or organizational structures, as these are open to permanent revolution. In many cases, this reflects the changing terrain of medical knowledge, where practices have to be updated on a regular basis to reflect the emergent, sometimes conflicting, research evidence.

In the new conditions of work in medicine, described in more detail below, there is a need for professionals to be literally more mobile, and metaphorically more flexible, in their working habits. This is a recurring theme throughout this book. The old structures of bounded teams and firms have given way to more flexible structures of multidisciplinary collaboration around patients. This means that traditional, bounded territories have to be relinquished in a new mode of 'deterritorializing'. Those who previously gained identities of consistency and stability within fixed territorial boundaries may now find themselves in the identity of the nomad, on short-term placements, temporary contracts, and working across disciplines.

In Deleuzian studies, three new academic approaches have been developed to articulate and analyse these lines of flight: micropolitics, rhizomatics, and cartography. Micropolitics discusses power relations, mediated by rules and roles, in local contexts. Identities are constructed out of such politics. In medicine, micropolitics will typically involve confirmations of identity through retreat to the uniprofessional role—maintaining strong boundaries between doctors and others. Deleuzian micropolitics map out how identities shift as a result of breakdown in traditional 'silo' structures. For example, what happens when traditional vertical hierarchies in the operating theatre, based on knowledge and skill levels, are challenged in a focus upon shared practices in communication for patient safety (Henderson et al., 2007)? Indeed, it is often the case that where communication skills are the focus, nurses are better at this than doctors or surgeons (Bleakley, 2006b).

The line of flight introduced by research in patient safety, linking safety to quality of communication and collaboration within and across teams, introduces the need for new identities of 'expert collaborator' and 'interprofessional'. The same argument applies to a shift from paternalistic medicine to patient-centred practice. The line of flight of patient-centredness cuts across traditional identities and requires a new micropolitical climate of democratic practices informed by dialogue. Again, *the identity shift from 'being an autocrat' to 'becoming a democrat' is absolutely central to the emergence of a new medical professional for the twenty-first century.*

Rhizomatics is micropolitics without the power implications. It describes the distributed cognitive architecture underpinning practices. Just what are the horizontal structures of a new democracy in medicine? Rhizomatics describes such structures. Nobody has been more productive in this field than Yrjö Engeström (2008) who has coined, or sometimes recovered and reworked, a new vocabulary to describe collaborative practices. Rather than problematic (and abstract) terms such as 'teams', which also describe static states ('norms') and imply fixed identities ('leaders', 'facilitators'), Engeström, as we have seen, shifts the focus to concrete activities of collaboration—teeming, swarming, collaborative intentionality, wildfire activities, cognitive trailing, knotworking, networking, meshworking, and so forth.

Identity is therefore implicated in the activity. The medical professional is no longer 'a good communicator' or 'a people person', implying some (segmented) structure of character or agency, but rather participates expertly in fighting wildfires, swarming, knotworking, meshworking, and networking. An example of this is the necessity for members of a clinical group collaborating around a patient to set up the distributed cognitive structure of 'situation awareness', where a common mental model of activity is generated, practitioners are aware of others' roles, and this mental model is projected into the future in mapping the day's work. The commonly held model will, ideally, be rechecked at regular intervals through briefing and debriefing. As described in previous chapters, the cognitive architecture of such a model is what Adrian Cussins (1992) calls 'cognitive trails'—similar to the 'song-lines' of Australian Aboriginals. These trails are laid down as aspects of expertise in collective memory, into which newcomers must be initiated to know the territory of their work. The trails are, however, refreshed, beaten anew. Such a dynamic, shared tacit expertise, a 'cognitive unconscious' (Reber, 1993), is, again, the heart of 'becoming a medical professional' and is shared collectively within the medical community as a set of 'cognitive scripts' informing diagnoses (Eva, 2005).

Cartography shifts attention from the actor to the activity and its context. Now we study just what and where the wildfire is, where it is burning, and how strongly. What 'net' or 'mesh' or 'knot' is 'worked' in, say, a multidisciplinary hospital oncology or community mental health meeting? How are knots both tied and untied? How are territories and their boundaries articulated and mapped, and how is deterritorializing achieved, for example, through 'boundary crossing' (Kerosuo & Engeström, 2003)? Boundary crossing is an activity shaped by the contours of the context and produces the identity of the 'boundary crosser' according to context. For example, a 'professional' boundary-crossing activity notes all the usual precautions of having identity papers at the ready, being sensitive to local customs and so forth. Just as doctors complain of nonclinical managers' boundary crossing literally and inappropriately into clinical spaces, so managers may complain of clinicians' boundary crossing into resources or funding meetings without an understanding of the values of the management culture.

Cartography is essential to our understanding of the becoming of the medical professional where it maps the spaces in which legitimation of activity occurs. On an international scale, this area has become one of the most sensitive yet under-researched in medicine and medical education. In identity models based on the 'selfsame', differences are often ignored, trodden on, or overwhelmed by the assumed superiority of the 'selfsame'. Thus, doctors in paternalistic and autocratic mode take over the experiences of their patients (Coulter, 2002) and often assume superiority over other health-care professions (Allard, Bleakley, Hobbs, & Vinnell, 2007), while surgeons assume superiority within the medical hierarchy (Cassell, 1991, 2000). On a global level, this can result in a neo-imperialism or neocolonialism, in which a certain brand of medical education (Western metropolitan) is exported to cultures where such methods of learning (e.g. 'self-direction' or 'small-group led') may be alien (Bleakley, Brice, & Bligh, 2008). Foucault (1976) traces this authority to the powerful legitimating force of the 'clinic'. It is because of this space and its rules that doctors can perform intimate or invasive acts of examination and investigation that would not be allowed in other spaces, such as the patient's home or in public.

Becoming a Diagnostician

The 'becoming' of the medical professional is not a diffuse or hazy pulse or flow. There are clear markers of shifts in identity that correlate with development of expertise. The key marker is 'becoming a diagnostician' or 'symptomatologist' (Smith, 2005) that can also be described as the development of expertise in connoisseurship of symptoms. This has been conventionally described as the achievement of a professional status within a clinical specialty (Becker et al., 1980) through acquisition of a certain level of expertise that is both formally examined and recognized by peers.

In Foucault's (1976) terms, the doctor is socialized into a particular kind of 'gaze' that is legitimated within the structure of the clinic (discussed in more detail below) and successfully negotiates a number of passages of 'examination' or surveillance, both technically and professionally (ethically), in a shaping or forming of an ethical self. In Erving Goffman's (1990) terms, the doctor adopts a role through expert performance as an actor, gradually learning the script and managing 'front stage' and 'backstage' self-presentations. In psychological terms, identity is achieved through mastery, outwardly displayed as performance based on developing a certain cognitive architecture. As more 'cases' are encountered, so doctors learn to recognize patterns, and they lay down cognitive structures or 'scripts' that allow for rapid judgment, bringing together scientific knowledge and sense-based judgment (Eva, 2005).

While other areas of health-care have their own methods of clinical judgment (Higgs, Jones, Loftus, & Christensen, 2008), and these may interact with, and support, the clinical reasoning of doctors (Gao & Bleakley, 2008), medical professionalism is characterized by both its breadth (range) and depth (intensity or power) of clinical reasoning. While doctors and surgeons are increasingly involved in preventive medicine, their daily work is curing illness and relieving symptom—making a diagnosis, offering a prognosis, and setting out a treatment plan or regime. This is done with attention to patients' needs (patient-centred practice) and sensitivity to collaborating effectively with colleagues around patient care pathways. The former is 'professional' work, while the latter is 'interprofessional' work (Bleakley, Boyden, Hobbs, Walsh, & Allard, 2006).

The Undoing of the Modern Clinical Gaze

Michel Foucault's (1976) *The Birth of the Clinic*, first published in 1963, describes the genesis of modern medicine—coincidentally with the European Enlightenment in the late eighteenth and early nineteenth century—as the development of a particular kind of 'gaze' upon the patient's body. Previously, medicine had fitted patients into preset systems of classification (such as the four humours) and treated them based on what can now be seen as a spurious system of diagnosis through the odour and colour of urine, the consistency of stools, and so forth, related to an abstract set of categories.

The new clinical gaze was based on close, empirical observation of the individual patient, including intimate examination combined with auscultation, palpation, and percussion. This was matched to a growing epidemiological knowledge of the frequency and distribution of illnesses. Where patients were traditionally visited at home, learning was restricted, but when medical education was established at the bedside in the hospital setting, as a teaching clinic, this legitimated intimate physical examination in a way that had not been possible in family home settings.

The medical gaze was educated through looking literally into the depths of bodies through cadaveric dissection and pathological anatomy and translating this deep looking, metaphorically, across to the surface examination of patients. The doctor's diagnostic gaze was a transposition of anatomical and pathological knowledge into the unseen depths of the patient's body, guided by the text of surface symptoms. The invention of the stethoscope by Laënnec in 1816 increased the power of the clinical gaze as it provided a necessary 'moral distancing' from the patient. The clinician's gaze into the body was then further augmented by Roentgen's discovery of the X-ray in 1895, and in time, more sophisticated radiological imaging. However, these augmentations have gradually come to replace, rather than amplify, the clinician's personal gaze (Bleakley & Bligh, 2009).

The medical gaze described by Foucault has operated as the dominant discourse of medicine for the past 200 years, but as we progress into the new millennium, it can be argued that a new discourse is emerging in medicine that is just as radical as the break that Foucault described. This new discourse is educating a different kind of medical gaze—as suggested above, one that is 'distributed', rather than focused and penetrating. This gaze is creating the conditions for the emergence of a new identity structure for doctors.

By a 'gaze' Foucault meant two things—first, a literal looking and seeing. Modern medicine is empirical—based upon close noticing and physical examination of symptoms as a basis to diagnosis, prognosis, and treatment plan. But also, Foucault describes a twin 'seeing and saying' that is metaphorical rather than literal. As the doctor gazes at the patient's outward symptoms, and asks about onset, duration, pain levels, and so forth and then continues to examination, that doctor is metaphorically—at the same time—gazing into the interior anatomy, which is known from anatomical atlases and dissection. The personal gaze is then augmented (and increasingly replaced, rather than supplemented) through tests and radiological imaging.

Also, the doctor, in the identity of the 'interprofessional' rather than the 'professional', is now more closely implicated in a network of services around a patient, where the medical professional is no longer autonomous. Clinical reasoning is both augmented and dispersed not only by instruments but also by a range of other health-care professionals and scientists, such as nurses, pharmacists, and biochemists. The personal medical gaze described by Foucault is fractured and multiplied to such an extent that Foucault's era of modern medicine, that has lasted 200 years, is now eclipsed.

Kenneth Ludmerer (1999) describes a crisis in medicine, concerning a widespread loss of faith by the public in doctors, leading to a reconsideration of the profession's level of autonomy. Doctors were judged to be unable to self-regulate adequately enough to inspire public confidence. The profession was also seen to refuse transparency, traditionally closing ranks to cover poor practice. This has led to the introduction of a monitory democracy (Keane, 2009) as a series of quality assurance mechanisms, including appraisal and appraisal-based revalidation in some countries. Where patients are also gradually acquiring greater powers and confidence in both challenging and collaborating with doctors, so traditional paternalism has been eroded. Finally, the need for change in the way that doctors share the uncertainties of their practices with patients and colleagues is being addressed.

What does this raft of changes mean for the 'becoming' of the doctor? In short, doctors must now be democrats rather than autocrats. They must shift allegiance from traditional vertical, hierarchical structures, to horizontal and dialogical collaborative working patterns; recognize the importance of nontechnical (communication) factors in patient safety; and engage with the democratic process whereby a professional community accounts publicly for its activities through assembly and representative democracies (Keane, 2009). In short, they must become citizens in medicine just as they are citizens in public life.

As I argued in Chap. 3, paradoxically many doctors working in, and supporting, democracies fail to reproduce such democratic structures in their own work settings. Democracy may still be a global experiment despite its many historical incarnations (where only 14 % of the world's population live in countries exercising full democracies, yet 35 % live in countries with authoritarian regimes), but research evidence clearly shows the advantages of collaboration-based democratic work patterns in health-care over autocratic structures.

If the doctor is now a social being, medical education must switch its attention away from individualistic learning theories to social learning theories; while in the area of expertise the doctor is no longer just achieving technical proficiency, but also nontechnical proficiency, modelling productive communication and interpersonal behaviour. Indeed, the doctor's work is not just about producing health or repair, but also about producing the social conditions of communication through which a patient's safety is guaranteed during a period of care. An outcome of a doctor's work now includes the production of social and affective capital (effective relationships with patients and colleagues) (Engeström, 2008).

Finally, the doctor must move beyond reflective practice, or self-direction, to accommodate to the reality of an embodied cognition that is distributed or affords a collective mind (Clark, 1997, 2009). The doctor's 'mind' is also 'in' an array of artifacts—computers, clinical reasoning software, paperwork, patient records, instruments, monitors, test results, syringes, drips, radiological images, sophisticated technologies, research papers, research and audit data, and so forth and 'in' the social, potentially collaborative, context in which his or her work occurs. Cognitive embodiment in these distributed resources makes it impossible to talk about a singular medical gaze in Foucault's terms and demands that we employ learning theories—such as communities of practice approaches, actor-network theory, and cultural–historical activity theory—that comprehend this fractured, multiple and (supple)mented gaze that is now social. Importantly, Deleuze's work helps us to appreciate the origins of the postmodern, distributed medical gaze as an example of the birth of a new line of flight, one that is desegmented or nomadic at birth.

Such eruption of a new line of flight also confounds traditional pedagogical maps—used to stabilize, segment, domesticate, and house—such as reflective practice. Traditional reflective practice models describe reflection as inner-directed and not social, privileging introspection over dialogue (Schön, 1990). This is safe territory for the conventionally autonomous and monological physician, working against the grain of the social, dialogical being that the physician must become for authentically 'safe' practice showing high levels of patient safety awareness. Rather, the doctor must become a reflexive practitioner (Findlay & Gough, 2003)—a full participant in a dialogical democracy (Bleakley, 1999), where practitioners must transparently account for professional values, practices, communications, and thinking process. This reflexive accounting for becoming a professional has led to new forms of textual practices that afford identity construction, as discussed below. The reflexive taxis is one that follows a line of flight not to return it to the nest but to trace its potential trajectory.

Becoming Medical Professionals Through New, Work-Based Textual Practices

A body of empirical research in work settings shows that medical and health-care work 'is changing' leading to 'problematizing identity' (Iedema & Scheeres, 2003, p. 316), offering what Jackson (2000) calls a 'new textualization' of work. Due to the implementation of new work settings—such as multidisciplinary clinical care pathways—doctors, surgeons, allied health professionals, and health-care workers are talking to each other in new ways (first text); talking to patients in new ways (second text); educating in new ways (third text); and talking about this work to academic researchers in new ways (fourth text). Also, doctors are talking to themselves (reflexively) in new ways about these emergent work conditions (fifth text), in shaping new identities through aesthetic and ethical self-forming, following Foucault's descriptions of an inner-directed governmentality and care of the self, discussed earlier.

Where reflection-in-practice and reflection-on-practice have become established ways of identity construction as a medical professional (Schön, 1990)—involving self-monitoring—reflection-as-practice, or critical reflexivity, is now becoming a desired practice. Here, doctors account publicly for their profession and its value through a variety of textual practices. In this section, I describe a first level of such practices in the context of doctors working with a wider range of colleagues and within an authentic patient-centred approach. In the following section, this is widened to second- and third-level reflexive practices, in accounting for medicine's wider identity as a profession through writing about medicine and through media representations of medicine and doctors, particularly television soap operas.

In adopting new ways of doing things (practices), and describing them to others and to oneself (reflection on practices), a shift in identity occurs. Sometimes, this shift offers not a fine-tuning of practices and the values that inform them, but a reinvention. In this case, reflection shifts to 'reflexivity'—a critical re-examination of what doctors do, why they do it one way and not another, and importantly 'who am I?' as a doctor engaging in these new forms of work.

In the process of negotiating new ways of relating that require new activities (e.g. leading a brief or a debrief on a ward or in an operating theatre), doctors and surgeons now have to renegotiate their identities as they recount, through speaking and writing, to a wider variety of other people (including patients) why they are doing what they are doing, in ways that were previously unfamiliar. This need not be seen as a product of political correctness, bureaucratic management, or surveillance, but as a new way of accounting for work.

Examples include clinically situated work such as multidisciplinary meetings, now including accountability to colleagues through practices of equality and equity; accountability to patients through collaborative practices such as briefing and debriefing; and what may be termed extra-clinical work, such as incident and accident reporting, appraisal, audit, and a range of educational activities. These activities radically expand and democratize the previously insular, restricted practices of closed mortality and morbidity departmental meetings.

In new, unstable and fluid work settings, doctors must speak from positions for which they have uncertain authority, little practice, or do not yet 'know the texts', especially in the nontechnical realms of practice that have now been shown to be central to maintaining patient safety (systems of communication, interpersonal skills, situation awareness).

Uncertainty is created where identity is destabilized by fluid work settings, such as work-about-work or new modes of work-within-work that transcend 'communities of practice' boundaries, such as patient care pathway interdisciplinary team meetings. Here, subjectivities are not given, expressed, and exercised, but are formed through the negotiations that go on within these new textualities of 'speaking about' oneself in relation to a complex of 'others', the details of whose work are actually unknown. Where it was once acceptable for the doctor to assume what the nurse or physiotherapist did, and to not have to account for professional behaviour to them, now doctors must sit down—as interprofessionals—to learn with, from and about 'others', as they are also accountable to others and to self. In this process, what counts as 'professional behaviour' is also redefined according to changing contexts for work.

Further, where paternalism towards patients was the norm, such behaviour is rapidly becoming challenged, indeed, unacceptable (Coulter, 2002), as doctors must now collaborate with patients. These are new forms of democracies, requiring the exercise of authentic democratic participation (assembly democracy), producing the new identity of the doctor as 'medical citizen'. In opening up such possibilities, contemporary doctors are recovering a long established tradition of learning from the patient, including getting the diagnosis from within the patient's story (Groopman, 2007).

As Iedema and Scheeres (2003, p. 334) suggest, such new work settings are 'volatile, political, and confronting'. This challenges the conventional certainties of a doctor's role and places traditional identity at risk. The common textual practices in medicine of 'telling' and informing' (monologue) that Atkinson (1995) described as 'the liturgy of the clinic' are being replaced by conversing, negotiating, collaborating, and supporting—again, participative dialogue or engagement rather than authoritative monologue or telling.

How are work modes changing? As noted earlier, there is, first, a wholesale shift from stable medical teams with continuity to ad hoc constitution of teams. In parallel, traditional apprenticeship 'family' structures of 'firms' have dissolved so that junior doctors must learn to be nomads rather than members of a stable 'house'. As Richard Sennett (quoted in Bauman, 2004, pp. 30–31) suggests: 'A flexible workplace is unlikely to be a spot in which one would wish to build a nest'. Rather, we are seeing the rise of 'cloakroom communities' that are 'patched together for the duration of the spectacle and promptly dismantled again once the spectators collect their coats from their hooks in the cloakroom'.

'Routine' work, based on stable groups, suggests Sennett, is crumbling across all sectors, not just health-care. As described earlier, Engeström (2008) suggests that new professional work settings are even seeing the dissolution of what we have habitually come to call 'team' structures. Rather, we are entering an era of 'collaborative intentionality' and 'negotiated knotworking', of rapidly pulsating work, where groups of people come together for connected and collaborative tasks and where, as argued in previous chapters, there is no stable 'centre', or the centre does not hold. Thus, there is no development of identity as a team member in the sense of passage (and staggered socialization) through the typical stages of group development ('norming', 'storming', 'performing', and 'mourning'). Perhaps 'mourning' is now the default position.

Knotworked sets of professionals (ad hoc 'teams') must tune to the 'pulse' of the work and move straight to 'performing', as threads of activity are tied, re-tied, and untied, again with no particular centre that holds. This new, dynamic work pattern—that takes technical proficiency as a given in its organic formation of work groups, but has no such faith in nontechnical proficiency, such as skill in communication—suggests that while work itself may have an object or be goal oriented (benefit to, care of, and safety for the patient; sensitivity to colleagues), identity may not be goal oriented but means oriented. In other words, you work creatively with what you have, not with a planned team where identities are fixed by hierarchy and role.

In these shifting work modes, again medicine mirrors the wider culture. Andy Hargreaves (2003, p. 25) describes a shift in society from 'sustained family conversations and relationships' to 'episodic strings of tiny interactions', and this has also occurred, as noted above, in medicine's transformation of the 'family' or 'firm' structures to more open, complex, and fluid arrangements.

Where the centre no longer holds, anarchy does not necessarily break loose. Rather, practices and identities are reinvented dynamically. Such changes mirror the wider runaway world, where mastery and control seem impossible, and adaptation, flexibility, and tolerance of uncertainty are paramount. For example, the new wave of iatrogenic diseases—hospital-acquired infections—seems runaway, monsters, almost impossible to control, as do new viral infections that evade cures. This does not stop us from attempting to master or nail these runaway objects, but we must recognize that stabilization is sometimes impossible and adaptive strategies are necessary. Medicine is a culture of both high need for control and high risk and uncertainty.

The emphasis upon collaborative work practices and consequent identity production requires the application of theories to explore and explain such new work contexts. Again, social learning theories (communities of practice, cultural–historical activity theory, and actor-network-theory) offer the most powerful explanations. Of these, communities of practice frameworks (Lave & Wenger, 1990; Wenger, 1998) are typically interested in how professional identities are stabilized. Novices enter a community of practice legitimately but peripherally, and as central participation is gradually achieved through recognition and application of expertise, so an identity emerges and stabilizes. Learning is a meaningful act of participation in a community of practice.

This model can be seen as a restatement of anthropological rites of passage and socialization models of the sort reported earlier, where engagement with a community invites initiation into the shared repertoire or history of that community and consequent identity construction through membership. Cultural histories include stories, rituals, humour, styles of working, effectiveness with key and local artifacts, and initiation into local knowledge. The communities of practice model differ from such traditional ethnographic models where it moves beyond description to prescription. The model prescribes the ideal community—as receptive, where communication is horizontal or nonhierarchical and engagement is mutual or reciprocated by experts (experts do not humiliate or harass). This is a gentle process 'that confers a sense of belonging', but 'more significantly, an increasing sense of identity as a master practitioner' (Lave & Wenger, 1990, p. 111). The tone of the communities of practice model, even in prescribing ideal, horizontal, forms of engagement, is undoubtedly tender-minded. It prescribes reciprocal partnerships between novice and expert and not judgmental initiations. For this reason alone, the model is readily open to scepticism from the characteristically tough-minded medical community, although the notions of learning by engagement or participation are second nature to such a community.

Where the 'communities of practice' model focuses upon progressive stabilization of identity, however, it does not have explanatory power to address the new complex, dynamic, unstable work contexts described above as liquid and runaway. Further, the model does not adequately describe how, for example, a doctor's social mind is constructed as it is mediated through artifacts (computers, patients' notes, drug charts, drips, syringes, and so forth) and collaborative practices. Actor-network-theory and cultural–historical activity theory can be seen to be particularly responsive to these issues. While I have devoted separate chapters to these approaches, let us refresh our memories about their purposes and foci, as this relates to our theme of identity construction of the doctor as a 'becoming'.

Actor-network-theory, in refusing personal agency and stability of systems, focuses upon how connections are made between persons and the material and symbolic worlds of artifacts. Bruno Latour (2007), the key figure in the field, suggests that abstract, high level, descriptors such as 'social' are limited. What are needed are specific descriptors for specific assemblages—ways of coming together, or connecting, and ways of disconnecting. Stabilization of notions such as 'professionalism' is also refused, where 'professionalism' is neither a prior category nor an aim, but a set of instants—or the dynamic making and unmaking of assemblages. Professionalism is an effect of rapidly pulsing moments in work contexts in which assemblages and connections are made and unmade.

Where learning theories describe interactions with the material world, such as learning a skill with an instrument (e.g. an endoscope), they stress human mastery rather than the interaction between person and artifact. Actor-network-theory specifically places people (actors) in networks (other actors and 'actants' or material objects such as computers), where person and artifact are considered to be in dialogue and mutually engaged. This is not a form of animism. Any practitioner will tell you how the instrument, such as an endoscope or a scalpel, 'speaks back' to the hand and guides the strength of grip or pressure in the feed or cut.

For actor-network-theory, we experience the world as a set of rapidly pulsing and changing associations, over which we attempt to gain mastery. This offers a working definition of clinical medicine. A sense of identity does not emerge out of the mastery, however, but out of the quality of association that is made between person and mediating material artifact as 'types of connections'—ties, bonds, aggregates, forces, and assemblages (Latour, 2007, p. 5). A doctor does not 'learn' through mastery of tasks informed by knowledge, but makes the right kinds of connections between the material and the human world or puts things together in a way that creates both meaning and function. This is the heart of diagnosis or symptomatology. In this sense, through bringing form and function into dialogue, the doctor is as much an artist as a scientist. This aesthetic identity offers a further platform for consideration of becoming a medical professional. In short, a medical education should place emphasis upon how the material world 'speaks back' to doctors as they work with it, shaping awareness and senses.

Cultural–historical activity theory (Engeström, 1987, 2008) sees activity systems (such as a community of practice) as inherently unstable and transformative—adaptive, complex, and dynamic systems. Such systems achieve temporary stability through agreement about common objects (aims) for the activity (such as patient care and safety), where identity is stabilized temporarily as an interaction between roles (division of labour) and rules (protocols) within the work system, such as a ward or family practice. However, this stabilization is temporary, as the activity system is inherently expansive, where the production and consumption of new artifacts and community structures are common.

Activity theory describes a collective capacity to carry out work, rather than an individual agency and identity at work. Groups of people create transformations and innovations in concert with artifacts, established rules (protocols), and work roles, and this affords identity and meaning. Identity is then an emergent property of the activity system, not a given condition, such as a character trait. Identity, however, is constructed as a performing and becoming—again, an activity not an essence— under conditions of dynamic process and transformation based on tensions inherent to a system and working across systems. Division of labour already means that members of the activity system have different subgoals and agendas, so that how they achieve the shared object of the activity, and how they translate rules and protocols, may produce conflict.

Identity formation is not then, as the communities of practice models suggests, necessarily about gradual stabilization within a community through increasingly meaningful (peripheral to central) participation, but may result from perturbation, resistance, and conflict and reflects this as the continual emergence of multiple and fractured sets of identities, achieving only temporary stability.

In acquiring a 'boundary-crossing' mentality—advertised by flexibility and tolerance—the origins of identity are again not grounded in 'selfsame' (identification with my professional group) but in 'difference' (I know myself in the mirror of the 'other'). Characteristically, selfsame identities exclude the other (intolerance), where identities grounded in difference respect that difference and value the other (tolerance). As argued previously, a powerful example of tolerance of difference is the ability for a doctor to recognize the patient as a guest in the household of medicine and to offer that patient unconditional hospitality (Bleakley, 2006b).

Bounded communities of practice, the basic unit of analysis of which is the 'team', are problematic according to Engeström (2008). Teams present a 'puzzle' as we have seen from previous chapters. Where exactly 'is' the team? What practitioners experience on the ground is, in Wenger's term, 'participation' and in activity theory, 'intent' to collaborate (although this usually sticks at a lower level of coordination or cooperation). At the level of what Wenger calls 'participation' and Engeström 'activity', abstract knowledge ('reification' in Wenger's term) or theory is secondary to work experience. A 'team' is an abstraction or reification. Rather, what is experienced are concrete, dynamic forms such as 'teeming', 'swarming', 'knotworking', 'meshworking', 'networking', and 'wildfire activities'. Becoming a doctor is then not becoming a team member, but becoming adept at varieties of collaborative activities and performances, such as networking and knotworking.

This new vocabulary for participation and activity attempts, metaphorically, to grasp what actually happens on the ground in work contexts, in dynamic terms. This may appear to be reactive to situations rather than proactive, but this would be a misunderstanding. Proactivity is inherent to an activity system, as is instability. Proactivity attempts to maintain activity and complexity in the face of instability, in what Searle (1990) calls 'we-intentions' and Engeström (2005) 'collaborative intentionality'. Such potential is achieved, again, through open dialogue, the hallmark of a democratic power structure.

For Ciborra (2000), powerful and successful work collectives do not, paradoxically, so much seek control over their collaborative work as understanding and meaning (returning us to the heart of Wenger's argument about an effective community of practice that generates meaning out of learning and learning out of meaning). Rather, collectives, in Ciborra's view, need not resort to top-down control (the knee-jerk reaction of autocracies) but generate good work practices from 'drift, care, hospitality, and cultivation' (in Engeström, 2008, p. 202). Collaborative activity produces affect or emotional capital, and this provides the conditions of possibility for further collaboration. Sceptics may ask: 'where is the leadership in such structures?' Leadership is *distributed*, according to the changing foci of work activities within an overall collaboration. The 'knot' in knotworking has no single centre or leader, but still holds appropriately to ensure collaboration and the realization of a common object or intention.

'Medutainment': Reflexive Accounting in the Public Realm

In this final section, I briefly describe how two further levels of textual practices are emerging, as characteristic aspects of the postmodern condition of medical practice—first, doctors are inventing a new genre of social-realist literature in writing about their practices and experiences for the public, as auto-ethnographies and second, doctors' identities are 'preformed' for public consumption through media representations in television soap operas ('medi-soaps'). The latter moves identity construction away from the high modernist territory of authentic expression of self, with a focus on essences and being, towards the territory of simulation and the simulacrum, where 'becoming' a medical professional—a twenty-first-century doctor—is now governed partly by public expectations shaped by media representations.

These virtual textual practices offer new territory for the management of professional identity by doctors, where the ongoing process of professional becoming can no longer be explored simply in terms of peripheral to central participation in a community of practice (the stabilization of a medical identity within a mixed community of doctors and surgeons and within defined communities of specialists), but the medical professional's becoming is literally serial—situated in a series of encounters with patients and colleagues that has been transposed to a series of books about doctoring and television soap opera series.

Perhaps eclipsing, rather than supplementing, the ethnographic studies described at the beginning of this chapter, there is a rich seam of autobiographical and auto-ethnographic accounts by doctors themselves of what they do and how their culture may be characterized. Richard Selzer (1996), writing since the early 1970s, has led the way in this social-realist genre. A new generation of physicians and surgeons writing on medicine and surgery (e.g. Edwards, 2007; Gawande, 2002, 2007; Lam, 2006; Patterson, 2007; Verghese, 1998, 2009; Weston, 2009) are doing something quite different from the previous generation of writers such as Selzer.

Selzer, while in a humane manner, lauds surgery, where a writer such as Atul Gawande admits to its limitations, uncertainties, hubris, and pitfalls (while, productively, suggesting remediation); and, in the context of emergency medicine, Nick Edwards brings the black humour characterizing that culture to the general public for scrutiny. Gawande in particular—surgeon, educator, researcher, and also staff writer on medicine for *The New Yorker*—offers the public education service that the historian of medical education, Kenneth Ludmerer (1999), had demanded as a primary responsibility of twenty-first-century medicine.

As mentioned earlier, Ludmerer, in a North American context, suggested that medicine, as a previously self-regulating profession, had to win back the faith of the public, lost through its inability to disclose or admit to error, close ranks in cases of poor practice, and find a productive way to discuss uncertainty with patients. Gawande—in sharp contrast to this legacy—openly shares such issues with his reading audience. In doing so, he sets out a new agenda for surgical educators, intimately linked with the construction of identity as 'surgical educator' focused first on learning with, from, and about patients.

The previously insular worlds of emergency medicine and the operating theatre in particular are now the subject of almost prurient public interest—however distorted the representation—through television medical soap operas such as *E.R.* and *Grey's Anatomy* in the USA and *Holby City* and *Casualty* in the UK. Whatever clinicians think of these representations, they are increasingly being used as 'infotainment' or 'edutainment' ('medutainment') to provide the public with opportunities to glimpse into worlds to which they previously would not have had easy access. It can be argued that these virtual representations offer, collectively, another form of monitory democracy, an emerging 'democracy of democracies', a superordinate governance arrangement that no longer allows the previously self-regulating body of medical professionals to engage in restrictive or closed practices.

The self-regulating clinic, described by Foucault as both the literal and cognitive architecture that legitimated the clinical gaze, has now become other directed and porous, as doctors increasingly come to write about their work as quasi-academic auto-ethnographies or through social-realist or fictional genres; where television soap operas offer educational and informational services; and the Internet clinic remains permanently open. Times have changed radically, and we can already judge how becoming a doctor of the future will be different from the outcome of a medical education, established through Abraham Flexner's (1910) report, that had changed little in basic structure over the last century. Deleuze has often been referred to as the philosopher who has best described the horizon that is the emerging millennium (DeLanda, 2002). His ideas provide a rich framework for understanding what it is to become a doctor of the future.

The reader may think that I have strayed from the work of Gilles Deleuze, but what I have done towards the close of this chapter is to further demonstrate how much we need Deleuzian thinking to understand the unfolding new world of liquid medical work. Foucault himself predicted that the twenty-first century would be the age of Deleuze, and indeed, while the neologisms and extensive vocabulary of Deleuze's vitalism may be a burden for some, it actually provides an articulation of the world that Deleuze saw as a vitalist. Challenging philosophies based on 'lack' and 'compensation', such as traditional psychoanalysis, Deleuze saw the world—and the social world—as inherently and primarily abundant and productive. So much so that our task as humans is partly to segment, striate, or order this world. However, this must not be reductive, turning abundance into lack. First, we must appreciate the vitality of this abundance and attempt to live its presence in ways of 'becoming', attentive to lines of flight.

Throughout the chapters in the second half of this book, dealing with team-based, institutional level communication, I have stressed the importance of thinking in terms of adaptive, complex, dynamic systems that are often at maximum complexity at the edge of chaos and show emergent properties. In short, we cannot apply linear thinking (teams as 'jigsaws'; teams with regular developmental patterns or phases) to team-based communication. We must now think local systems or systems in context. However, up to now, I have not provided a formal account of current thinking in complexity theory as applied to 'team' dynamics. The following chapter addresses this gap, linking the celebration of abundance and uncertainty in this chapter, undersigned by Deleuze, with a cautionary note to avoid unnecessary reduction of communication in medicine to simplistic explanations. This returns us to the warning in the first chapters of the book concerning the reduction of professional communication to instrumental skills practiced virtually, lists of competencies acting as potential dead-ends (and resisting lines of flight), and flimsy protocols—like cheap garden fences unable to manage the onslaught of the real and marauding weather of clinical practice that is uncertainty's favoured climate.

Chapter 15
Team Process and Complexity Theory: Blunting Occam's Razor

Learning as a Complex Activity

I have mentioned complex, adaptive systems thinking many times in this book. In this chapter, I clarify and explore precisely what I mean by systems thinking and the importance that such thinking has for understanding communication in medicine.

The third to fourth century BCE Chinese philosopher Zhuangshi said: 'A good butcher changes his knife once a year, because he slices flesh. A mediocre butcher changes his knife once a month, because he hacks at bone' (Jullien, 2007, pp. 88–89). Close observation of a skilled artisan at work, such as a master butcher, reveals an internal coherence to the execution of the skill. It is economical, fluid, elegant, and—paradoxically—restrained. The knife's edge seems to 'fall' into the meat. The best artisans are at one with their tools and the objects of their work—they do not force. Indeed, there is a sense of minimal interference from the hands, a kind of 'lifting off', where the tool does the work. Paradoxically, while 'grip' may seem key to control tools, it is 'release' that distinguishes the expert from the novice. The novice's grip is taut and fearful, where the master butcher shows 'ease and relaxation' in the heat of work. It is to this level of expertise that every novice aspires, in any trade or profession.

At first sight, it might seem that the butcher is learning as an individual, but this overlooks the fact that not only is the craftsman embedded in an immediate context including artifact (cleaver) and carcass, both of which 'speak back' or afford information, but also stands in the stream that is a historical and cultural tradition of a community of practice. To isolate the learner from context—describing learning psychologically—is to miss half the story. As we have seen, learning is not just the mastery of skills and knowledge, but offers legitimate entry into a community of practice or the gaining of an identity (Bleakley, 2006c; Engeström, 2008; Lave & Wenger, 1990; Wenger, 1998). Further, the artifacts (tools) with which a person works and through which he or she learns embody histories and come to inscribe learning through cultural wisdom (Latour, 2007; Law & Hassard, 1999). Divorcing

A. Bleakley, *Patient-Centred Medicine in Transition: The Heart of the Matter*,
Advances in Medical Education 3, DOI 10.1007/978-3-319-02487-5_15,
© Springer International Publishing Switzerland 2014

learning from context is reductive and misrepresents the learning experience that may be better understood through complexity theory.

Surgery, once a high form of butchery, was radically transformed by anaesthesia—and now by scopes, robotics, and lasers—into a highly sophisticated activity spawning subspecialties. As Richard Sennett (2008, p. 197) points out, the evolution of skill needed for modern surgery is intimately linked with development of sophisticated metal instruments, where once 'Medieval doctors used cooking knives for dissection'. Surgery, once limited to use of dull iron instruments, was transformed when the means of sharpening those instruments changed from varieties of composite stone (often combined with lubrication such as oil) to leather straps and then through the development of sharp steel blades and customized handles.

In tracing the history of the scalpel, Sennett notes how, in seventeenth-century Europe, it took three generations, moving into the eighteenth century, to embed mastery of the effective use of scalpels for dissection and surgery. A variety of scalpels were developed for particular purposes, such as sharp at the tip for slicing through delicate membranes or hooked and dulled to lift tissue or the double-sided, sharp pointed blade—the lancet—for efficiency. In that set of scalpels is also an example of a distributed cognition at work across differing communities—surgeons, barbers, blacksmiths, designers, engineers, metallurgists, and industrial steelworkers experimenting, sharing knowledge, deepening expertise, and widening the range of application.

As we move into an era of laser surgery, we will see a further radical transformation of activity shaped by that technology to illustrate what Yrjo Engeström (1987, 2008), the leading figure in contemporary cultural–historical activity theory, calls 'learning by expanding'. Learning is understood through complexity theory as a cross-community social activity involving large numbers and intensities of interactions of elements over time.

Inevitably, the conservative, core aspect of apprenticeship—passing down values, knowledge, and skills unchanged through transmission and reception—is reformulated, as apprenticeships become more complex in the professions, involving high-level creative and skilled work. In this reformulation, knowledge production is possible alongside information reproduction, as communities of practice become interested in their own processes, investigating and reflexively accounting for their own purposes, histories, traditions, and futures, or expanding their work from doing it to talking about it and researching it (Engeström, 2008; Iedema & Scheeres, 2003). Where members of such practice communities go beyond reflection on their own work to concerns about what gives value and meaning to work in the wider social sense, this reflexivity or metacognition again changes the level of complexity as further dimensions to a system come into play.

As scalpels became progressively lighter and sharper, so they became more difficult to master, introducing greater instability and uncertainty into the system. But dynamic, complex systems are both adaptive and open. As new properties emerge so the now highly unstable system may reorder at a higher level of complexity. The challenge for surgeons was first to unlearn habitual techniques acquired for cruder, heavier, instruments, which required particular arm and shoulder coordination not unfamiliar to the master butcher. Focus now shifted to fine-hand control, the mark of the expert surgeon—first finger and thumb coordination and fingertip control in particular—as the new, lighter scalpels amplified clumsy or gross movements. For example, in using a flat surface of the scalpel to lift tissue, the fourth and fifth finger muscles have to be contracted to offer counterpoise to the movement of thumb, forefinger, and second finger. Also, the scalpel needs to be 'lifted off'—an application of restraint, of minimum force.

For the expert, the scalpel, or any tool, teaches the hand how to best use it. Skill emerges as a conversation between the user and the instrument. Learning is always relational, whether it is forming a relationship with tools or instruments, languages, and codes or with persons in and across specific practice communities—early modern surgeons talking with blacksmiths and modern surgeons talking with scrub nurses who come to know the particular blades that individual surgeons prefer as they deliberately lay out the instrument sets.

Learning Theory at the Cutting Edge

A Close Shave with Occam's Razor

And so to another blade—'Occam's (or Ockham's) razor', attributed to the fourteenth-century English Franciscan friar William of Ockham, is the idea that the simplest solution is the best, or entities should not be multiplied beyond necessity. Such thinking characterizes the dominant Enlightenment tradition that merges logical positivism with analytic philosophy to shape the method of empirical science. Occam's razor began as a rule of thumb, but has been elevated to the status of logical operation or scientific principle.

In contrast to reductive science with its attraction to simplicity, quantum mechanics in physics, systems-based biology, and studies of dissipative structures in chemistry have together brought about a well-documented paradigm shift in scientific thinking, celebrating complexity and holism as explanatory and exploratory models (Kauffman, 1995; Prigogene & Stengers, 1985). Models of complexity—based on sharp imaginations and preferring elegance to simplicity—necessarily dull or blunt Occam's razor and reveal its rhetorical purpose as an old saw persuading us to champion the supposed virtue of simplicity.

Contrasting Approaches to Complexity Theory

Contemporary medicine, including surgery, is a complex, often messy and uncertain, practice that needs to be understood through rich, productive theory, and there is indeed an impressive international body of work applying complexity theory to medicine, health-care, and health policy (Greenhalgh, Plsek, Wilson, Fraser, & Holt, 2010; Holt & Marinker, 2010; Paley, 2010; Plsek & Greenhalgh, 2001; Plsek, Sweeney, and Griffiths, 2002; Sweeney, 2006). Such application is contested and has led to an academic spat between those who see complexity theory as having wide application—including the social and cultural spheres of human life—and those who see this widening of application as a dilution, or indeed corruption, of complexity theory's origins in mathematical or computational modelling of natural phenomena.

The former, liberal interpretation of complexity theory's reach describes productive convergence between various holisms such as systems, chaos, and network theories. The latter purists see computational complexity theory as distorted by psychological approaches widely used in the literature applying complex systems thinking to the human face of health-care (Greenhalgh et al., 2010; Plsek & Greenhalgh, 2001), claiming that complexity has been appropriated as 'a variation on democratic, collaborative, "bottom-up" methods for the management of change in systems' (Paley, 2010, pp. 59–61).

In this chapter, I explicitly follow the liberal line in seeing wide application for complexity models—including the political—and indeed extend this reading by aligning complexity theory with social learning theories to better understand medical education. With notable exceptions (Dickey, Girard, Geheb, & Christine, 2004; Dornan, 2010; Mennin, 2010; Regehr, 2010) applications of complexity theory are rare in the field of medical education, rather than medicine, health-care organization, or the field of education studies (Davis & Sumara, 2006). There are good reasons for this, discussed later. Complexity is still a relatively unfamiliar way of imagining and understanding the terrain of learning in medical education and requires engagement with an unfamiliar vocabulary.

Three Approaches to Learning as a Complex Social Phenomenon

As we have seen in several contexts throughout this book, contemporary social learning theories include three main approaches: communities of practice or situated learning (Crook, 2002), actor-network-theory (Latour, 2007), and cultural–historical activity theory (Engeström, 2008). Such theories stress the importance of both context (learning is situated) and process (learning is dynamic). Where traditional learning theories focus upon what is learned or accumulated by an individual and how that is retained and reproduced, social learning theories focus upon processes of collaboration, means of access to distributed knowledge, how knowledge acquires legitimacy and meaning, knowledge production rather than reproduction, socialization as a process of learning, and identity construction as a learning outcome.

Social learning theories can be seen as species of complexity thinking, where complexity describes the nature of the phenomenon (such as interaction between several clinical teams around a patient with multiple, chronic illnesses) (Engeström, 2004, 2008; Engeström, Engeström, & Kerosuo, 2003), and learning theory offers a way of explaining and exploring that phenomenon at a certain level of analysis. Social learning theories may also be seen as a family, often engaging in implicit rather than explicit reference to each other through the key, binding notions of communities, activities, and networks (Edwards, Biesta, & Thorpe, 2009).

We have seen that actor-network-theory in particular, originating within the sociology of science, sets out to describe how scientific facts and practices associated with the generation of those facts circulate and gain legitimacy within scientific communities. Serendipitously, actor-network-theory provides a powerful account of work-based learning in describing how knowledge is a product of interactions between actants (artifacts: instruments, materials, and symbols) and actors (practitioners), where material and cultural worlds are given equal status. Such interactions produce networks that provide temporary stability for knowledge or in which knowing is enmeshed. Knowledge is not then in persons but is an effect of relations or interactions within networks, engaging both the material world (artifacts) and persons (Fox, 2009).

Tamsin Haggis (2009) describes these three social learning theories as bound by two main principles of complexity theory—difference and process. By 'difference', Haggis means a radical situatedness. A particular system—such as a neural network, a family group, or a community—is nested, related to and affected by other systems. However, the emergent properties of that system will be unique to its particular level of dynamic, generated by the number, quality, and intensity of interactions of elements. Further, while each system is different, its difference is known only in relation to another system—there is no essential identity to the system. By 'process', Haggis means that every system is dynamic and is best appreciated as fluid and unfolding, where properties emerge in non-linear, often unpredictable ways.

We have seen that a situated learning or communities of practice model describes learning not as sedimentation of knowledge but as cultural participation. Learners gain entry into a community of practice as a form of identity construction through legitimation of role that is also a means of gaining temporary stability within a dynamic system. Recall surgeons embedding skills of scalpel use over three generations as metallurgy technologies afforded widespread experimentation with varieties of instruments. The complex system of the surgical community and its learning processes are fluid, as new practices and sub-communities emerge, but temporary stabilities are necessary to embed practices, as expert practitioners become reflexive about their work, or gain insights into its dynamic (Iedema & Scheeres, 2003). The mark of the expert, in achieving legitimate central, rather than peripheral, participation is then to innovate within the community, to produce rather than reproduce knowledge. Such practitioners are themselves emergent properties of the complex system, who have insight into the dynamics of the system or are reflexive.

I have also described how cultural–historical activity theory focuses upon the mediation of learning by artifacts and communities, describing learning by expanding, where not only is knowledge distributed but also knowing becomes progressively wider in a social sense through expanding and more intensive participation in learning networks. This does not signal that bigger is better, but rather signals greater complexity. Activity theory describes activity systems, such as clinical teams, as sharing a common object (for example patient care or safety) and displaying some kind of boundary, albeit highly permeable. Differing activity systems may interact across these boundaries (Kerosuo & Engeström, 2003). The level of interaction is regulated by boundary objects—such as a shared patient or item of equipment, a protocol or a common management structure.

What Unit of Analysis?

Bleakley (2006a, 2006b, 2006c) has argued that contemporary social learning theories provide a more powerful explanation of how learning can occur through a collaborative medical education than the currently dominant learning theories that focus upon the individual. The unit of analysis for learning then shifts from individual cognition to complex system to include distributed cognition. Importantly, this shift can be described as a political event, moving from privatized knowledge to shared knowledge realized democratically or collaboratively. The key shift in thinking is from connectionist and retrospective (analysis of events as if static and private) to dynamicist and prospective (synthesis of events as moving through time and becoming public). Individualistic approaches to learning may inadvertently feed the heroic archetype that prevents medicine from developing an authentic citizenry. How can collaboration and democracy sit easily with autonomy—which tends to autocracy?

Individualism can conveniently ignore contexts and their complexities. To return to the surgeon at work in conversation with artifacts such as scalpels, this describes a complex system in which other systems such as toolmakers are implicated. There are enough potential interactions to produce a significant level of complexity. As we move this to the wider surgical team and their artifacts (surgeons, anaesthetists, anaesthetic assistants, scrub nurses, circulating nurses, and patients), this provides a more complex system through multiplying up the number of potential interactions. This level offers the typical activity system unit of analysis. Typically, this activity system in a day's work will cross the boundaries of several other systems, such as a recovery team, a ward team, a team of hospital porters, a team of radiographers, and so forth. If we take each of these practitioners and place them in the context of their professional groups (surgeons, nurses, anaesthetists) and situate them in the histories of such groups, this level offers the typical unit of analysis of the community of practice.

If we now change the focus of the level of complexity by introducing both the built environment (the operating theatre, the anaesthetic room, the hospital ward, the recovery room, the community clinic) and the organizational structure, we radically increase the potential number of interactions and the complexity of the system. We can describe these various levels of complexity or systems as nested, and we are now far from learning being confined to the cognition of the individual.

Instead of thinking about practitioners learning and practicing autonomously, the surgical team, for example, shares an ecology of practice (teams working around patients with a variety of artifacts) generating a common intelligence and affect as collaborative process, with practitioners often working at maximum complexity at the edge of chaos. Intersubjective understanding and interprofessional collaboration potentially replace intrasubjectivity, habitual patterns of autonomy, and reluctant multiprofessional coordination and cooperation.

Attractors and Dissipative Structures

Connectionist thinking would be concerned to delineate just where clinical teams begin and end (boundaries), but complexity thinking imagines such spatial issues differently, describing fuzzy boundaries, topologies (teams aggregating in space), and state spaces (teams passing through time, where distributed cognition assumes differing patterns), addressing the reality of uncertainty and ambiguity experienced by such teams. State spaces can be mapped as all the possible transitions a working team may move through in a set period. Topologies can also be mapped—not as the peaks and troughs in an individual's work or related to specific locations (corridor talk or briefing room meeting), but rather as processes such as territorializing and deterritorializing (Deleuze & Guattari, 2004a, 2004b)—the imperialistic conquering of spaces (a doctor or surgeon rules the roost) or the democratizing of spaces (a doctor is one member of a health-care team sharing a common wealth).

Rather than defining boundaries we can use the term attractors to describe areas (space) and periods (time) in the state space towards which a trajectory of activity will be drawn, such as the attention of an anaesthetic team during an equipment malfunction. Why a term such as attractor is important is that it orients us to the work of the environment-shaping activity rather than to the cognition of practitioners dictating events. This shift in apprehension is necessary if one is to understand cognition as distributed (Crook, 2002).

As team activity moves through time, sometimes coordinated, sometimes uncoordinated, so perturbations and unexpected or ambiguous periods will occur, to which the team must adapt if it is not to fall into chaos. These emergent properties offer learning opportunities that are quite different from the planned learning outcomes that define contemporary, formal medical education programmes. Such learning outcomes offer a known and non-negotiable horizon. Horizon thinking in complex systems is quite different, where the horizon is partly unknown and unknowable—hence, systems are adaptive. Where traditional ergonomics plans to compensate for the unknown through design, complexity thinking sees transients—uncertain, often temporary, perturbations—as potential opportunities rather than threats to the stability of a system.

Dissipative (open) structures (Prigogene & Stengers, 1985) reformulate as they pass into higher orders of complexity, but their transitional phases are unsettling. Practitioners must collaboratively exercise tolerance of uncertainty during such transitions as their horizon thinking adjusts. Where the autonomous practitioner tries to engage with the system through self-direction, those who think complexity will also think coupling—where no part of the system changes without other parts also changing. For example a key member of a clinical team reports in sick and there is no backup—how will that team adapt? Coupling is the central dynamic in an activity system, such as a clinical team, where the key elements (practitioners, shared object(s) of the activity, artifacts, community, roles, and rules) are in constant interaction to dynamically form and reform the system. Coupling describes the process of interaction and relation of elements in a system, including emergent factors as the system moves through time, attempting to adapt as it works far from equilibrium. The clinical team, as system, is open or dissipative, attempting to regulate itself through feedback, organization, and set roles, rules, protocols, and adaptation. But it is inherently unstable and must be able to tolerate the ambiguity that this instability affords.

Patterns of Resistance to the Values Advertised by Complexity Theory

There are good reasons why complexity theory as an informing framework and social learning theories as explanatory models have not become dominant in medical education. The values they represent are alien to the clinical culture. Heroic individualism (Bellah et al., 2007; Ludmerer, 1999), autocracy, and meritocracy are still preferred modes to collaboration and democracy, despite the emergence of a new era of health-care that calls for interdisciplinary teamwork around patients. The dominant cultural mindset in medicine values self-directedness and self-reference over other-directedness, mirrored in personality and organizational structures that can broadly be termed authoritarian, characterized by intolerance of ambiguity.

Individualistic theories have their roots in Western capitalism, pragmatism, and cultures of self-help and self-sufficiency. Here, knowledge is privatized and treated as capital for self-interest. Social learning theories have their roots in Soviet collectivism, stemming from the work of Lev Vygotsky (Daniels, 2005) after the 1917 revolution. Here, knowledge as capital is shared and commonly owned. The Cold War prevented productive comparisons and cross-fertilization of these competing views. As the Cold War thawed, so knowledge of social learning theories gained a foothold in the capitalist world, appealing to that world's interest in social democracy and chiming with established, holistic views that recognized uncertainty as a resource rather than a threat, such as ecological systems modelling (Kauffman, 1995) and complexity theory.

As Haggis (2009) points out, however, we should not place social learning theories and individualistic theories in unproductive opposition. Rather, learning can be explored as nested levels of complexity or varieties of complex adaptive systems in various forms of relation. Here, the main issues are what do we mean by 'learning' and what is the most appropriate unit of analysis for any one example of learning? Each complex system—at the level of neuronal networks, persons, groups and teams, cultures and languages, and histories—provides a unit of analysis. Complexity thinking then focuses us upon differences (relations) between systems and kinds of systems as appropriate units of analysis.

Complexity theory, describing nested systems with their unique internal dynamics, offers deep difference or radical situatedness. Complexity theory prompts us to ask: at what level of complex organization is the phenomenon under investigation operating in relation to other systems? Further, how will systems best adapt within ecologies? This is often framed in negative Darwinian terms as survival of a system, but we might think rather that systems interacting in certain ways with other systems do not simply adapt or merely survive, but flourish and innovate. Systems are also not constituted by other systems (the social imperative) but bear qualities and forms, such as intensities, of relations to other systems (Smith, 2005).

Learning Defined

Learning can then be thought of as the overall process by which a system's emergent properties are transformed into adaptive innovations. Researchers of learning will focus upon important emergent properties, choose appropriate units of analysis to describe those properties, and describe the dynamic system in relation to other systems. This resonates with the definition of learning derived from complexity theory offered by Davis and Sumara (2006), where learning is the process by which the unit of analysis (person, institution) is 'constantly altering its own structure in response to emergent experiences'. The focus of a complexity theory approach to learning can then be distinguished from individualistic and social constructionist approaches, where learning is not how individuals create meanings, or how meanings are socially constructed and transmitted, but rather how meanings emerge from complex process.

As an illustrative example, within social learning approaches, cultural–historical activity theory has itself undergone historical transformation as a complex system, as it sets out to study how learning occurs in other complex systems, such as primary health-care (Engeström, 2008). Activity theory has acted as a responsive learning organization in Davis and Sumara's definition 'constantly altering its own structure in response to emergent experiences' and has followed its own imperative of learning by expanding. The first wave of activity theory, drawing on original Russian theorists such as Vygotsky and Leontiev, focused on the mediation of learning by artifacts and communities. A second wave focused upon defining shared objects that constituted an activity system such as a clinical team, including inherent paradoxes such as what may happen when practitioners working in the same activity system have differing objects of concern. A third and current phase now focuses upon relations between numbers of activity systems sharing the same object—such as a number of clinical teams working around a patient in the community—and what happens at the highly flexible and permeable borders of those systems. Thus, activity theory as an explanatory framework has itself become more complex where its focus has shifted to a new level of complexity—the relations between several activity systems. In this move, it has also come to be more reflexive about its history as an emergent community of practice.

The Conditions of Possibility for the Emergence of Complexity Theory as an Explanatory Model in Medical Education

Unfortunately for advocates of complexity thinking, complex may not describe the imaginations of those who are nevertheless embedded daily in complex systems. Rather, they may universally apply Occam's razor as a default method and reductionism as a default value. While complexity theory and related social learning theories may offer excellent models for understanding both medical practice and the education of that practice, this still leaves the issue unaddressed of receptivity of such theories within a community of practice such as medical education, whose primary body is not academic but clinical. This standing body may remain sceptical, showing active resistance towards learning theories that do not accord with dominant values, even where such theories draw from models that are, as explained earlier, well established in medicine but absent from its pedagogy.

Medical education has characteristically preferred reductive, instrumental explanations for dynamic phenomena that may be better appreciated through complexity theory. It may be that a condition of possibility for the emergence of complexity science in medical education has to be established, such as the dialogical imagination, described by Mikhail Bakhtin (1981). A monological mindset is characterized by habitual self-reference or interest in the 'selfsame' rather than 'difference'. The shift from the values of a monological to a dialogical imagination may be crucial in preparing the ground for adoption of social learning theories as examples of complexity thinking.

Despite the common root of 'hospital' and 'hospitality', doctors and surgeons habitually revert to identification with their own values (that of the wider medical or surgical culture), or the values of their specialty, at the expense of authentic understanding of and tolerance for the values of another culture, such as nursing or clinical psychology. An imagination of difference, or a dialogical mindset of reciprocity and hospitality, works quite differently (Bleakley, 2002). The assumption here is not that I accommodate an Other to my viewpoint (the basis of imperialism and colonialism), but that I tolerate the difference between myself and the other, see this difference, however ambiguous, as a resource and come to learn from this.

Bakhtin (1981) defines dialogism as 'a constant interaction between meanings'. Meanings are context-defined and inherently ambiguous precisely because they are relational. Democratic structures exist to allow for plural voices but also to find ways to come to agreements about activity. As Stewart Mennin (2010) points out, knowledge production is relational, and understanding is a process of transaction and translation.

A condition of possibility for the establishment of complexity theory as a dominant discourse in medical education is the valuing of relational production of learning, knowledge, and innovation. The primary pattern of resistance to this is offered by the discourse of the heroic individual and the associated cult of personality and uncritical role modelling. In political terms, such a model resists the establishment of democratic or participatory teamwork for either hierarchical meritocracies or autocracies. Hierarchical and monological imagination in clinical teams can be seen as a typical pattern of resistance against complexity and emergent democracy and is characterized by intolerance of ambiguity—the primary characteristic of the authoritarian.

Adorno, Frenkel-Brunswik, Levinson, and Sanford's (1950) classic study of the authoritarian personality type described intolerance of ambiguity as a key characteristic. This can be generalized to collectives, where medicine (and surgery in particular) has traditionally shown intolerance of uncertainty and ambiguity or the desire to reduce, or defend against, uncertainty as a key strategy (Cassell, 1991; Fox, 1997/1959). Medicine traditionally works in hierarchies or autocratic and meritocratic vertical authority structures, resisting horizontal, democratic structures. In order to establish an imagination of complexity, nourishing application of social learning theories, medical education must model a democratic culture tolerant of ambiguity that can improvise and innovate like expert jazz musicians and does not need to retreat to safety by marching to a regular beat. Democratic structures are structures of complexity.

A typical act of resistance to developing democratic habits is to maintain medicine as a permanent state of 'warfare', hostility, conflict, and emergency. This, as pointed out in an earlier chapter, chimes with medicine's characteristic militaristic metaphors such as 'waging war on disease' and the 'fight against cancer'. A state of exception or emergency (such as crisis or warfare) outside the norms of democratic life allows politicians to make autonomous, autocratic decisions without due democratic process. Those who resist democratic process in medicine may maintain a permanent state of exception, such as hostilities between professions. This reflects a monological rather than dialogical imagination and will frustrate engagement with complexity theory as a potentially democratizing presence.

I have now completed a blueprint for a revolution in communication in medicine, where medicine must be democratized to provide the conditions of possibility for the emergence of safe care for patients. This requires a reconceptualization of medical education for the future, focused on collaborative teamwork practices and based around live experiences with patients. Such education must be carefully designed to gain the best possible learning experiences in the field of communication with patients, colleagues, and organizational members such as management. We can borrow the methods of briefing, and feedback through debriefing, now being employed in clinical work to inform work-based learning.

Beyond a reconceptualization (mobilizing epistemologies) of medical education for non-technical or communication practices, there are two further requirements: considerations of ontological and axiological issues. Ontological issues involve understanding how multiple identity constructions for professional practitioners may occur and be managed. I have argued that the epistemological issues of communication in medicine cannot be separated from ontological considerations. Finally, underpinning both theories of knowledge and ways of being are forms of value. Practice must engage the moral imagination and moral indignation exercised as forms of resistance such as *parrhesia*. Without the moral dimension, communication practices are merely technical and not humane.

There is one further substantial issue to consider—how will communities of practice in medical education research the emerging world of complex, liquid team-based communication *as they reflexively apply the principles of collaborative, team-based activities to that research enterprise*? The following chapter addresses this question.

Chapter 16
Building a Collaborative Community of Practice in Medical Education Research

What Is a 'Collaborative' Community of Medical Education Researchers?

The project outlined in this book is to address the problem of communication hypocompetence at the structural level of democratizing the institution of medicine. This is a long-term goal of medical education that will hopefully show in better patient safety practices of future generations of doctors. However, I have also pointed out that acquiring democratic habits and literacy in democracy as this applies to patient care and collaboration with colleagues is complex. Importantly, the best available evidence must shape this project. It would be incongruous if the medical education *research* culture did not follow the same trajectory, to move from individual and isolated research to collaborative and programmatic research. This chapter provides a blueprint for furthering the formation of collaborative communities of medical education researchers, asking also how researchers become legitimate members of such communities.

Glenn Regehr's (2004) thematic synopsis of trends in medical education research, referencing 140 articles, asks what we might mean by 'advancement' in the field. His view is that the medical education research community suffers from both a lack of focus upon theory and a lack of systematic endeavour and will not advance until these two areas are positively addressed. This calls for a radical shift in medical education culture to:

- Move away from parallel research activity to interactivity
- Embrace programmatic rather than simply thematic research
- Generate theory rich research within the medical education community rather than outside that community

Regehr suggests that the explosion of interest in researching clinical decision-making expertise some years ago was a 'parallel' research activity that did not lead to those researchers collaborating within a medical education research community

A. Bleakley, *Patient-Centred Medicine in Transition: The Heart of the Matter*, Advances in Medical Education 3, DOI 10.1007/978-3-319-02487-5_16, © Springer International Publishing Switzerland 2014

and generating theory within such a community, but led to dispersal to other communities of practice (such as psychology or education studies). The call is for coordinated effort to develop a dedicated and bounded medical education research community. In other words, to ensure that legitimacy can be achieved within a medical education research community for those who may feel that their legitimate place is in another research community, such as a pure social science group.

Would it be possible, for example, to legitimize social science subgroups within a medical education research community? Some may think that this has already been achieved, but there are many counter-indications. For example, a journal such as *Social Science and Medicine* is more readily aligned with a social science community than with a medical education community. A 'medical sociologist' identity construction is more likely to occur within a sociology community of practice than within a medical education community of practice.

How might we identify the 'community' of medical education researchers? Regehr says that his article offers 'an examination of *our* literature' (emphasis mine), assuming identification with a community, but here the notion of 'community' is problematic. Because people engage in the same activities, does this make them a community? Do they need, as the originator of 'community psychology', Alfred Adler (Adler and Brett, 2009/1938) suggested, 'fellow feeling' (*gemeinschaftsgefühl*), a sense of community spirit and, if so, how is this established? While commentators call for collaboration in research and for the development of common identity, how can this be achieved in the face of the deliberate engineering of an academic environment based on competition for scarce resources and personal hostility disguised as 'critique?' Such values are reinforced by competitive academic funding structures such as the UK Research Excellence Framework (REF) (previously the Research Assessment Exercise or RAE).

Paradoxically, Albert (2004) and Albert, Hodges, and Regehr (2007) already contradict the notion of community as a shared perspective through careful articulation of the tension between a community of academics and a community of clinicians in the wider field of medical education research. This suggests that reference to a cohesive community of research may be a convenient fiction. Indeed, how membership of such a community is defined is problematic and raises issues about how an identity of 'researcher' may be constructed. For example, how much and what kind of 'research' does a medical educator have to carry out before he or she is identified as, or takes on the identity of, a 'researcher?' Does a medical educator gain 'legitimate peripheral participation' (Lave & Wenger, 1990) in a community of practice of medical education researchers if he or she is primarily a clinical teacher who engages in occasional scholarship of teaching (Bleakley, Bligh, & Browne, 2011)?

Regehr's (2004) proposal for 'communal effort' towards success in future medical education research has three components: collaboration within the culture, communal theory building, and programmatic research leading to knowledge building. But again, these suggestions are built on an assumption of 'community'. Given the deep splits (and consequent spats) that are common within the academic community—often based on discipline allegiances or arcane theoretical positioning within disciplines and within the medical and surgical communities, with subspecialty identifications, consequent 'silo' effects, and difficulties in boundary crossing—is a communal effort in medical education research a bridge too far? A pessimistic view is that this would be a community of convenience or, worse, a community of those who have little in common (Lingis, 1994).

Three Platforms for Collaboration

In order to build a genuinely collaborative research community, three platforms have to be established. First, the philosophy of 'fellow feeling' must be established around a common concern. The primary concern is the patient, the heart of the matter, where 'fellow feeling' equates with patient-centredness. A community of medical education researchers may be identified by a common aim: to improve patient care in systematic ways. This would be the shared outcome of the activity system (Engeström, 2008) that is a medical education research community. Where clinicians work around issues of patient-centredness on a daily basis, academics (who are 'ideas-centred') do not. One way in which academic and clinical communities can establish 'fellow feeling' (authentic collaboration) is for academics to also learn patient-centredness. Where patient-centredness is learned from patients, then those engaged in research in medical education without clinical experience could undergo appropriate socialization into clinical contexts, gaining experience around patients.

The second platform on which a medical education research community can be built is 'interdisciplinarity'. This is discussed in depth below. Establishing networks of interdisciplinarity means shifting the focus of power from sovereign power (certain disciplinarians want to discipline others through their disciplines or retreat to conventions of hierarchy) to capillary power (power runs through the network as forms of collaborative knowledge).

The third platform on which a medical education research community can be built is the establishment of stable identities of 'interdisciplinary researchers'. As interdisciplinary practices of research are inhabited, or indwelt, so 'self-forming' (Foucault, 2002) occurs. Here, the focus of the identity formation is also the locus, as the research team establishes itself as a household, a local ecology under one roof. The roof is not literal, but is the binding metaphor—the commitment to genuine collaboration. The local ecology works on the biological principle of adaptation and can be modelled as an adaptive, complex system within a finite resource environment.

I fully support Regehr's (2004) argument that the quality of medical education research will remain stunted unless we develop programmatic and systematic research, and this is best done collaboratively, internationally, and across networks. Implementation of such a plan could involve the three platforms discussed above (clinically focused patient-centredness, academic interdisciplinarity, and the construction of identity of researcher as 'interdisciplinarian') as a basis for development of genuine collaborative research communities grounded in 'fellow feeling'.

Below, I look at these three platforms in a slightly different way, to emphasize that the establishment of interdisciplinarity requires alignment of knowledge (epistemological alignment), values (axiological alignment), and relationships (ontological alignment), in the face of potential threat of disruption through wider policy directives based on seemingly compulsive, short-term, management-led cycles of reorganization of health services (a threat to the stability of the local ecology of clinicians engaged in research).

For medical education research, the sticking point in the development of collaborative communities may well be that awkward gap between the academic research community and the clinical community, highlighted by Albert (2004) and Albert et al. (2007). Albert (2004) discusses the tension between academic research communities and the clinical communities they inform, where academic researchers will probably continue to exercise their collective autonomy, as they demand more research sophistication from clinicians, while clinicians will continue to hold a 'conservation' view in which they resist the world of academia in an effort to promote research that is 'useful'. This historical gap between the needs of the two communities is difficult to bridge.

For Albert, a research culture is not formed out of the will of a few interested individuals, but is shaped by larger social forces. Research is a social practice, and methods are seen as 'legitimate' within the relative, but not arbitrary, codes of practice of research cultures. Also, subjectivities (such as the identity of the 'researcher') are constructed through the accepted social practices of the research culture. Albert asks who shall decide on the quality of medical education research. Clinicians call for relevant, applied knowledge to improve practice, but are often naïve about the range and sophistication of research methodologies and their informing conceptual frameworks. Academics must publish or perish and wish to contribute to knowledge so that research for them may emphasize meaningfulness over relevance, and they may alienate those who are often the subjects of, or allies in, their research—clinicians.

A key tension in medical education research occurs as pragmatic clinicians seek direct, 'quick and dirty', applications for research, where more theoretically inclined academic researchers want to build theory, cherish ideas, and take pride in research for its own sake. At its best, this tension is productive, creating dialogue and exchange of ideas between the two cultures. At its worst, the academic community may pursue idiosyncratic research satisfying its own internal demands such as publication and conferencing outputs, while the culture of clinicians may appear to be merely adding to their reputation of anti-intellectualism.

Here, I progress the perceptive observations of Albert et al. to develop a model of a collaborative research community building on the three platforms articulated above, as a creative knowledge environment (CKE) (Hemlin, Allwood, & Martin, 2004). Building a genuine collaborative research community as a CKE depends upon four factors:

1. Developing genuine interdisciplinarity, while creatively meeting the implementation challenge to the development of that interdisciplinarity—where, for example, the 'permanent revolution' of health service policy reorganizations does not allow time to embed practices and may spurn evidence for practice change

2. Aligning epistemologies (theories of knowledge) across communities that support theoretically informed research (cognitive alliance)
3. Aligning axiologies (values) across communities to develop potentials for collaboration grounded in common understandings (values alliance) and moral engagement
4. Aligning ontologies (conditions of being) across communities that allow for the affective development of collaboration and identities (social alliance)

Conditions for Collaboration

Developing Interdisciplinarity

Collaborative research communities necessarily need to learn to work in interdisciplinary ways. Interdisciplinarity does not just happen, but must be learned (and earned). More importantly, for interdisciplinarity to work as a basis to collaborative research, disciplinarity has to be 'unlearned', or aspects of disciplinarity have to be suspended.

Dalke, Grobstein, and McCormack (2006, p. 2) suggest that there are 'risks' in interdisciplinary collaboration, but that the benefits far outweigh the risks. Diana Rhoten's (2004) review of interdisciplinary research centres in the sciences shows that weaker collaborative associations are more common than genuinely interdisciplinary collaborations. The history of the establishment of interprofessional education and associated research provides a good historical model for interdisciplinarity. Many activities aspiring to 'interprofessionalism' remain at the level of 'multiprofessionalism', where interprofessionalism is defined as 'learning with, from, and about other profession(al)s'.

Multiprofessionalism remains at the level of learning (and working) with other professionals, where professional silos are reinforced and boundaries are not crossed. Why this transition is important is because a growing body of evidence demonstrates that patient care and patient safety both significantly improve where clinical teams work interprofessionally, rather than remaining at the level of multiprofessional activity, as detailed throughout this book.

It is, of course, easy to map levels of interdisciplinarity but hard to realize these in practice. Again, learning to work in an interdisciplinary way also requires parallel unlearning and suspension of disciplinary habits that work at cross purposes with interdisciplinary collaborations. Couturier, Gagnon, Carrier, and Etheridge (2008) offer an excellent introduction to theorizing interdisciplinarity and propose a developmental model that is progressed here.

In *disciplinarity* we work within an identified discipline, its historical traditions, conventions, and habits. Of course, disciplinarity can be creative and interdisciplinarity does not so much require the avoidance of a discipline position as its judicious application and suspension. *Pluridisciplinarity* brings together disciplines that still remain highly disciplined and bounded. *Multidisciplinarity* introduces discipline *negotiations*, where the object or subject of study or activity, such as a patient, becomes the focus and collaboration is weak or guarded. *Interdisciplinarity* introduces a genuine level of collaboration where interests of single disciplines are suspended for interest of the 'object' of the activity, such as the patient. As discipline boundaries are crossed, the complex adaptive system of the 'interdiscipline' offers emergent properties that would not be gained if boundaries were maintained. However, higher levels of risk are now introduced, and the system has to be closely managed to gain benefit.

The system is inherently unstable. Disciplines are now transformed, and discipline identities are constructed as 'interdisciplinarians' or interdisciplinary researchers. We might characterize this transition to interdisciplinarity as a deterritorialization (Deleuze & Guattari, 2004a). New geo-cognitive challenges emerge, such as how one occupies the 'interspace', the difference between disciplines that is now tolerated and what this space can generate in the way of new knowledge.

Couturier and colleagues (2008, p. 342) note that the *National Register of Scientific and Technical Personnel* for 2007 records 'more than 8,000 disciplines'. The authors explain this extraordinary figure as a consequence of 'the modern, positivistic conviction that the fragmentation of objects will make the world more intelligible'. Actually, this also makes the world more visible. Discipline tags are like signs on the landscape that let us know we are in a 'garden', in 'woodland', in 'undergrowth', and so forth, while we can just as readily collapse this back to the generic 'landscape'. The exponential growth in the number of disciplines is a symptom of the need for specialist rather than generic descriptors of work and of resistance to interdisciplinary approaches.

Disciplines 'discipline'—they focus and bring the world into order so that saying and seeing become the same thing. As we increase the size of the catalogue, so we generate varieties of analytic ways of seeing and acting. The antidote to this atomization is the overview, the holistic grasp, generic seeing. This offers synthetic ways of seeing. A team of specialists working around a patient 'sees', or constructs, that patient according to how each of those practitioners has been disciplined. This leads to multiple ontologies within the same workspace (Mol, 2008). However, contemporary clinical teamwork aims to offer holistic and integrated care around the patient. The overall vision of the team, reflected in their 'situation awareness', or how well attuned they are to the work and perspectives of the other team members, draws disciplines together and then transcends disciplinarity. This is one of the models of patient-centredness generated earlier in this book—the team-based approach.

I have argued in the opening chapters that we now have a good body of evidence to suggest that such an approach enhances the safety of the patient by reducing the possibility of medical error grounded in team miscommunications. However, as Couturier and colleagues (2008) argue, 'interdisciplinarity' has been applied to health-care work before the notion has been carefully thought through. This has led to evidence being accrued from studies where conflicting models of 'interdisciplinarity' are at work. It is important to work towards conceptual clarification.

For Couturier and colleagues, interdisciplinarity is first an epistemological problem—a problem of knowledge—and second a practice problem or an issue of translation of knowledge. However, because of the pragmatic drive in health-care and the need for quick fixes, practice solutions are privileged. Indeed, implementation may outrun investigation, where management promotes cycles of practice change without practitioners having time to bed in the previous round and without a full evidence base for efficacy. Thus, effort is put into encouraging on the ground 'collaboration' in team work without first really setting out what is meant by an interdisciplinary collaboration, as a 'profound transformation in the very activity of knowing'. What Couturier and colleagues mean by this is that education for inter-disciplinarity has focused upon the relational and affective dimensions of collaboration on the ground, at the expense of 'the meeting of epistemologies', or the clash of worldviews that so clearly occurs when, for example, differing medical special-ists and health-care practitioners work around a patient.

Now we are in a position to be able to address the conceptual difficulties raised by the question 'how do we establish "fellow feeling" in a community of research-ers?' The world of interprofessional education has struggled with how to translate models of collaboration into effective practice for patient benefit and safety and then has struggled with how to evaluate and research such practices. However, signifi-cant progress has recently been made in the field.

Conceptual clarification of multiprofessionalism and interprofessionalism has helped to inform research. Where learning 'with, from, and about' other profession-als is translated into work-based learning, we have key markers, such as the emer-gence of situation awareness and 'boundary crossing', that can be tracked in research (Engeström, 2008; Kerosuo & Engeström, 2003). As we translate this work into the field of collaborative research in medical education, our key transitions are from multidisciplinarity to interdisciplinarity to trans- and circumdisciplinarity.

The key cognitive emergent property in such transition is shared cognition and the key affective property is 'fellow feeling'. The paradox of this emphasis upon the relational aspects of interdisciplinarity (and interprofessionalism) is that it increases the already burdensome workload of practitioners. This effect is doubled where both new learning and unlearning of old habits are invoked. However, the long-term benefits include greater efficiency in teamwork and, more importantly, potential improvement in patient safety.

Again, such benefits emerge only if the knowledge and skills needed for the new collaborative teamwork have time to bed in or become tacit. One important set of knowledge and skills is research of practice by practitioners themselves, usually in collaboration with academic researchers. While learning self-research knowledge and skills, such as collaborative inquiry, again adds to the work burden, there are long-term benefits, including the establishment of audit and appraisal cultures.

Marjorie Garber (2003) notes that 'interdisciplines' work around the edges of established disciplines, forming, as it were, a connective tissue between those disci-plines. Their place is to offer a 'transgressive' possibility that conventional single-discipline study would not provide. Hence, suggests Garber, interdisciplines will not become 'centres' of the academy. Dalke et al. (2006) disagree with Garber, suggesting that interdisciplinary study is already at the centre of academic life. This does not stop interdisciplinarity from offering an intellectual edge or transgressive possibilities. What concerns me about both these views is the continued use of the metaphor of the 'centre'.

I have already argued for patient-centredness without a centre. This is not just play on words, but a key aspect of systems thinking. A systems approach to interdisciplinarity would see the power of bringing several disciplines together as transforming static centres into dynamic attractors suspended in a temporary network (Bleakley, 2010). Interdisciplinary research might transcend the need for 'centres' in a 'liquid' world—also challenging our current dominant funding models based on establishing centres of excellence, rather than excellent, responsive, and transformative networks or webs. The centre need not hold because it is the quality of the network that matters, based also on responsive not working.

Where disciplinarity is still strong, there are dangers of new forms of colonialism, as discussed later. These are resisted by interdisciplinarity, which is the postcolonial position of 'Empire' or globalization, where traces of disciplinarity still linger. In what can be called *profound interdisciplinarity*, efforts are made by all concerned to engage in axiological, epistemological, and ontological conversations for collaboration. In what can be called *faux interdisciplinarity*, the smell of colonialism lingers and knowing and being are not transformed, as some wish to colonize and the colonized engage in patterns of resistance, from outright challenge to more subtle forms such as gently mocking the tactics of the colonized in limited imitation. These unfortunate arrangements are wholly unproductive of collaboration, as discipline differences are not respected.

From profound interdisciplinarity, there are two more transformative possibilities. Interdisciplinarity can morph into *transdisciplinarity*, where nagging boundary residues are now dissolved and researchers are thinking and acting as 'interdisciplinarians'. The danger here is that researchers believe that they have reached an ideal condition, a higher state. But 'utopia' literally means 'no place', and the better descriptor for a transdisciplinarity is *circumdisciplinarity*, where members of a collaborative research team cycle back to previous issues to evaluate how these have now been managed and how the research collaboration may proceed. Indeed, if this is a 'task/finish' group, the focus may be upon how to dissolve the collaboration. Further, circumdisciplinarity involves all stakeholders.

Ted Wong (2002) points to an intra-discipline battle within science, between 'observational' scientists interested primarily in empirical data and 'theoretical' scientists interested primarily in modelling and theory. In some ways, these echo, respectively, the interests of the clinical community and the academic research community in medical education research. Wong characterizes the observational scientists as working with metonymy, where the theoretical scientists work with metaphor. As previously discussed, Roman Jakobson (1992) famously set out this distinction in language usage from work on aphasics, and the distinction has been applied as a way of describing a theoretical tension in knowledge communities.

Those with a metonymic orientation like to work with contiguity and association or linkages and repetition. Traditional scientific observation works this way, through replication of results in repeated experimentation. A typical linkage might be 'wand–staff–sceptre–ruler'. Those with a metaphoric bent prefer substitution to contiguity. When somebody says 'alarm bells were ringing' or 'I smell a rat', they do not literally hear the bells or smell the animal. The metaphor collapses complex associations into a succinct image. The image substitutes for the concrete object.

Dalke et al. (2006) take Wong's model and apply it generally to the development of interdisciplinary research. Every research culture develops a 'metonymic landscape' as its own position of research. Typically, for a science culture, this will be a set of related ideas around how to maintain 'objectivity' and for a humanities culture, around ideas such as 'expression', 'subjectivity', 'interpretation', and 'narrative'. Each culture will also have a guiding metaphor such as 'detachment' for science and 'indwelling' for the humanities. Interdisciplinarity requires 'grappling with the metaphors' of another culture in order to change 'our own metonymic landscapes'. In this process, both guiding metaphors and the nature of the research landscapes we inhabit are transformed, elaborated, and doubled.

I will now offer a development of this line of thinking about interdisciplinarity. So far, I have described an epistemological exchange and promised transformation. In developing collaborative research cultures, the problem, suggests Couturier and colleagues (2008, p. 346), is not the affective work of how professionals shall get on with each other in team settings, but rather overcoming historical epistemological barriers. 'Working together' in a research community is then secondary to establishing an 'epistemological dialogue' within the reality of an uncomfortable aggregation of differing knowledge communities (such as the clinical and the academic).

While this epistemological gap must be addressed, 'circumdisciplinarity' may never be achieved if the affective, relational nature of collaborative research communities is not addressed at the same time as the epistemological issues. This relational work is fundamental to setting up a 'community'. In light of the above discussion, we can carry out the work of establishing a metonymic landscape of research as an epistemological concern (deciding, e.g. on the relative status of evidence-based and narrative approaches to knowledge). However, this work will not progress if we cannot discuss it without interpersonal stress, tension, and the resulting danger of collapse of negotiation.

An ontological community has to be established as the framework for the epistemological discussion. Transitions from cooperation through coordination to collaboration must be set up in the face of the deeply divisive competitive atmospheres generated by policy, such as the UK higher education culture's REF, mentioned above. The policy rhetoric of such frameworks calls for collaboration between research centres. The reality, as Rhoten (2004) shows, is that collaboration remains at a weak level and disciplinary tensions remain unresolved. We suggest that this is because ontological work has to be done, where affective, interpersonal issues shape research effectiveness.

In the new interdisciplinary (and circumdisciplinary) climates, epistemological families may be created, inviting hybridization of research. However, such research families will remain dysfunctional and never mature into long-standing collaborative communities if ontological families are not established, leading to positive identity constructions as 'interdisciplinary' researchers.

I have suggested that the epistemological *and* ontological transformations required to establish genuine research communities turn linear research teams or groupings into non-linear, complex dynamic systems, generating greater potential but greater risk. With this dynamic change comes the promise of innovation. As this transformation is established, old models of research leadership and management will be transformed into models of emergent and distributed leadership. Cognition in such research collaborations will be shared or distributed, and members will have to learn how to access distributed cognition that is also 'nomadic' or always on the move. These new collaborative structures transform hierarchies into networks and territorialization or boundary setting (familiar from discipline-based practices) into deterritorialization and boundary crossing.

Collectively, this constitutes a paradigm shift in medical education research. As Merleau-Ponty (1968) describes a qualitative shift from inhabiting the 'known body' to the 'lived body', so we see the transformation of the weakly collaborative 'known' research community into a strongly collaborative 'lived' research community. This community is characterized by epistemological transformation (shared knowledge) *and* ontological transformation (fellow feeling), bounded by an axiological transformation (shared values and moral concerns).

As introduced earlier, working within a climate of managerial and political 'permanent revolution' policy directives frustrates the embedding of practices by not giving enough time for new practices to become tacit before such practices are displaced. Collaborative research must be embedded. If researchers are learning new values, knowledge, and skills (interdisciplinarity to circumdisciplinarity, as genuine collaboration) in both epistemological and ontological realms, they need time for practice so that expertise can be gained. One of Regehr's (2004) main observations concerning the current state of the medical education research community is the lack of research expertise. The model of collaboration promoted in this book demands gaining expertise, but there are fundamental blocks to this possibility.

Sennett (2008) observes that skills needed in contemporary health-care are not allowed to embed because of the excessive nature of organizational change. For example, the UK National Health Service (NHS) has undergone four major reorganizations, along Fordist management lines, in the past decade and a fifth is in process, where general practitioners will manage a front line service for the sale of health products to consumers (patients) within a capitalist market system.

A good example of a recent change is the introduction of clinical teamwork practices that are gradually dissolving stable teams for ad hoc teams. Old fashioned Fordist production line practices demand that 'teams' are constituted from a pool of workers as protection against collaborative resistance to the 'owners' of the means of production (in the NHS this means 'management'). Practitioners must become adaptable 'team players'. As team formations are demanded, basic team work practices, such as briefing and debriefing, have not been introduced, so that clinical 'teams' have the same status as 'research communities' in our discussion above. As we noted above, competitive and divisive research policies linked to funding also work against embedding collaborative activities.

Aligning Epistemologies, Axiologies, and Ontologies

By alignment, I mean creating productive conversation between positions, as well as adopting common positions. Aligning knowledge communities, such as the academic and clinical, rarely happens spontaneously. First, such communities have differing epistemological outlooks. This is further complicated by differences within academic and clinical communities. Broadly, the clinical community represents its primary epistemological interest as science, but admits to narrative practices in patient encounters. The academic medical education research community has epistemological interests in both scientific and narrative approaches, but the science approach of social scientists often has quite a different feel to the science approach of the clinical community. In short, there is a complicated conversation to be had about epistemological territory prior to assuming that a collaborative knowledge community can develop within medical education research.

Such potential cognitive alliance will only develop to full collaboration if it is informed by understanding of distributed cognition as an effect not just of learning in research activity but of unlearning (Rushmer & Davies, 2004). Part of the unlearning process is a letting go, or tempering, of the ideology of individualism to embrace social learning. How can research collaboration be genuine if it is not understood as an act of shared learning and cognition leading to the establishment of a research community of practice, where both knowledge and information have a 'social life' (Brown & Duguid, 2000)?

Collaborative epistemological positions, discussed briefly above, and ontological positions, discussed briefly below, are held in place by shared values. Knowing and being (identity) will not converge or engage in dialogue across differing research communities of practice unless there are shared values. While the clinical and academic research communities, for example, may differ in what kind of research they value—from the pragmatic, applied end of the scale to the pure, conceptual end—a shared value should be beneficial to the patient. I have outlined several approaches to patient-centredness and suggested that academic researchers would benefit from clinically sited experience in which the 'patient' becomes a phenomenological, lived reality for the researcher and not simply an object of study.

Where I go further is to suggest that the 'hospitality' that medicine promises ('hospital' becoming a metaphor for all clinics, consultations, pharmacies, and clinically based research) is literalized, where patient-centred values are realized in clinical hospitality and this extends also to working with colleagues. The exercise of such hospitality across colleague teams, such as clinical researchers collaborating with academic researchers, calls for alignment of ontologies. Ontology is the study of 'existence' or 'being' and is intimately tied with identity construction. Ontologies also introduce issues of human relationship and affect. Simply, members of collaborative research communities do not just have to work through knowledge differences, but have to do this interpersonally, socially. As we have said, communities are not communities without the development of 'fellow feeling'.

Finally, the patient must enter the research community as a valued member. The epistemological, axiological, and ontological alignments between clinical and academic members of the medical education research community discussed above must now extend to patients. Research funding bodies will now encourage patient involvement in planning, implementation, governance, and evaluation of research, and there are a number of organizations, such as INVOLVE in the UK that have sophisticated models of patient involvement and illustrative case studies at hand. But collaborating with patients in medical education research is in its infancy and will remain stilted where the medical education research community remains weak in its understanding of collaborative research models such as action research and collaborative inquiry (Heron, 2001; Reason & Bradbury, 2006).

In the models of new forms of relationship and collaboration discussed so far in this book, I have often cited Hardt and Negri's (2001, 2006, 2009) developmental model of post-imperialism—where an emergent new world order is described—as a framework through which we may better understand communication in medicine as an aspect of medical education and medical education research. The first phase of this is 'Empire', where, in the wake of the demise of the old imperialisms and subsequent decolonizing, a global capitalism emerges as 'globalization'. This wave is characterized by conflict based on identification with exclusive value systems, recognizing only the 'selfsame' as valid and returning to the safety of bounded disciplines. The second wave, yet to come, is that of the 'Multitude', a democratic world order based on tolerance of difference. Here, boundaries are crossed as the Other is faced. The third wave, a horizon possibility, is the realization of a 'common wealth' in which radical alterity or difference is accommodated. Here, interdisciplinarity matures to trans- and circumdisciplinarity. In Levinas's (1969) view, this is not simply the accommodation of the Other's views to one's own, but the realization of self-identity only in the mirror of the Other (the patient, the work colleague) to whom one offers genuine hospitality.

In this radical move, medicine, medical education, and medical education research produce 'patients' of a different order than the consumer of services through 'ontological production'—the production of new forms of relationship and identities. In medicine and health-care, the patient is no longer treated as a passive item on a production line, where efficiency and throughput are the markers of medical excellence, but as the central participant in a relational medicine and as a key component of a distributed cognition in clinical reasoning and treatment. In medical education, the patient is realized as coeducator of the medical student and doctor or surgeon in training. In medical education research, the patient can be collaborator at various levels—in planning, implementation, ethical approval, governance, and management and evaluation.

In such models of collaboration—doctors in dialogue with both academic researchers and patients with new identities—performance of doctors is not judged in terms of throughput, as generation of units or numbers of patients treated within set time limits for identified activities, but in terms of quality of provision. Importantly, where a certain level of technical competence amongst doctors is assumed, patient care and safety is dependent upon the quality of nontechnical factors—relationships, teamwork, and communication. Through such ontological work, doctors can restore public faith in medicine (Ludmerer, 1999).

Through new, horizontal teamwork arrangements with colleagues, more collaborative patterns of education with students and juniors in training and dialogue with patients, medicine may become genuinely democratic. Such emerging democracy in turn may be peer regulated for quality through evidence accruing from medical education research. In these two cycles of activity, we move towards a new horizon of meaning for relational medicine with the patient as, and at, the heart of the matter.

Part III
A Brief but Provocative Conclusion

Chapter 17
Conclusion: Professing Medical Identities in the Liquid World of Teams

Putting Medicine on the Couch

In this book, I have laid out some of the current issues to be considered and addressed in the broad field of communication in medicine—working with patients and with colleagues mainly in clinical team settings. 'Communication' also implies communicating with oneself—acknowledging technical and professional limits, reflecting in and on practice, and becoming critically reflexive about the values that inform practice. This must mesh with self-care. Communication and professionalism are not about the instrumental following of protocols but about wise practice that Aristotle called *phronesis*, where practice is adapted to context.

Much of this book considers current ills in medical practice within the realms of communication and professionalism. Such ills are expressed as symptoms—most importantly, the unacceptably high rate of medical error associated with 'communication hypocompetence' that has been described as an iatrogenic epidemic.

A second, often unacknowledged, set of symptoms can be readily recognized in doctors' socialized 'patient speak'. What do I mean by this? Patients properly complain when doctors talk at them in technical terms that the patient does not understand ('hypotensive', 'atherosclerotic', 'haematoma'), and every communications skills training programme attempts to address this issue. However, what socialization into medical culture achieves (by medical students and junior doctors or interns imitating the styles and manners of their teachers, down through the generations) is a 'patient speak' that can be demeaning, even insulting, for patients. This includes a number of stock phrases, such as 'this may be a little uncomfortable' (where an intervention is potentially painful); making an embarrassing intimate examination sound innocuous: 'could you just "pop off" your clothes and "hop on" the bed?' This is neither technical nor professional language, but a kind of in-house talk that only serves to confuse.

A third important area for symptom production is from limited self-knowing and self-caring, such as the relatively high rates of suicide, burnout, depression, and

A. Bleakley, *Patient-Centred Medicine in Transition: The Heart of the Matter*, Advances in Medical Education 3, DOI 10.1007/978-3-319-02487-5_17, © Springer International Publishing Switzerland 2014

drug and alcohol abuse amongst doctors in relation to other professions. Some readers may think that my account is biased towards such ills and does not adequately praise contemporary medical practice and doctors. Let me assure you that I have the greatest respect for what medicine and doctors have achieved technically. I am not interested in either 'doctor bashing' or 'clinical team bashing' and have benefitted personally from sophisticated medical interventions and good health-care. However, the focus of this book is on the non-technical aspects of doctoring, where there is still much to be achieved. I also recognize that patients—people—have a responsibility to act considerately and respectfully towards doctors and other health-care professionals. I have said nothing in this book of violent, abusive, uncooperative, resistant, and arrogant patients!

My own practice has been in psychoanalytic psychotherapy, and so I tend to read phenomena for their depths and for what is not immediately expressed. I also spot behaviours as often symptomatic of deeper, underlying, and unaddressed issues. Symptom is sometimes dangerous if left untreated or unattended. On the other hand, symptoms can also serve useful purposes and sometimes are best listened to closely, or noticed ('attended to', which is the root meaning of 'therapy'), rather than 'treated'. For example, the symptom of so-called 'empathy decline' may in fact be protective. Doctors cannot be open, and raw, to all their patients, because medicine deals so much with suffering and death. Doctors must have ways of defending themselves against meeting so much suffering in one day. Limits to empathy may indicate that those defences are functioning well. However, this is different from defences becoming so hardened that the doctor becomes cynical or uncaring.

In this final chapter, before summing up, I will first put medicine on the couch in light of the warnings given in the previous paragraph. Putting 'medicine' on the couch means analysing not just an individual doctor's ills (at the extreme end, what, e.g. motivated Harold Shipman as a serial murderer of his vulnerable patients?) but also medicine as an institution. I will briefly consider three levels of symptom: (1) at the level of the institution, (2) at the level of medical culture and subcultures, and (3) at the level of teams and individuals.

First, medicine as an institution shows a chronic symptom of mistrust of 'outsiders', historically justified as a claim to a high degree of professional autonomy. This can be read analytically as institutional paranoia. I have detailed how medicine as an institution has had to respond to the demands of its 'customers'—patients—for greater accountability. This includes a demand for transparency and collaboration not only with patients but also with doctors' employers, politicians, managers, and health-care colleagues.

One important product of this process of transparency and accountability has been the development of systems of appraisal and revalidation. However, such processes, because of their technical focus (problem-solving), have become overdetermined, so that politicians and managers have been seen to erode and undermine the professional autonomy of clinicians rather than form that autonomy (or temper it constructively). Analytically, the issue is how to treat the paranoia of medicine as an institution—in other words, why has the institution of medicine continued to distrust transparency and public accountability and, as a result, 'shut up shop'? The answer is clear from the third point considered below—medicine, and surgery in particular, was able to close ranks where it recognized that it had failed its patients through avoidable error. 'Never admit to error' became an unwritten law of medicine and surgery. Paranoia was then masked by hubris and arrogance.

The paranoia that I describe is a fear of failure, baldly the fear of admitting to the possibility of failure. This has long been linked in sociological studies of surgery with intolerance of ambiguity and uncertainty—surgeons and doctors have, historically, been unable to admit to (and embrace as a resource) the high levels of uncertainty that inhabit their work. This has two effects—to produce an authoritarian culture that is self-serving and readily closes ranks and to produce paranoia—the creeping fear that something really is rotten in the state of Denmark and that somebody may just expose the nature of the emperor's delusion concerning his 'new clothes'. Analytically, the emperor must know that he is naked and vulnerable and that support is available. Basically, paranoia describes a range of delusions. Medicine and surgery in particular have colluded as an institution to maintain delusions about levels of uncertainty and ambiguity in practice. Importantly, a sea change is now at work to address such institutional delusion, as this book suggests.

Second, patterns of socialization into medicine and surgery show symptoms. Analytically, these are anal and sadistic. In the same way that institutions such as the armed forces rationalize humiliation, long work hours including sleep deprivation, and hierarchy, as character building, this is also the case historically with medicine. This is also rapidly changing through measures such as the European Working Time Directive that demand more humane work schedules. While medicine has justified such punitive socialization as necessary for learning the range and depth of technical skill necessary for specialization, as well as building character, such regimes increase risk to patients as attention levels of doctors are compromised through fatigue.

'Sadistic', a seemingly harsh word, is however an appropriate description where those who exert authority seemingly gain pleasure from tactics such as humiliating juniors and resort to justifications for such tactics as 'it never did me any harm'. Of course such tactics do harm, as we have seen from the relatively high suicide, burnout, depression, and drug and alcohol abuse rates of doctors. 'Anal' describes the necessity of the culture to resort to rules and strict hierarchies in militaristic fashion ('anal retentive'), as if juniors were not able to self-regulate. In contrast, anal retention usually twins with 'anal expulsion'—the need for an individual or culture to explode irrationally, smearing others with such explosions. Again, historically, senior doctors and surgeons have been able to get away with aggressive and verbally abusive outbursts that would not be tolerated in other contexts, but are, irrationally, justified as 'character building'—tempering or hardening in the furnace.

In a traditional psychoanalysis, anality is expected to mature to genitality, or adult relationships that relinquish the desire for control and humiliation to shared concerns, collaboration, and democratic encounters. The main argument of this book can then be recast psychoanalytically—medicine's and medical education's necessary transformation from autocratic to democratic methods, to improve patient safety through better communication, is a shift from 'anal' concerns to 'genital' concerns. The unresolved early history of medicine as an institution fostering control, autonomy, and socialization through humiliation has resulted in medicine being stuck in an anal phase. Medicine has yet to mature into a 'sexual' adult with desires for collaborative and equal exchange to promote shared satisfaction.

There are many forces at work to change this institutional pattern of control—referred to earlier as 'status asymmetry', or the inappropriate translation of meritocracy into autocracy—notably the increase in the number of women entering medicine. The feminizing of medicine (Bleakley, 2013a)—that may lead to transformation from a tough-minded to a tender-minded culture—may be the single most significant cultural shift seen in the profession, but as explored earlier, there is a fear that the reach of this feminizing potential may not seriously affect medical education (which is failing to recruit women doctors in numbers) or the top ranks of medical practice (senior consultants and senior clinician managers). However, the emergence of a tender-minded culture echoes the movement of medical culture from valorizing heroic individualism to promoting collaborative practices.

Finally, I have explored how doctors and surgeons *as a community* suffer from communication hypocompetence, evidenced in the levels of unnecessary risk that patients are exposed to. If poor communication is the symptom, what is the cause? Analysis suggests light levels of autism—a kind of Asperger's syndrome (the light end of the autism spectrum) as an inability to form satisfying or complete social relationships, linking back to difficulties in moving from an anal to a genital stage of development. While a light level of defence against intimacy is necessary, hardening to fall short of an adequate level of communication with patients and colleagues is symptomatic of an underlying neurosis.

While, in medical education, we are increasingly discussing the study of medicine as gaining legitimate entry into a community of practice and forming an identity as a doctor, we rarely discuss the instabilities and neuroses of that community of practice (and its sub-communities). Are we continuing to support medical students' legitimate entry into a psychologically unstable community of practice, so that they form fractured identities?

It is easy to bandy labels about, and readers should be cautious of reading these psychological labels too literally. My frail diagnoses are made purely as a platform, a stimulus to discussion about what can now be done in the way of intervention. The basic intervention that I argue for, again, is the democratizing of medical practice and medicine as an institution—a structural challenge beyond the education of individual medical students and doctors. Literacy in democracy can be equated with effective communication and support practices with patients, colleagues, and self. This is not a technical practice, limited to learning skills, but one exercising the moral imagination.

Professing Medicine

The new era of health-care promises collaborative, team-based, patient-centred practice. Medical culture has some way to go to fully embrace this democratic ideal, where meritocracy so readily translates into autocracy, realized in hierarchical work practices. At the height of the communication hypocompetence epidemic in 2000, in one report, medical error was estimated as the third biggest killer after cancer and heart disease in North America (Starfield, 2000) and quality of clinical team process was at an all-time low, rejecting the democratic habits that North America so famously values as its primary cultural export. The figures in such reports are still hotly disputed and often employed rhetorically, and risk is inevitable in medicine and especially surgery. I do not wish to add fuel to that controversy. A wider range of studies is reported in the opening chapters of this book. Collectively, they cannot be ignored, showing that medical error is a significant source of unnecessary deaths that can be addressed and substantially reduced.

While medicine may now be at the beginning of the long road to achieving democracy in communication, the medical education culture urgently needs to politicize its research programme—to stop putting so much energy into reactive, data-farming studies that are complicit with unproductive practices compromising patient care and safety, and to become proactive in stimulating culture change in medicine. Medical culture patently needs to democratize at a faster rate, and medical education can provide that democratizing force and tune its intensity, drawing on politically aware, cutting-edge thinking across a range of disciplines, including the humanities. For example, understanding of both 'identity' and 'teamwork' has radically progressed over the past 30 years as modernist paradigms have been challenged by postmodern thinking and practice, yet little of this sea change has registered in medical education, which remains strangely conservative.

I have argued for fresh thinking in medical education to respond to a new wave of work practices in health-care, embedded in wider cultural flux. Transition to 'liquid' times and a 'runaway' world' involves once routine work groups becoming what sociologists call 'cloakroom communities', such as work groups that have little or no continuity. We have seen that, in medicine, traditional territorial team structures—stable 'firms' and 'houses'—have been replaced by unstable, nomadic activities. Teamwork, described typically in terms of content and role ('how' things are done, habitually), must now be described in terms of process and accountability ('why' things are done, adaptively). Such team process has been described as 'teeming', 'negotiated knotworking', and 'collaborative intentionality', rapidly pulsating work that requires a variety of team players to come together temporarily for coordinated, cooperative, or collaborative activities, often in concert with other 'teams', in which situation awareness is best established through protocols such as briefing. Such emergent work patterns lead to new identity constructions.

It is not only the participants in these new activities who must unlearn and relearn practices but those who study such practices must learn a new vocabulary of appreciation and understanding of such practices: complexity, dynamic systems activity, emergent properties, boundary crossing, knotworking, networking, meshworking, translation, cognitive trails, rhizomatic and mycorrhizal structures, nomadism, deterritorializing, segmentation, and so forth. Reference to settled structures with centres fails to address the new nomadic, liquid, and runaway world of health-care.

Metaphors of the tree developing to fruition, as the long-standing emblem of vertical or hierarchical team structures and their related codes, or of pieces of the 'jigsaw' coming together to form a solution to a problem must be abandoned as inadequate in understanding a liquid world. Rather, we need problem-stating metaphors that encompass the unseen, the complex, and the horizontal in patterns of work. Such metaphors include the rhizome rather than the tree, an underground, horizontal root complex occasionally pushing up shoots, and tangled mycorrhizal structures symbiotic with other plants, to develop large complex, underground networks, signifying multi-team boundary-crossing negotiations as the key practices in future health-care.

Our understanding of identity construction will necessarily shift as medical work changes, to problematize identity through new textualizations of work. As I have described throughout this book, in the varied contexts of multidisciplinary, patient-centred care pathways, doctors and health-care workers are talking to each other in new ways (first text), talking to patients in new ways (second text), and talking to researchers in new ways about this work (third text). This complex of emergent and highly labile conditions demands a renegotiation of identities. Central to such renegotiation is a challenge to the traditional forms of gaining an identity through social inclusivity (entry into the profession) as this generates social exclusivity (exit or exile from other communities of practice).

Rather, this inclusivity–exclusivity dynamic is now reversed, or irreversibly interrupted, as doctors supplement and subvert their traditional identities as specialist diagnosticians in becoming interprofessionals, advocates, and teachers, while patients, for example, become diagnosticians (experts in their own conditions) and 'medical citizens' (politicized, in terms of demanding democratization of health-care practices, including participation in decision-making within an assembly democracy). In an era of transparency and accountability (monitory democracy), doctors have to recount to a wider variety of people, and in a wider variety of ways, why they do what they do. Doctors now have to speak and write in new ways that question conventions of what it means to be and speak like a doctor. 'Bedside' and 'consulting room' manner should no longer vacillate between obfuscating technical language, and 'this won't hurt a bit' condescension, or 'just pop off your clothes' chumminess. Neither of these styles attempts empathy.

As the repertoire of the doctor widens in collaborative team settings, to include peer and patient input into appraisal and revalidation, incident reporting, multidisciplinary audit, shared teaching, and team-based diagnostic work, so identities multiply and shift, in transformative states of 'becoming' rather than fixed states of 'being', again problematizing identity. Becoming 'part of the team' must now be reconceptualized as 'part of the teeming', where doctors' liquid professional identities include that of 'interprofessional team player' working around the pulse of the patient, who is the heart of the matter.

These are exciting times for medical education, as the status and value of communication in medicine has now come into sharp and alarming focus. Medical educators must respond to the challenge of forming a 'commonwealth' out of practitioner and patient resources to democratize medical practice.

References

Abse, D. (2008). *Serving two gods. Acumen*. Academy of Medical Educators. Retrieved September 17–21, 2008, from http://www.medicaleducators.org/

Accreditation Council for Graduate Medical Education. (2005). *Advancing education in interpersonal and communication skills*.

Adler, A. (2009/1927). *Understanding life: An introduction to the psychology of Alfred Adler*. Oxford, England: Oneworld.

Adler, A., & Brett, C. (2009/1938). *Social interest: Adler's key to the meaning of life*. Oxford, England: Oneworld.

Adorno, T. W., Frenkel-Brunswik, E., Levinson, D. J., & Sanford, R. N. (1950). *The authoritarian personality*. New York: Harper and Row.

Agamben, G. (1998). *Homo sacer: Sovereign power and bare life*. Palo Alto, CA: Stanford University Press.

Agency for Healthcare Research and Quality (AHRQ). (2008). *National healthcare quality report*. Rockville, MD: US Department of Health and Human Services.

Ainley, P., & Rainbird, H. (Eds.). (1999). *Apprenticeship: Towards a new paradigm of learning*. London: Routledge.

Akrich, M. et al. (2002). The key to success in innovation part I: The art of interessement. *International Journal of Innovation Management, 6*, 187–206.

Albanese, M. A., Snow, M. H., Skochelak, S. E., Huggett, K. N., & Farrell, P. M. (2003). Assessing personal qualities in medical school admissions. *Academic Medicine, 78*, 313–321.

Albert, M. (2004). Understanding the debate on medical education research: A sociological perspective. *Academic Medicine, 79*, 948–954.

Albert, M., Hodges, B., & Regehr, G. (2007). Research in medical education: Balancing service and science. *Advances in Health Sciences Education Theory and Practice, 12*, 103–115.

Allard, J., Bleakley, A., Hobbs, A., & Coombes, L. (2011). Pre-surgery briefings and safety climate in the operating theatre. *BMJ Quality and Safety*, published online ahead of print July 2011. doi:10.1136/bmjqs.2009.032672.

Allard, J., Bleakley, A., Hobbs, A., & Vinnell, T. (2007). 'Who's on the team today?': Collaborative teamwork in operating theatres should include briefing. *Journal of Interprofessional Care, 21*, 189–206.

Ambady, N., Koo, J., Rosenthal, R., & Winograd, C. H. (2002). Physical therapists' nonverbal communication predicts geriatric patients' health outcomes. *Psychology and Aging, 17*, 443–452.

Anon. (2010). *Actor-network theory*. Memphis, TN: Books LLC.

Apple, M. (2004). *Ideology and curriculum* (3rd ed.). New York: RoutledgeFalmer.

Applebee, A. N. (1996). *Curriculum as conversation: Transforming traditions of teaching and learning*. Chicago: University of Chicago Press.

A. Bleakley, *Patient-Centred Medicine in Transition: The Heart of the Matter*,
Advances in Medical Education 3, DOI 10.1007/978-3-319-02487-5,
© Springer International Publishing Switzerland 2014

Arnold, L., & Stern, D. T. (2006). What is medical professionalism? In D. T. Stern (Ed.), *Measuring medical professionalism* (pp. 15–37). Oxford, England: Oxford University Press.

Arthur, H., Wall, D., & Halligan, A. (2003). Team resource management: A programme for troubled teams. *Clinical Governance, 8*, 86–91.

Ashley, C. (1944). *The Ashley book of knots.* London: Doubleday.

Ashley, P., Rhodes, N., Sari-Kouzel, H., Mukherjee, A., & Dornan, T. (2009). 'They've all got to learn'. Medical students' learning from patients in ambulatory (outpatient and general practice) consultations. *Medical Teacher, 31*, e24–e31.

Atkins, S., & Ersser, S. J. (2008). Clinical reasoning and patient-centred care. In J. Higgs, M. A. Jones, S. Loftus, & N. Christensen (Eds.), *Clinical reasoning in the health professions* (3rd ed., pp. 77–88). Philadelphia: Butterworth Atkins.

Atkinson, P. (1995). *Medical talk and medical work: The liturgy of the clinic.* London: Sage.

Bachelard, G. (1968/1934). *The philosophy of no: A philosophy of the new scientific mind.* New York: Viking Press.

Bakhtin, M. M. (1981). *The dialogic imagination: Four essays.* Austin, TX: University of Texas Press.

Barr, H. (2007). *Interprofessional education in the United Kingdom: 1966 to 1997.* London: Higher Education Academy.

Barron, K., Atkins, C., Bone, P., Dowd, J., Gidley, S., Hesford, S., et al. (2009). *House of Commons health committee patient safety: Sixth report of session, 2008–09.* Retrieved from http://www.publications.parliament.uk/pa/cm200809/cmselect/cmhealth/151/151i.pdf

Bate, P. (2000). Changing the culture of a hospital: From hierarchy to networked community. *Public Administration, 78*, 485–512.

Bauman, Z. (2000). *Liquid modernity.* Cambridge, England: Polity Press.

Bauman, Z. (2004). *Identity.* Cambridge, England: Polity.

Bauman, Z. (2007). *Liquid times: Living in an age of uncertainty.* Cambridge, England: Polity.

Bauman, Z. (2008). *Globalization: The human consequences.* Cambridge, England: Polity.

Beach, M. C., & Inui, T. (2006). Relationship-centered care. A constructive reframing. *Journal of General Internal Medicine, 21*(Suppl. 1), S3–S8.

Becker, H. S., Geer, B., Hughes, E. C., & Strauss, A. L. (1980). *The boys in white: Student culture in medical school.* New York: Transaction Publishers.

Beckman, H. B., & Frankel, R. M. (1984). The effect of physician behavior on the collection of data. *Annals of Internal Medicine, 101*, 692–696.

Beger, H. G., & Arbogast, R. (2006). The art of surgery in the 21st century: Based on natural sciences and new ethical dimensions. *Langenbecks Archives of Surgery, 391*, 143–148.

Bellah, R. N., Madsen, R., Sullivan, W. M., Swidler, A., & Tipton, S. M. (2007). *Habits of the heart: Individualism and commitment in American life* (3rd ed.). Berkeley, CA: University of California Press.

Benbassat, J., & Baumal, R. (2009). A proposal for overcoming problems in teaching interviewing skills to medical students. *Advances in Health Sciences Education: Theory and Practice, 14*, 441–450.

Benson, J., & Britten, N. (2003). Patients' views about taking antihyperintensive drugs: Questionnaire study. *British Medical Journal, 326*, 1314–1315.

Bhabha, H. (1994). *The location of culture.* London: Routledge.

Black, A. E., & Church, M. (1998). Assessing medical student effectiveness from the psychiatric patient's perspective: The medical student interviewing performance questionnaire. *Medical Education, 32*, 472–478.

Bleakley, A. (1992). Greens and greenbacks. *Spring, 52*, 68–71.

Bleakley, A. (1999). From reflective practice to holistic reflexivity. *Studies in Higher Education, 24*, 315–330.

Bleakley, A. (2000a). Adrift without a lifebelt: Reflective self-assessment in a post-modern age. *Teaching in Higher Education, 5*, 405–418.

Bleakley, A. (2000b). Writing with invisible ink: Narrative, confessionalism and reflective practice. *Reflective Practice, 1*, 11–24.

Bleakley, A. (2001). From lifelong learning to lifelong teaching: Teaching as a call to style. *Teaching in Higher Education, 6*, 113–116.

Bleakley, A. (2002). Teaching as a gift: The gendered gift and teaching as hospitality. In G. Howie & A. Tauchert (Eds.), *Gender, teaching and research in higher education*. London: Ashgrove.

Bleakley, A. (2006a). 'You are who I say you are': The rhetorical construction of identity in the operating theatre. *The Journal of Workplace Learning, 18*, 414–425.

Bleakley, A. (2006b). A common body of care: The ethics and politics of teamwork in the operating theater are inseparable. *Journal of Medicine and Philosophy, 31*, 1–18.

Bleakley, A. (2006c). Broadening conceptions of learning in medical education: The message from teamworking. *Medical Education, 40*, 150–157.

Bleakley, A. (2009). Curriculum as conversation. *Advances in Health Sciences Education: Theory and Practice, 14*, 297–301.

Bleakley, A. (2010). Blunting Occam's razor: Aligning medical education with theories of complexity. *Journal of Evaluation in Clinical Practice, 16*, 849–855.

Bleakley, A. (2011a). Becoming a medical professional. In L. Scanlon (Ed.), *"Becoming" a professional: An interdisciplinary analysis of professional learning* (pp. 129–152). Dordrecht, Netherlands: Springer.

Bleakley, A. (2011b). *Unpublished audit: Close call reports*. Truro, England: Royal Cornwall Hospitals Trust.

Bleakley, A. (2012a). The proof is in the pudding: Putting actor-network-theory to work in medical education. *Medical Teacher, 34*, 462–467.

Bleakley, A. (2012b). Establishing patient safety nets: How actor-network-theory can inform clinical education research. In V. Cook, C. Daly, & M. Newman (Eds.), *Socio-cultural perspectives on work-based learning in clinical practice*. Oxford, England: Radcliffe.

Bleakley, A. (2012c). The humanities offer a democratizing force for medical education. *Ars Medica, 9*, 1–6.

Bleakley, A. (2012d). The curriculum is dead! Long live the curriculum! Designing an undergraduate medicine and surgery curriculum for the future. *Medical Teacher, 34*, 543–547.

Bleakley, A. (2013a). Gender matters in medical education. *Medical Education, 47*, 59–70.

Bleakley, A. (2013b). Working in 'teams' in an era of 'liquid' healthcare: What is the use of theory? *Journal of Interprofessional Care, 27*, 18–26.

Bleakley, A., Allard, J., & Hobbs, A. (2013). 'Achieving ensemble': Communication in orthopaedic surgical teams and the development of situation awareness—An observational study using live videotaped examples. *Advances in Health Sciences Education: Theory and Practice, 18*, 33–56.

Bleakley, A., & Bligh, J. (2008). Students learning from patients: Let's get real in medical education. *Advances in Health Sciences Education: Theory and Practice, 13*, 89–107.

Bleakley, A., & Bligh, J. (2009). Who can resist Foucault? *Journal of Medicine and Philosophy, 34*, 368–383.

Bleakley, A., Bligh, J., & Browne, J. (2011). *Medical education for the future: Identity, power and location*. Dordrecht, Netherlands: Springer.

Bleakley, A., Boyden, J., Hobbs, A., Walsh, L., & Allard, J. (2006). Improving teamwork climate in operating theatres: The shift from multiprofessionalism to interprofessionalism. *Journal of Interprofessional Care, 20*, 461–470.

Bleakley, A., Brice, J., & Bligh, J. (2008). Thinking the post-colonial in medical education. *Medical Education, 42*, 266–270.

Bleakley, A., Farrow, R., Gould, D., & Marshall, R. (2003a). Making sense of clinical reasoning: Judgment and the evidence of the senses. *Medical Education, 37*, 544–552.

Bleakley, A., Farrow, R., Gould, D., & Marshall, R. (2003b). Learning how to see: Doctors making judgments in the visual domain. *Journal of Workplace Learning, 15*, 301–306.

Bleakley, A., Hobbs, A., Boyden, J., & Walsh, L. (2004). Safety in operating theatres: Improving teamwork through team resource management. *Journal of Workplace Learning, 16*, 414–425.

Bleakley, A., & Marshall, R. (2012). The embodiment of lyricism in medicine and Homer. *Medical Humanities, 38*, 50–54.

Bleakley, A., & Marshall, R. (2013). Can the science of communication inform the art of the medical humanities? *Medical Education, 47*, 126–133.

Bleakley, A., Marshall, R., & Brömer, R. (2006). Toward an aesthetic medicine: Developing a core medical humanities undergraduate curriculum. *Journal of Medical Humanities, 27*, 197–214.

Bligh, J., & Bleakley, A. (2006). Distributing menus to hungry learners: Can learning by simulation become simulation of learning? *Medical Teacher, 28*, 606–613.

Bligh, J., & Brice, J. (2008). What is the value of good medical education research? *Medical Education, 42*, 652–653.

Boerma, W. G., & van den Brink-Muinen, A. (2000). Gender-related differences in the organization and provision of services among general practitioners in Europe: A signal to health care planners. *Medical Care, 38*, 993–1002.

Bordo, S. (1993). *Unbearable weight: Feminism, western culture, and the body*. Berkeley, CA: University of California Press.

Boreham, N. (2004). A theory of collective competence: Challenging the neo-liberal individualization of performance at work. *British Journal of Educational Studies, 52*, 5–17.

Borrill, C. S., Carletta, J., Carter, A. J., Dawson, J. F., Garrod, S., Rees, A., et al. (2000). *The effectiveness of health care teams in the national health service*. Birmingham, England: University of Aston, Aston Business School, Aston Centre for Health Service Organization Research.

Boulis, A. K., & Long, J. A. (2004). Gender differences in the practice of adult primary care physicians. *Journal of Women's Health (Larchmt), 13*, 703–712.

Bourdieu, P. (1977). *Outline of a theory of practice*. Cambridge, England: Cambridge University Press.

Bourdieu, P., & Passeron, J.-C. (1977). *Reproduction in education, society and culture*. Beverly Hills, CA: Sage.

Boyle, D., Dwinnell, B., & Platt, F. (2005). Invite, listen, and summarize: A patient-centered communication technique. *Academic Medicine, 80*, 29–32.

Branch, W. T. (2001). Small-group teaching emphasizing reflection can positively influence medical students' values. *Academic Medicine, 76*, 1171–1172.

Branch, W. T. (2006). Viewpoint: Teaching respect for patients. *Academic Medicine, 81*, 463–467.

Brill, N. I. (1976). *Teamwork: Working together in the human services*. Philadelphia: Lippincott.

British Medical Association. (2007). *Doctors' health matters 08 May 2007*. Retrieved from http://www.bma.org.uk/doctors_health/doctorshealth.jsp?page=6

British Medical Association. (2008). *Role of the patient in medical education*. British Medical Association Medical Education Subcommittee. Retrieved from http://www.bma.org.uk/images/roleofthepatient_tcm27-175953.pdf

Britten, N. (2003). Commentary: Does a prescribed treatment match a patient's priorities? *British Medical Journal, 327*, 840.

Britten, N. (2008). *Medicines and society: Patients, professionals and the dominance of pharmaceuticals*. Basingstoke, England: Palgrave MacMillan.

Brown, J. (2008). How clinical communication has become a core part of medical education in the UK. *Medical Education, 42*, 271–278.

Brown, J. S., & Duguid, P. (2000). *The social life of information*. Boston, MA: Harvard Business School Press.

Bruner, J. (2002). *Making stories: Law, literature, life*. New York: Farrar, Straus and Giroux.

Buddeberg-Fischer, B., Klaghofer, R., Abel, T., & Buddeberg, C. (2003). The influence of gender and personality traits on the career planning of Swiss medical students. *Swiss Medical Weekly, 133*, 535–540.

Bunker, J. P. (2001). *Medicine matters after all*. London: Nuffield Press.

Buszewicz, M., Pistrang, N., Cape, J., & Martin, J. (2006). Patients' experiences of GP consultations for psychological problems: A qualitative study. *British Journal of General Practice, 56*, 496–503.

Butt, A. R. (2010). Medical error in Canada: Issues realting to reporting of medical error and methods to increase reporting. *McMaster University Medical Journal (Clinical Review), 7*, 15–18.

Calman, K. C. (2007). *Medical education past, present and future: Handing on learning*. Edinburgh, Scotland: Elsevier.

Canguilhem, G. (1991). *The normal and the pathological*. New York: Zone Books.

Carlisle, A. J., Parker, R. M., Cantey, P., Wolf, M. S., & Moore, J. R. (2010). Medicine and compassion: Exploring and teaching the art of medicine in Italy. *The New Physician, 59*. Retrieved June 21, 2011, from http://www.amsa.org/AMSA/Homepage/Publications/TheNewPhysician/2010/1210medicine_and_compassion.aspx

Carothers, T. (2006). The backlash against democracy promotion. *Foreign Affairs, 85*, 55–68.

Cartledge, P. (2009). *Ancient Greek political thought in practice*. Cambridge, England: Cambridge University Press.

Carvajal, D. (2011, March 8). The changing face of Western medicine. *International Herald Tribune*, p. 1.

Carvel, J. (2002, April 11). Concern as women outnumber men in medical schools. *The Guardian*.

Cassell, J. (1991). *Expected miracles: Surgeons at work*. Philadelphia: Temple University Press.

Cassell, J. (2000). *The woman in the surgeon's body*. New Haven, CT: Harvard University Press.

Centre for the Advancement of Interprofessional Education. Retrieved from http://www.caipe.org.uk/about-us/defining-ipe/

Chaiklin, S., Hedegaard, M., & Jensen, U. J. (2003). *Activity theory and social practice: Cultural historical approaches*. Aarhus, Denmark: Aarhus University Press.

Chambers, T. (1999). *The fiction of bioethics: Cases as literary texts*. New York: Routledge.

Charon, R. (2011). The novelization of the body, or, how medicine and stories need one another. *Narrative, 19*, 33–50.

Chatwin, B. (2005). *The songlines*. London: Vintage.

Christakis, N., & Fowler, J. (2010). *Connected: The amazing power of social networks and how they shape our lives*. London: HarperPress.

Christianson, C. E., McBride, R. B., Vari, R. C., Olson, L., & Wilson, H. D. (2007). From traditional to patient-centered learning: Curriculum change as an intervention for changing institutional culture and promoting professionalism in undergraduate medical education. *Academic Medicine, 82*, 1079–1088.

Ciborra, C. (2000). A critical review of the literature on the management of corporate information infrastructure. In C. Ciborra (Ed.), *From control to drift: The dynamics of corporate information infrastructure* (pp. 15–40). Oxford, England: Oxford University Press.

Cixous, H. & Clément, C. (1986). *The Newly Born Woman*. Minnesota: University of Minnesota Press.

Cixous, H. (1991). *Coming to writing and other essays*. Cambridge, MA: Harvard University Press.

Cixous, H. (Ed.). (2004). *The Hélène Cixous reader*. London: Routledge.

Clark, A. (1997). *Being there: Putting brain, body, and world together again*. Cambridge, MA: The MIT Press.

Clark, A. (2009). *Supersizing the mind: Embodiment, action, and cognitive extension*. Oxford, England: Oxford University Press.

Clearihan, L. (1999). Feminisation of the medical workforce. Is it just a gender issue? *Australian Family Physician, 28*, 529.

Cohen, L., Manion, L., & Morrison, K. (2000). *Research methods in education* (5th ed.). London: RoutledgeFalmer.

Cole, T. R., & Carlin, N. (2009). The suffering of physicians. *The Lancet, 374*, 1414–1415.

Colliver, J. A., Conlee, M. J., Verhulst, S. J., & Dorsey, J. K. (2010). Reports of the decline of empathy during medical education are greatly exaggerated: A reexamination of the research. *Academic Medicine, 85*, 588–593.

Colquhoun, G. (2007). *Playing god: Poems about medicine*. London: Hammersmith Press Ltd.

Cooke, M., Irby, D. M., & O'Brien, B. C. (2010). *Educating physicians: A call for reform of medical school and residency*. San Francisco: Jossey-Bass/Carnegie Foundation for the Advancement of Teaching.

Coulter, A. (2002). *The autonomous patient: Ending paternalism in medical care*. London: The Nuffield Trust/The Stationery Office.

Couturier, Y., Gagnon, D., Carrier, S., & Etheridge, F. (2008). The interdisciplinary condition of work in relational professions of the health and social care field: a theoretical standpoint. *Journal of Interprofessional Care, 22*, 341–351.

Crook, C. (2002). Learning as cultural practice. In M. R. Lea & K. Nicoll (Eds.), *Distributed learning: Social and cultural approaches to practice* (pp. 152–169). London: Routledge/Falmer.

Culler, J. (1997). *Literary theory: A very short introduction.* Oxford, England: Oxford University Press.

Cumming, A. (2002). Good communication skills can mask deficiencies. *British Medical Journal, 325,* 676.

Cussins, A. (1992). Content, embodiment and objectivity: The theory of cognitive trails. *Mind, 101,* 651–688.

Dalke, A., Grobstein, P., & McCormack, E. (2006). Exploring interdisciplinarity: The significance of metaphoric and metonymic exchange. *Journal of Research Practice, 2,* Article M3. Retrieved August 1, 2011, from http://jrp.icaap.org/index.php/jrp/article/view/43/54

Daniels, H. (2005). *An introduction to Vygotsky.* London: Routledge.

Daniels, H., Edwards, A., Engeström, Y., Gallagher, T., & Luvigsen, S. R. (Eds.). (2009). *Activity theory in practice.* London: Routledge.

Daston, L., & Galison, P. (2007). *Objectivity.* New York: Zone Books.

Davis, B., & Sumara, D. (2006). *Complexity and education.* Mahwah, NJ: Lawrence Erlbaum Associates.

De Cossart, L., & Fish, D. (2005). *Cultivating a thinking surgeon: New perspectives on clinical teaching, learning and assessment.* Harley, England: TFM Publishing.

DeLanda, M. (1997). *A thousand years of nonlinear history.* New York: Swerve Editions.

DeLanda, M. (2002). *Intensive science and virtual philosophy.* London: Continuum.

DeLanda, M. (2006). *A new philosophy of society: Assemblage theory and social complexity.* London: Continuum.

Deleuze, G. (1991). *Bergsonism.* New York: Zone Books.

Deleuze, G. (1993). *The fold: Leibniz and the Baroque.* Minneapolis, MN: University of Minnesota Press.

Deleuze, G., & Guattari, F. A. (2004a). *A thousand plateaus.* London: Continuum International Publishing Group Ltd.

Deleuze, G., & Guattari, F. (2004b). *Anti-Oedipus: Capitalism and schizophrenia.* London: Continuum International Publishing Group Ltd.

Deleuze, G., & Parnett, C. (2007). *Dialogues* (2nd ed.). New York: Columbia University Press.

Denekens, J. P. (2002). The impact of feminisation on general practice. *Acta Clinica Belgica, 57,* 5–10.

Derese, A., Kerremans, I., & Deveugele, M. (2002). Feminisation, the medical profession and its education. *Acta Clinica Belgica, 57,* 3–4.

Derrida, J. (1967). *Of grammatology.* Baltimore: Johns Hopkins University Press.

Diamond, L. (2008). The democratic rollback. *Foreign Affairs, 87,* 36–48.

Dickey, J., Girard, D. E., Geheb, M. A., & Christine, K. (2004). Using systems-based practice to integrate education and clinical services. *Medical Teacher, 26,* 428–434.

Dornan, T. (2010). On complexity and craftsmanship. *Medical Education, 44,* 2–3.

Doukas, D. J., McCullough, L. B., & Wear, S. (2010). Reforming medical education in ethics and humanities by finding common ground with Abraham Flexner. *Academic Medicine, 85,* 318–323.

Dyrbye, L. N., Thomas, M. R., Massie, F. S., Power, D. V., Eacker, A., Harper, A., et al. (2008). Burnout and suicidal ideation among U.S. medical students. *Annals of Internal Medicine, 149,* 334–341.

Eco, U. (1999). *Kant and the platypus: Essays on language and cognition.* London: Secker & Warburg.

Edwards, N. (2007). *In stitches: The highs and lows of life as an A & E doctor.* London: Friday Books.

Edwards, R., Biesta, G., & Thorpe, M. (Eds.). (2009). *Rethinking contexts for learning and teaching: Communities, activities and networks.* London: Routledge.

Engel, G. L. (1977). The need for a new medical model: A challenge for biomedicine. *Science, 196,* 129–136.

Engeström, Y. (1987). *Learning by expanding: An activity-theoretical approach to developmental research.* Helsinki, Finland: Orienta-Konsultit.

Engeström, Y. (1999). *Learning by expanding: Ten years after* (Introduction to the German edition). Retrieved July 12, 2010, from http://lchc.ucsd.edu/MCA/Paper/Engestrom/expanding/intro.htm

Engeström, Y. (2000). Activity theory as a framework for analyzing and redesigning work. *Ergonomics, 43*, 960–974.

Engeström, Y. (2004). New forms of learning in co-configuration work. *Journal of Workplace Learning, 16*, 11–21.

Engeström, Y. (2005). Knotworking to create collaborative intentionality capital in fluid organizational fields. In M. M. Beyerlein, S. T. Beyerlein, & F. A. Kennedy (Eds.), *Collaborative capital: Creating intangible value* (pp. 307–336). Amsterdam: Elsevier.

Engeström, Y. (2008). *From teams to knots: Activity-theoretical studies of collaboration and learning at work.* Cambridge, England: Cambridge University Press.

Engeström, Y., Engeström, R., & Kerosuo, H. (2003). The discursive construction of collaborative care. *Applied Linguistics, 24*, 286–315.

Engeström, Y., Engeström, R., & Vähääho, T. (1999). When the center does not hold: The importance of knotworking. In S. Chaiklin, M. Hedegaard, & U. J. Jensen (Eds.), *Activity theory and social practices* (pp. 345–374). Aarhus, Denmark: Aarhus University Press.

Engeström, Y., & Middleton, D. (Eds.). (1998). *Cognition and communication at work.* Cambridge, England: Cambridge University Press.

Eva, K. W. (2005). What every teacher needs to know about cognitive reasoning. *Medical Education, 39*, 98–106.

Fadiman, A. (1997). *The spirit catches you and you fall down: A Hmong child, her American doctors, and the collision of two cultures.* New York: Farrar Straus Giroux.

Fanon, F. (2001/1961). *The wretched of the earth.* Harmondsworth, England: Penguin.

Farrell, C., Towle, A., & Godolphin, W. (2006). *Where's the patient's voice in health professional education?* Vancouver, British Columbia, Canada: University of British Columbia. Retrieved from http://www.chd.ubc.ca/dhcc/sites/default/files/documents/PtsVoiceReportbook.pdf

Fenwick, T., & Edwards, R. (2010). *Actor-network theory in education.* London: Routledge.

Findlay, L., & Gough, B. (2003). *Reflexivity: A practical guide for researchers in health and social sciences.* Oxford, England: Blackwell.

Finn, R. (2008). The language of teamwork: Reproducing professional divisions in the operating theatre. *Human Relations, 61*, 103–130.

Finn, R., & Waring, J. J. (2006). Organizational barriers to architectural knowledge and teamwork in operating theatres. *Public Money and Management, 26*, 117–124.

Flexner, A. (1910). *Medical education in the United States and Canada.* New York: Carnegie Foundation for the Advancement of Teaching.

Flin, R., O'Connor, P., & Crichton, M. (2008). *Safety at the sharp end: A guide to non-technical skills.* Aldershot, England: Ashgate.

Flynn, T. (1987). Foucault as parrhesiast: His last course at the College de France. *Philosophy and Social Criticism, 12*, 213–229.

Foucault, M. (1975). *Discipline and punish: The birth of the prison.* New York: Random House.

Foucault, M. (1976). *The birth of the clinic.* London: Tavistock.

Foucault, M. (1987). The ethic of care for the self as a practice of freedom. *Philosophy and Social Criticism, 2*, 112–131.

Foucault, M. (1989a). *The order of things.* London: Routledge.

Foucault, M. (1989b). *The birth of the clinic: An archaeology of medical perception.* London: Routledge.

Foucault, M. (1990). *The care of the self.* London: Penguin Books.

Foucault, M. (2001). *Fearless speech.* New York: Semiotext[e].

Foucault, M. (2002). *Power: The essential works of Michel Foucault 1954-1984* (3rd ed.). Harmondsworth, England: Penguin.

Foucault, M. (2005a). *The hermeneutics of the subject: Lectures at the College de France 1981–1982.* New York: Picador.

Foucault, M. (2005b). *The hermeneutics of the subject*. New York: Picador.

Fox, R. C. (1957). Training for uncertainty. In R. K. Merton, G. Reader, & P. Kendall (Eds.), *The student-physician*. Cambridge, MA: Harvard University Press.

Fox, R. (1997/1959). *Experiment perilous: Physicians and patients facing the unknown*. New Brunswick, NJ: Transaction.

Fox, S. (2009). Contexts of teaching and learning: An actor-network view of the classroom. In R. Edwards, G. Biesta, & M. Thorpe (Eds.), *Rethinking contexts for learning and teaching: Communities, activities and networks* (pp. 31–43). London: Routledge.

Franěk, J. (2006). Philosophical parrhesia as aesthetics of existence. *Continental Philosophy Review, 39*, 113–134.

Frank, A. W. (1999). Relations of power and 'informed choice': Commentary on Rose Weitz's 'watching Brian die'. *Health, 3*, 239–246.

Franks, A., & Rudd, N. (1997). Medical student teaching in a hospice—What do the patients think about it? *Palliative Medicine, 11*, 395–398.

French, J. R. P., & Raven, B. (1959). The bases of social power. In D. Cartwright & A. Zander (Eds.), *Group dynamics*. New York: Harper and Row.

Friedson, E. (1970). *Profession of medicine*. New York: Harper and Row.

Frode, H. (2010). Multidisciplinary collaboration as a loosely coupled system: Integrating and blocking professional boundaries with objects. *Journal of Interprofessional Care, 24*, 19–30.

Funnell, M. M., & Anderson, R. M. (2004). Empowerment and self-management of diabetes. *Clinical Diabetes, 22*, 123–127.

Fysh, T. H., Thomas, G., & Ellis, H. (2007). Who wants to be a surgeon? A study of 300 first year medical students. *BMC Medical Education, 19*, 2.

Gabbay, J., & Le May, A. (2011). *Practice-based evidence for healthcare: Clinical mindlines*. London: Routledge.

Gao, L., & Bleakley, A. (2008). Developing 'thinking as a doctor': What is the influence of other healthcare professionals upon the early learning of medical students? *International Journal of the Humanities, 6*, 65–74.

Garber, M. (2003). *Academic instincts*. Princeton, NJ: Princeton University Press.

Garfinkel, H. (1967). *Studies in ethnomethodology*. Englewood Cliffs, NJ: Prentice-Hall.

Gaskell, G., & Bauer, M. W. (2000). Towards public accountability: Beyond sampling, reliability and validity. In M. W. Bauer & G. Gaskell (Eds.), *Qualitative researching with text, image and sound*. London: Sage.

Gawande, A. (2002). *Complications: A surgeon's notes on an imperfect science*. London: Profile Books.

Gawande, A. (2007). *Better: A surgeon's notes on performance*. London: Profile Books.

Gawande, A. (2009). *The checklist manifesto: How to get things right*. London: Profile Books.

Gawande, A. A., Zinner, M. J., Studdert, D. M., & Brennan, T. A. (2003). Analysis of errors reported by surgeons at three teaching hospitals. *Surgery, 133*, 614–621.

General Medical Council. (2006). *Good medical practice*. London: GMC.

General Medical Council. (2007). *The new doctor*. London: GMC.

General Medical Council. (2009). *Tomorrow's doctors 2009: Outcomes and standards for undergraduate medical education*. London: GMC.

Genn, J. M. (2001). Curriculum, environment, climate, quality and change in medical education—A unifying perspective. *Medical Teacher, 23*, 337–344 (Part 1), 445–454 (Part 2).

Giddens, A. (1991). *Modernity and self-identity*. Cambridge, England: Polity.

Giddens, A. (2002). *Runaway world*. London: Profile.

Giddings, A. E. B., & Williamson, C. (2007). *The leadership and management of surgical teams*. London: The Royal College of Surgeons of England.

Ginsburg, S., & Lingard, L. (2006). Using reflection and rhetoric to understand professional behaviors. In D. T. Stern (Ed.), *Measuring medical professionalism* (pp. 195–212). Oxford, England: Oxford University Press.

Goffman, E. (1971). *The presentation of self in everyday life*. London: Penguin.

Goffman, E. (1990). *The presentation of self in everyday life*. Harmondsworth, England: Penguin.

Goffman, E. (1991). *Asylums: essays on the social situation of mental patients and other inmates*. London: Penguin.

Goodman, P. (1964). *Compulsory mis-education*. New York: Horizon Press.

Goodman, N. (1978). *Ways of worldmaking*. Indianapolis, IN: Hackett.

Graban, M. (2011). *Statistics on healthcare quality and patient safety problems—Errors and harm*. Retrieved May 26, 2011, from http://www.leanblog.org/author/admin/

Graber, M. L., Franklin, N., & Gordon, R. (2005). Diagnostic error in internal medicine. *Archives of Internal Medicine, 165*, 1493–1499.

Greenberg, C. C., Regenbogen, S. E., Studdert, D. M., Lipsitz, S. R., Rogers, S. O., Zinner, M. J., et al. (2007). Patterns of communication breakdowns resulting in injury to surgical patients. *Journal of the American College of Surgeons, 204*, 533–540.

Greenblatt, S. (1980). *Renaissance self-fashioning*. Chicago: University of Chicago Press.

Greene, G. (1993). *The ministry of fear: An entertainment*. Harmondsworth, England: Penguin Books.

Greenhalgh, T., Plsek, P., Wilson, T., Fraser, S., & Holt, T. (2010). Response to 'the appropriation of complexity theory in health care'. *Journal of Health Services Research & Policy, 15*, 115–117.

Groopman, J. (2007). *How doctors think*. Boston, MA: Houghton Mifflin Company.

Gruppen, L. D., Branch, V. K., & Laing, T. J. (1996). The use of trained patient educators with rheumatoid arthritis to teach medical students. *Arthritis Care Research, 9*, 302–308.

Gschwandtner, S. (2006). A brief history of string—From the *eruv* to the *quipu*. *Cabinet, 23*, 38–42.

Guattari, F. (1995). *Chaosmosis: An ethico-aesthetic paradigm*. Sydney, New South Wales, Australia: Power Publications.

Guattari, F. (2008). *The three ecologies*. London: Continuum.

Guelich, J. M., Singer, B. H., Castro, M. C., & Rosenberg, L. E. (2002). A gender gap in the next generation of physician-scientists: Medical student interest and participation in research. *Journal of Investigative Medicine, 50*, 412–418.

Guggenbuhl-Craig, A. (1983). *Power in the helping professions*. Dallas, TX: Spring Publications.

Hafferty, F. (2006). Measuring professionalism: A commentary. In D. T. Stern (Ed.), *Measuring medical professionalism* (pp. 281–306). Oxford, England: Oxford University Press.

Haggis, T. (2009). Beyond 'mutual constitution': Looking at learning and context from the perspective of complexity theory. In R. Edwards, G. Biesta, & M. Thorpe (Eds.), *Rethinking contexts for learning and teaching: Communities, activities and networks* (pp. 44–60). London: Routledge.

Haidet, P., Dains, J. E., Paterniti, D. A., Hechtel, L., Chang, T., Tseng, E., et al. (2002). Medical student attitudes toward the doctor-patient relationship. *Medical Education, 36*, 568–574.

Halpern, J. (2001). *From detached concern to empathy: Humanizing medical practice*. Oxford, England: Oxford University Press.

Hamberg, K. (2003). Gender perspective relevant in many medical school subjects. Essential to perceive men and women holistically. *Lakartidningen, 100*, 4078–4083.

Hampton, J. R., Harrison, M. J., Mitchell, J. R., & Seymour, C. (1975). Relative contributions of history-taking, physical examination, and laboratory investigation to diagnosis and management of medical outpatient. *British Medical Journal, 2(5969)*, 486–489.

Harden, S. W. (2011, March). Surgeons and teamwork. *AAOS Now*. Retrieved from http://www.aaos.org/news/aaosnow/mar11/managing3.asp

Hardt, M., & Negri, A. (2001). *Empire*. Cambridge, MA: Harvard University Press.

Hardt, M., & Negri, A. (2006). *Multitude: War and democracy in the age of empire*. Harmondsworth, England: Penguin.

Hardt, M., & Negri, A. (2009). *Commonwealth*. Cambridge, MA: Harvard University Press.

Hare, I., & Weinstein, J. (Eds.). (2009). *Extreme speech and democracy*. Oxford, England: OUP.

Hargie, O., Boohan, M., McCoy, M., & Murphy, P. (2010). Current trends in communication skills training in UK schools of medicine. *Medical Teacher, 32*, 385–391.

Hargie, O., Dickson, D., Boohan, M., & Hughes, K. (1998). A survey of communication skills training in UK schools of medicine: Present practices and prospective proposals. *Medical Education, 32*, 25–34.

Hargreaves, A. (2003). *Teaching in the knowledge society: Education in the age of insecurity.* Milton Keynes, England: Open University Press.

Harman, G. (2009). *Prince of networks: Bruno Latour and metaphysics.* Melbourne, Victoria, Australia: Re-press.

Hartz, M. B., & Beal, J. R. (2000). Patients' attitudes and comfort levels regarding medical students' involvement in obstetrics-gynecology outpatient clinics. *Academic Medicine, 75*, 1010–1014.

Hasnain, M., Bordage, G., Connell, K. J., & Sinacore, J. M. (2001). History-taking behaviors associated with diagnostic competence of clerks: An exploratory study. *Academic Medicine, 76*(10 Suppl), S14–S17.

Haug, M., & Lavin, B. (1983). *Consumerism in medicine: Challenging physician authority.* Beverly Hills, CA: Sage.

Hawhee, D. (2004). *Bodily arts: Rhetoric and athletics in ancient Greece.* Austin, TX: University of Texas Press.

HealthGrades Quality Study. (2004). *Patient safety in American hospitals.* Health Grades, Inc.

HealthGrades Quality Study. (2008). *The eleventh annual healthgrades hospital quality in America study October 2008.* Health Grades, Inc.

Heisler, M., & Resnicow, K. (2008). Helping patients make and sustain healthy changes: A brief introduction to motivational interviewing in clinical diabetes care. *Clinical Diabetes, 26*, 161–165.

Helman, C. (2006). *Suburban Shaman: Tales from medicine's front line.* London: Hammersmith Press.

Hemlin, S., Allwood, C. M., & Martin, B. R. (2004). Conclusions: How to stimulate creative knowledge environments. In S. Hemlin, C. M. Allwood, & B. R. Martin (Eds.), *Creative knowledge environments: The influences on creativity in research and innovation* (pp. 193–220). Cheltenham, England: Edward Elgar.

Henderson, S., Mills, M., Hobbs, A., Bleakley, A., Boyden, J., & Walsh, L. (2007). Surgical team self-review: Enhancing organisational learning in the Royal Cornwall Hospital Trust. In M. Cook, J. Noyes, & Y. Masakowski (Eds.), *Decision making in complex environments* (pp. 259–270). Aldershot, England: Ashgate.

Heron, J. (2001). *Helping the client: A creative practical guide* (5th ed.). London: Sage.

Higgs, J., Jones, M. A., Loftus, S., & Christensen, N. (Eds.). (2008). *Clinical reasoning in the health professions* (3rd ed.). Amsterdam: Elsevier.

Hillman, J. (1981). *The thought of the heart.* Ascona, Switzerland: Eranos Foundation.

Hillman, J. (1994a). "Man is by nature a political animal", or: Patient as citizen. In S. Shamdasani (Ed.), *Speculations after Freud: Psychoanalysis, philosophy and culture* (pp. 27–40). London: Routledge.

Hillman, J. (1994b). *Healing fiction.* Dallas, TX: Spring Publications.

Hillman, J., & Ventura, M. (1993). *We've had a hundred years of psychotherapy and the world's getting worse.* San Francisco: Harper.

Hobbs, A. (2005, May 16–18). Team self-review: Improving teamwork and reducing error. In *Risk management: Health care risk report.*

Hobbs, A., & Bleakley, A. (2005, March 18–19). Close-call reporting. In *Risk management: Health care risk report.*

Hobsbawm, E. (2008). *On empire: America, war, and global supremacy.* New York: Pantheon Books.

Hodges, B. (2003). OSCE! Variations on a theme by Harden. *Medical Education, 37*, 1134–1140.

Hodges, B. (2010). *The objective structured clinical examination: A socio-history.* Saarbrücken, Germany: Lambert Academic Publishing.

Hojat, M., Gonnella, J. S., Mangione, S., Nasca, T. J., Veloski, J. J., Erdmann, J. B., et al. (2002). Empathy in medical students as related to academic performance, clinical competence and gender. *Medical Education, 36*, 522–527.

Hojat, M., Gonnella, J. S., Nasca, T. J., et al. (2002). Physician empathy: Definition, components, measurement, and relationship to gender and specialty. *American Journal of Psychiatry, 159*, 1563–1569.

Hojat, M., Louis, D. Z., Markham, F. W., Wender, R., Rabinowitz, C., & Gonnella, J. S. (2011). Physicians' empathy and clinical outcomes for diabetic patients. *Academic Medicine, 86*, 359–364.

Hojat, M., Mangione, S., Nasca, T. J., Rattner, S., Erdmann, J. B., Gonnella, J. S., et al. (2004). An empirical study of decline in empathy in medical school. *Medical Education, 38*, 934–941.

Hojat, M., Vergare, M. J., Maxwell, K., Brainard, G., Herrine, S. K., Isenberg, G. A., et al. (2009). The devil is in the third year: A longitudinal study of erosion of empathy in medical school. *Academic Medicine, 84*, 1182–1191.

Holt, T., & Marinker, M. (2010). *Complexity for clinicians*. Oxford, England: Radcliffe.

Howe, A. (2001). Patient-centered medicine through student-centered teaching: A student perspective on the key impacts of community-based learning in undergraduate medical education. *Medical Education, 35*, 666–672.

Iedema, R. (Ed.). (2007). *The discourse of hospital communication: Tracing complexities in contemporary health care organizations*. Basingstoke, England: Palgrave Macmillan.

Iedema, R., & Scheeres, H. (2003). From doing work to talking work: Renegotiating knowing, doing, and identity. *Applied Linguistics, 24*, 316–337.

Ikegami, E. (2005). *Bonds of civility: Aesthetic networks and the political origins of Japanese culture*. Cambridge, England: Cambridge University Press.

Illich, I. (1975). *Limits to medicine: Medical nemesis—The expropriation of health*. Harmondsworth, England: Penguin Books.

Institute of Medicine (IOM). (2003). *Patient safety, achieving a new standard of care*. Washington, DC: Institute of Medicine of the National Academies. Retrieved from http://iom.edu/Reports/2003/Patient-Safety-Achieving-a-New-Standard-for-Care.aspx

Irigaray, L. (1993). *je, tu, nous: Toward a culture of difference*. New York: Routledge.

Irvine, D. (2003). *The doctor's tale: Professionalism and public trust*. Abingdon, England: Radcliffe Medical Press.

Jackson, N. (2000). Writing-up people at work: Investigation of workplace literacy. *Literacy and Numeracy Studies, 10*, 5–22.

Jackson, A., Blaxter, L., & Lewando-Hundt, G. (2003). Participating in medical education: Views of patients and carers living in deprived communities. *Medical Education, 37*, 532–538.

Jagsi, R., Shapiro, J., & Weinstein, D. F. (2005). Perceived impact of resident work hour limitations on medical student clerkships: A survey study. *Academic Medicine, 80*, 752–757.

Jakobson, R. (1992). *On language*. Boston, MA: Harvard University Press.

Jason, H. (2000). Communication skills are vital in all we do as educators and clinicians. *Education for Health, 13*, 157–160.

Jefferson Demographics. (2005). *Jefferson longitudinal study of medical education* (Paper 10). Retrieved from http://jdc.jefferson.edu/jlsme/10

Jencks, C. (2007). *Critical modernism—Where is post modernism going?* London: Wiley Academy.

Joint Commission on Accreditation of Healthcare Organisations. (2004). *Sentinel event statistics* (Updated 2011). Retrieved from http://www.jointcommission.org/sentinel_event.aspx

Joint Commission on Accreditation of Healthcare Organizations. (2001, December 5). A follow-up review of wrong site surgery. *Sentinel Event Alert, (24)*.

Jolly, B., & Rees, L. (Eds.). (1998). *Medical education in the millennium*. Oxford, England: OUP.

Jullien, F. (2007). *Vital nourishment: Departing from happiness*. New York: Zone Books.

Kane, R. A. (1975). *Interprofessional teamwork* (Manpower Monograph No. 8). New York: Syracuse University School of Social Work.

Kangasoja, J. (2002). Complex design problems—An impetus for learning and knotworking. In P. Bell, R. Stevens, & T. Satwicz (Eds.), *Keeping learning complex: The proceedings of the fifth international conference on the learning sciences (ICLS)* (pp. 199–205). Mahwah, NJ: Erlbaum.

Karl, R. C. (2009). Aviation. *Journal of Gatrointestinal Surgery, 13*, 6–8.

Kassab, S., Abu-Hijleh, M., Al-Shboul, Q., & Hamdy, H. (2005). Gender-related differences in learning in student-led PBL tutorials. *Education for Health, 18*, 272–282.

Katz, P. (2000). *The scalpel's edge: The culture of surgeons*. New York: Prentice Hall.

Kauffman, S. (1995). *At home in the universe: The search for the laws of self-organisation and complexity*. London: Viking.

Keane, J. (2009). *The life and death of democracy*. London: Simon & Schuster.

Kelly, D., & Wykurz, G. (1998). Patients as teachers: A new perspective in medical education. *Education for Health, 11*, 369–377.

Kennedy, J. (2013). 'In the Blood'. PhD thesis in progress. Falmouth University.

Kerosuo, H. (2007). Renegotiating disjunctions in interorganizationally provided care. In R. Iedema (Ed.), *The discourse of hospital communication: Tracing complexities in contemporary health organisation* (pp. 138–160). Basingstoke, England: Palgrave Macmillan.

Kerosuo, H., & Engeström, Y. (2003). Boundary crossing and learning in creation of new work practice. *Journal of Workplace Learning, 15*, 345–351.

Kilminster, S., Downes, J., Gough, B., Murdoch-Eaton, D., & Roberts, T. (2007). Women in medicine—Is there a problem? A literature review of the changing gender composition, structures and occupational cultures in medicine. *Medical Education, 41*, 39–49.

Kirklin, D., Duncan, J., McBride, S., Hunt, S., & Griffin, M. (2007). A cluster design controlled trial of arts-based observational skills training in primary care. *Medical Education, 41*, 395–401.

Klamen, D., & Williams, R. (2006). Using standardized clinical encounters to assess physician communication. In D. T. Stern (Ed.), *Measuring medical professionalism* (pp. 53–74). Oxford, England: Oxford University Press.

Kleinman, A. (1988). *The illness narratives: Suffering, healing and the human condition*. New York: Basic Books.

Klemola, U.-M., & Norros, L. (1997). Analysis of the clinical behaviour of anaesthetists: Recognition of uncertainty as basis for practice. *Medical Education, 31*, 449–456.

Klemola, U. M., & Norros, L. (2001). Practice-based criteria for assessing anaesthetists' habits of action: Outline for a reflexive turn in practice. *Medical Education, 35*, 455–464.

Klitzman, R. (2006). Improving education on doctor-patient relationships and communication: Lessons from doctors who become patients. *Academic Medicine, 81*, 447–453.

Kohn, L., Corrigan, J., & Donaldson, M. (Eds.). (1999). *To err is human: Building a safer health system*. Washington, DC: National Academy Press.

Kristeva, J. (1982). *Powers of horror: An essay on abjection*. New York: Columbia University Press.

Kumagai, A. K. (2008). A conceptual framework for the use of illness narratives in medical education. *Academic Medicine, 83*, 653–658.

Kumagai, A. K., Murphy, E. A., & Ross, P. T. (2009). Diabetes stories: use of patient narratives of diabetes to teach patient-centered care. *Advances in Health Sciences Education, Theory and Practice, 14*, 315–326.

Kurtz, S., Silverman, J., & Draper, J. (2004). *Teaching and learning communication skills in medicine* (2nd Rev. ed.). Oxford, England: Radcliffe Publishing Ltd.

Lacan, J. (1998). *The seminar: Book XX: On feminine sexuality, the limits of love and knowledge: Encore, 1972-1973*. New York: Norton.

LaCombe, M. A. (1993). Letters of intent. In H. M. Spiro, M. G. McCrea, E. P. Curnen, et al. (Eds.), *Empathy and the practice of medicine: Beyond pills and the scalpel* (pp. 54–66). New Haven, CT: Yale University Press.

Laidlaw, A., & Hart, J. (2011). Communication skills: An essential component of medical curricula. Part I: Assessment of clinical communication: AMEE guide No. 511. *Medical Teacher, 33*, 6–8.

Laine, C., & Davidoff, F. (1996). Patient-centered medicine: A professional evolution. *Journal of the American Medical Association, 275*, 152–156.

Laing, R. (1972). *Knots*. Harmondsworth, England: Penguin Books.

Lam, V. (2006). *Bloodletting and miraculous cures*. Toronto, Ontario, Canada: Doubleday Canada.

Lather, P. (1986). Issues of validity in openly ideological research: Between a rock and a soft place. *Interchange, 17*, 63–84.

Lather, P. (1991). *Getting smart: Feminist research and pedagogy with/in the postmodern*. London: Routledge.

Lather, P. (1993). Fertile obsession: Validity after poststructuralism. *The Sociological Quarterly, 34*, 673–693.

Latour, B. (1987). *Science in action: How to follow scientists and engineers through society*. Cambridge, MA: Harvard University Press.

Latour, B. (1993). *We have never been modern*. Hemel Hempstead, England: Harvester Wheatsheaf.

Latour, B. (1996). *Aramis or the love of technology*. Cambridge, MA: Harvard University Press.

Latour, B. (1999a). On recalling ANT. In J. Law & J. Hassard (Eds.), *Actor network and after* (pp. 15–25). Oxford, England: Blackwell.

Latour, B. (1999b). *Pandora's hope: Essays on the reality of science studies*. Cambridge, MA: Harvard University Press.

Latour, B. (2007). *Reassembling the social: An introduction to actor-network-theory* (2nd ed.). Oxford, England: Oxford University Press.

Latour, B. (2010). *On the modern cult of the factish gods*. Durham, NC: Duke University Press.

Laurance, J. (2004, August 2). The medical timebomb: Too many women doctors. *The Independent*.

Lave, J., & Wenger, E. (1990). *Situated learning: Legitimate peripheral participation*. Cambridge, England: Cambridge University Press.

Law, J. (2004). *After method: Mess in social science research*. London: Routledge.

Law, J., & Hassard, J. (1999). *Actor network theory and after*. Oxford, England: Blackwell.

Law, J., & Singleton, V. (2010). Object lessons. *Organization, 17*, 331–355.

Lempp, H., & Seale, C. (2004). The hidden curriculum in undergraduate medical education: Qualitative study of medical students' perceptions of teaching. *British Medical Journal, 329*, 770.

Levinas, E. (1969). *Totality and infinity*. Pittsburgh, PA: Duquesne University Press.

Levine, D., & Bleakley, A. (2012). Maximising medicine through aphorisms. *Medical Education, 46*, 153–162.

Levinson, W., Gorawara-Bhat, R., & Lamb, J. (2000). A study of patient clues and physician responses in primary care and surgical settings. *Journal of the American Medical Association, 284*, 1021–1027.

Lewis, N. J., Rees, C. E., Hudson, J. N., & Bleakley, A. (2005). Emotional intelligence in medical education: Measuring the unmeasurable? *Advances in Health Sciences Education, Theory and Practice, 10*, 339–355.

Lief, H. I., & Fox, R. C. (1963). Training for "detached concern" in medical students. In H. I. Lief, V. F. Lief, & N. R. Lief (Eds.), *The psychological basis of medical practice* (pp. 12–35). New York: Harper and Row.

Lingard, L. (2007). The rhetorical 'turn' in medical education: What have we learned and where are we going? *Advances in Health Sciences Education, Theory and Practice, 12*, 121–133.

Lingard, L., Garwood, K., Schryer, C. F., & Spafford, M. M. (2003). 'Talking the talk': School and workplace genre tension in clerkship case presentations. *Medical Education, 37*, 612–620.

Lingard, L., Hodges, B., MacRae, H., & Freeman, R. (2004). Expert and trainee determinations of rhetorical relevance in referral and consultation letters. *Medical Education, 38*, 168–176.

Lingard, L., Reznick, R., DeVito, I., & Espin, S. (2002). Forming professional identities on the healthcare team: Discursive construction of the 'other' in the operating room. *Medical Education, 36*, 728–734.

Lingard, L., Reznick, R., Espin, S., Regehr, G., & DeVito, I. (2002). Team communications in the operating room: Talk patterns, sites of tension, and implications for novices. *Academic Medicine, 77*, 232–237.

Lingard, L., Schryer, C. F., Garwood, K., & Spafford, M. M. (2003). A certain art of uncertainty: Case presentation and the development of professional identity. *Social Science & Medicine, 56*, 603–616.

Lingis, A. (1994). *The community of those who have nothing in common.* Bloomington, IN: Indiana University Press.

Lipkin, M., Putnam, S., & Lazare, A. (Eds.). (1995). *The medical encounter.* New York: Springer.

Ludmerer, K. M. (1999). *Time to heal: American medical education from the turn of the century to the era of managed care.* Oxford, England: Oxford University Press.

Luther, V. P., & Crandall, S. J. (2011). Commentary: Ambiguity and uncertainty: Neglected elements of medical education curricula? *Academic Medicine, 86,* 799–800.

Mandelbaum, M. (2007). Democracy without America: The spontaneous spread of freedom. *Foreign Affairs, 86,* 119–130.

Marshall, R., & Bleakley, A. (2009). The death of Hector: Pity in Homer, empathy in medical education. *Medical Humanities, 35,* 7–12.

Marshall, R., & Bleakley, A. (2011). Sing, muse: Songs in Homer and in hospital. *Medical Humanities, 37,* 27–33.

Marshall, R., & Bleakley, A. (2013). Lost in translation. Homer in English; the patient's story in medicine. *Medical Humanities, 39,* 47–52.

Marvel, M. K., Epstein, R. M., Flowers, K., & Beckman, H. B. (1999). Soliciting the patient's agenda: Have we improved? *Journal of the American Medical Association, 281,* 283–287.

Massumi, B. (1992). *A user's guide to capitalism and schizophrenia.* Cambridge, MA: The MIT Press.

Mauksch, L. B., Dugdale, D. C., Dodson, S., & Epstein, R. (2008). Relationship, communication, and efficiency in the medical encounter: Creating a clinical model from a literature review. *Archives of Internal Medicine, 168,* 1387–1395.

McGushin, E. (2007). *Foucault's askēsis: An introduction to the philosophical life.* Evanston, IL: Northwestern University Press.

McKeown, T. (1979). *The role of medicine: Dream, mirage or nemesis?* Oxford, England: Blackwell.

McKinstry, B., Colthart, I., Elliott, K., & Hunter, C. (2006). The feminization of the medical work force, implications for Scottish primary care: A survey of Scottish general practitioners. *BMC Health Services Research, 6,* 56.

McManus, I. C. (1997). Medical careers: Stories of a life. *Medical Education, 31*(Suppl 1), 31–35.

McMurray, J. E., Cohen, M., Angus, G., Harding, J., Gavel, P., et al. (2002). Women in medicine: A four-nation comparison. *Journal of American Medical Women's Association, 57,* 185–190.

McWhinney, I. R. (1988). Appendix VI: Through clinical method to a more humane medicine. In K. L. White (Ed.), *The task of medicine: Dialogue at Wickenburg* (pp. 218–231). Menlo Park, CA: The Henry J. Kaiser Family Foundation.

Mechanic, D., McAlpine, D., & Rosenthal, M. (2001). Are patients' office visits with physicians getting shorter? *The New England Journal of Medicine, 344,* 198–204.

Mennin, S. (2010). Self-organisation, integration and curriculum in the complex world of medical education. *Medical Education, 44,* 20–30.

Merleau-Ponty, M. (1968). *The visible and the invisible.* Evanston, IL: Northwestern University Press.

Miettinen, R. (1999). The riddle of things. Activity theory and actor network theory as approaches of studying innovations. *Mind, Culture, and Activity, 6,* 170–195.

Millenson, M. L. (1999). *Demanding medical excellence: Doctors and accountability in the information age* (2nd ed.). Chicago: University of Chicago Press.

Miller, J.-A. (2005). Lacan's later teaching. *Lacanian Ink 21.*

Millman, M. (1976). *The unkindest cut: Life in the backrooms of medicine.* New York: William Morrow.

Mishler, E. G. (1984). *The discourse of medicine (language and learning for human service professions).* New York: Ablex Publishing Corporation.

Mol, A. (1999). Ontological politics. A word and some questions. In J. Law & J. Hassard (Eds.), *Actor network theory and after* (pp. 74–89). Oxford, England: Blackwell.

Mol, A. (2002). *The body multiple: Ontology in medical practice.* Durham, NC: Duke University Press.

Mol, A. (2008). *The logic of care: Health and the problem of patient choice*. London: Routledge.

Mol, A., Moser, I., & Pols, J. (Eds.). (2010). *Care in practice: On tinkering in clinics, homes and farms*. Bielefeld, Germany: transcript Verlag.

Montgomery, K. (2006). *How doctors think: Clinical judgment and the practice of medicine*. Oxford, England: Oxford University Press.

Mortality statistics: every cause of death in England and Wales. *The Guardian*. Retrieved January 14, 2011, from http://www.guardian.co.uk/news/datablog/2011/jan/14/mortality-statistics-causes-death-england-wales-2009#data

Muller, D., & Kase, N. (2010). Challenging traditional premedical requirements as predictors of success in medical school: The Mount Sinai School of Medicine Humanities and Medicine Program. *Academic Medicine, 85*, 1378–1383.

Neighbour, R. (2004). *The inner consultation: How to develop an effective and intuitive consulting style* (2nd Rev. ed.). Oxford, England: Radcliffe Publishing Ltd.

Neumann, M., Edelhäuser, F., Tauschel, D., Fischer, M., Wirtz, M., Woopen, C., et al. (2011, June 10). Empathy decline and its reasons: A systematic review of studies with medical students and residents. *Academic Medicine*. doi:10.1097/ACM.0b013e318221e615 (e-publication ahead of print).

Norman, G. (2003). RCT = results confounded and trivial: The perils of grand educational experiments. *Medical Education, 7*, 582–584.

Norman, G. (2004). Editorial—Theory testing research versus theory-based research. *Advances in Health Sciences Education, Theory and Practice, 9*, 175–178.

Norman, G. R., & Eva, K. W. (2010). Diagnostic error and clinical reasoning. *Medical Education, 44*, 94–100.

Norstedt, M., & Davies, K. (2003). Medical education seemingly 'immune' to discussions on sex and gender. A study indicates that the gender perspective in teaching is limited. *Läkartidningen, 100*(2056–9), 2062.

Nussbaum, M. C. (1999). *Sex and social justice*. New York: Oxford University Press.

Nussbaum, M. C. (2010). *Not for profit: Why democracy needs the humanities*. Princeton, NJ: Princeton University Press.

O'Flynn, N., Spencer, J., & Jones, R. (1997). Consent and confidentiality in teaching in general practice: Survey of patients; views on presence of students. *British Medical Journal, 315*, 1142.

Orr, M. (2003). *Intertextuality: Debates and contexts*. Cambridge, England: Polity Press.

Ousager, J., & Johannessen, H. (2010). Humanities in undergraduate medical education: A literature review. *Academic Medicine, 85*, 988–998.

Owen, J. M. (2005). Iraq and the democratic peace. *Foreign Affairs, 84*, 122–127.

Padel, R. (1992). *In and out of the mind: Greek images of the tragic self*. Princeton, NJ: Princeton University Press.

Padel, R. (1995). *Whom gods destroy: Elements of Greek and tragic madness*. Princeton, NJ: Princeton University Press.

Paley, J. (2010). The appropriation of complexity theory in health care. *Journal of Health Services Research & Policy, 15*, 59–61.

Parsons, T. (1991/1951). *The social system*. London: Routledge.

Patterson, K. (2007). *Consumption*. Toronto, Ontario, Canada: Vintage.

Pauli, H. G., White, K. L., & McWhinney, I. R. (2000a). Medical education, research, and scientific thinking in the 21st century. *Education for Health, 13*, 15–26 (part one of three).

Pauli, H. G., White, K. L., & McWhinney, I. R. (2000b). Medical education, research, and scientific thinking in the 21st century. *Education for Health, 13*, 165–186 (parts two and three).

Payne, M. (2000). *Teamwork in multiprofessional care*. Basingstoke, England: Palgrave.

Pedersen, R. (2010). Empathy development in medical education—A critical review. *Medical Teacher, 32*, 593–600.

Pendleton, D., Schofield, T., Tate, P., & Havelock, P. (2003). *The new consultation: Developing doctor-patient communication* (2nd Rev. ed.). Oxford, England: Oxford University Press.

Petersen, A., & Bunton, R. (Eds.). (1997). *Foucault, health and medicine*. London: Routledge.

Pignatelli, F. (1993). Dangers, possibilities: Ethico-political choices in the work of Michel Foucault. *Philosophy of Education*.

Pilpel, D., Schor, R., & Benbassat, J. (1998). Barriers to acceptance of medical error: The case for a teaching programme. *Medical Education, 32*, 3–7.

Pinar, W. F. (2004). *What is curriculum theory?* Mahwah, NJ: Lawrence Erlbaum.

Pinar, W. F. (2006). *The synoptic text today and other essays: Curriculum development after the reconceptualization*. New York: Peter Lang.

Pinar, W. F., Reynolds, W. M., Slattery, P., & Taubman, P. M. (Eds.). (1995). *Understanding curriculum: An introduction to the study of historical and contemporary curriculum discourses*. New York: Peter Lang.

Plato. (1956). Meno trs. In W. K. C. Guthrie (Ed.), *Protagoras and meno*. Harmondsworth, England: Penguin Books.

Platt, F. W. (1979). Clinical hypocompetence: The interview. *Annals of Internal Medicine, 91*, 898–902.

Plsek, P., & Greenhalgh, T. (2001). Complexity science: The challenges of complexity in healthcare. *British Medical Journal, 323*, 625–628.

Plsek, P., Sweeney, K., & Griffiths, F. (2002). *Complexity and healthcare: An introduction*. Oxford, England: Radcliffe.

Price, R., Spencer, J., & Walker, J. (2008). Does the presence of medical students affect quality in general practice consultations? *Medical Education, 42*, 374–381.

Prideaux, D., & Bligh, J. (2002). Research in medical education: Asking the right questions. *Medical Education, 36*, 1114–1115.

Prigogene, I., & Stengers, B. (1985). *Order out of chaos: Man's new dialogue with nature*. London: Flamingo.

Pronovost, P., & Vohr, E. (2010). *Safe patients, smart hospitals: How one doctor's checklist can help us change health care from the inside out*. New York: Hudson Street Press.

Quirk, M. (2006). *Intuition and metacognition in medical education*. New York: Springer.

Rabinow, P. (1994). Modern and countermodern: Ethos and epoch in Heidegger and Foucault. In G. Gutting (Ed.), *The Cambridge companion to Foucault* (pp. 197–214). Cambridge, England: Cambridge University Press.

Rahe, P. A. (2010). *Soft despotism, democracy's drift: Montesquieu, Rousseau, Tocqueville, and the modern prospect*. New Haven, CT: Yale University Press.

Reason, P., & Bradbury, H. (Eds.). (2006). *Handbook of action research*. London: Sage.

Reber, A. (1993). *Implicit learning and tacit knowledge: An essay on the cognitive unconscious*. Oxford, England: Oxford University Press.

Regehr, G. (2004). Trends in medical education research. *Academic Medicine, 79*, 939–947.

Regehr, G. (2010). It's not rocket science: Rethinking our metaphors for research in health professions education. *Medical Education, 44*, 31–39.

Reinders, M. E., Blankenstein, A. H., van Marwijk, H. W. J., Knol, D. L., Ram, P., van der Horst, H. E., et al. (2011). Reliability of consultation skills assessments using standardised versus real patients. *Medical Education, 45*, 578–584.

Rhoten, D. (2004). Interdisciplinary research: Trend or transition. *Items and Issues (Social Sciences Research Council), 5*, 6–12.

Rich, B. (2006). Breeding cynicism: The re-education of medical students. *American Philosophical Association Newsletters, 6*.

Richardson, W. C., et al. (2001). *Crossing the quality chasm: A new health system for the 21st century*. Washington, DC: National Academy Press.

Rider, E. A., & Keefer, C. H. (2006). Communication skills competencies: Definitions and a teaching toolbox. *Medical Education, 40*, 624–629.

Riggs, G. (2010). Commentary: Are we ready to embrace the rest of the Flexner report? *Academic Medicine, 85*, 1669–1671.

Riley, R., & Manias, E. (2007). Governing the operating room list. In R. Iedema (Ed.), *The discourse of hospital communication: Tracing complexities in contemporary health care organizations* (pp. 67–89). Basingstoke, England: Palgrave Macmillan.

Rogers, C. (1957). The necessary and sufficient conditions of therapeutic personality change. *Journal of Consulting Psychology, 21*, 95–103.

Rogoff, B. (1990). *Apprenticeship in thinking: Cognitive development in social context*. Oxford, England: Oxford University Press.

Romanyshyn, R. (1989). *Technology as symptom and dream*. London: Routledge.

Roter, D., & Hall, J. (2006). *Doctors talking with patients/patients talking with doctors: Improving communication in medical visits* (2nd ed.). Westport, CT: Greenwood Publishing Group.

RPSGB and BMA. (2000). *Teamworking in primary health care: Realising shared aims in patient care* (p. 2000). London: Royal Pharmaceutical Society of Great Britain and the British Medical Association.

Rushmer, R., & Davies, H. T. O. (2004). Unlearning in health care. *Quality & Safety in Health Care, 13*(Suppl 2), ii10–ii15.

Ryan, C. A., Walshe, N., Gaffney, R., Shanks, A., Burgoyne, L., Wiskin, C. M. (2010). Using standardized patients to assess communication skills in medical and nursing students. *BMC Medical Education, 10*, 24.

Salter, R. H. (1996). Learning from patients—Unfashionable but effective. *Postgraduate Medical Journal, 72*, 385.

Sanders, L. (2010). *Diagnosis: Dispatches from the frontlines of medical mysteries*. London: Icon Books.

Sandhu, B., Margerison, C., & Holdcroft, A. (2007). Women in the UK medical academic workforce. *Medical Education, 41*, 909–914.

Sanfey, H. A., Saalwachter-Schulman, A. R., Nyhof-Young, J. M., Eidelson, B., & Mann, B. D. (2006). Influences on medical student career choice: Gender or generation? *Archives of Surgery, 141*, 1086–1094.

Sass, L. (1994). *Madness and modernism: Insanity in the light of modern art, literature and thought*. New Haven, CT: Yale University Press.

Savage, C., & Brommels, M. (2008). Innovation in medical education: How Linköping created a Blue Ocean for medical education in Sweden. *Medical Teacher, 30*, 501–507.

Scardamalia, M. (2002). Collective cognitive responsibility for the advancement of knowledge. In B. Smith (Ed.), *Liberal education in a knowledge society* (pp. 67–98). Chicago: Open Court.

Schatzki, T. R., Knorr-Cetina, K., & von-Savigny, E. (Eds.). (2001). *The practice turn in contemporary theory*. Abingdon, England: Routledge.

Schernhammer, E. (2005). Taking their own lives—The high rate of physician suicide. *New England Journal of Medicine, 352*, 2473–2476.

Scheurich, J. J. (1997). *Research method in the postmodern*. London: The Falmer Press.

Schön, D. A. (1990). *Educating the reflective practitioner: Toward a new design for teaching and learning*. San Francisco: Jossey-Bass.

Searle, J. R. (1990). Collective intentions and actions. In P. R. Cohen, J. Morgan, & M. E. Pollack (Eds.), *Intentions in communication* (pp. 401–415). Cambridge, MA: MIT Press.

Selzer, R. (1996). *Mortal lessons: Notes on the art of surgery* (2nd ed.). San Diego, CA: Harcourt, Harvest.

Sennett, R. (2008). *The craftsman*. London: Penguin Books.

Serry, N., Bloch, S., Ball, R., & Anderson, K. (1994). Drug and alcohol abuse by doctors. *Medical Journal of Australia, 160*(402–3), 406–407.

Sexton, J. B., Helmreich, R. L., Neilands, T. B., Rowan, K., Vella, K., Boyden, J., et al. (2006). The safety attitudes questionnaire: Psychometric properties, benchmarking data, and emergency research. *BMC Health Services Research, 6*, 44.

Shakespeare, W. (2013, 2nd ed./ 1611). *The Tempest*. Cambridge: Cambridge University Press.

Shapiro, J. (2008). Walking a mile in their patients' shoes: Empathy and othering in medical students' education. *Philosophy, Ethics, and Humanities in Medicine, 3*, 10–22.

Sharpe, M. (2007). A question of two truths? Remarks on parrhesia and the 'political-philosophical' difference. *Parrhesia, 2*, 89–108.

Shaw, S. N. (2008). More than one dollop of cortex: Patients' experiences of interprofessional care at an urban family health centre. *Journal of Interprofessional Care, 22*, 229–237.

Silverman, J., Kurtz, S., & Draper, J. (2004). *Skills for communicating with patients* (2nd Rev. ed.). Oxford, England: Radcliffe.

Simons, P. R. J. (1999). Transfer of learning: Paradoxes for learners. *International Journal of Educational Research, 31*, 577–589.

Singer, P. (1983). *Hegel.* Oxford, England: Oxford University Press.

Singh, H., Thomas, E. J., Petersen, L. A., & Studdart, D. M. (2007). Medical errors involving trainees: A study of closed malpractice claims from 5 insurers. *Archives of Internal Medicine, 167*, 2030–2036.

Smith, R. (2003). What doctors and managers can learn from each other. *British Medical Journal, 326*, 610–611.

Smith, D. W. (2005). Critical, clinical. In C. J. Stivale (Ed.), *Gilles Deleuze: Key concepts* (pp. 182–193). Stocksfield, England: Acumen.

Snadden, D. (2006). Clinical education: Context is everything. *Medical Education, 40*, 97–98.

Sontag, S. (1978). *Illness as metaphor.* New York: Farrar Strauss & Giroux.

Sorensen, R., & Iedema, R. (Eds.). (2008a). *Managing clinical processes in health services.* Sydney, New South Wales, Australia: Mosby, Elsevier.

Sorensen, R., & Iedema, R. (Eds.). (2008b). *Managing clinical processes in health care.* London: Elsevier.

Sox, H. C., Jr., & Woloshin, S. (2000). How many deaths are due to medical error? Getting the number right. *Effective Clinical Practice, 3*, 277–283.

Spencer, J., Blackmore, D., Heard, S., McCrorie, P., McHaffie, D., Scherpbier A., et al. (2000). Patient-oriented learning: A review of the role of the patient in the education of medical students. *Medical Education, 34*, 851–857.

Spiro, H. M., McCrea Curnen, M. G. Peschel, E., & St James, D. (Eds.). (1993). *Empathy and the practice of medicine: Beyond pills and the scalpel.* New Haven, CT: Yale University Press.

Starfield, B. (2000). Is US health really the best in the world? *Journal of the American Medical Association, 284*, 483–485.

Stern, D. T. (Ed.). (2006a). *Measuring medical professionalism.* Oxford, England: Oxford University Press.

Stern, D. S. (2006b). A framework for measuring professionalism. In D. T. Stern (Ed.), *Measuring medical professionalism* (pp. 3–14). Oxford, England: Oxford University Press.

Stewart, M. (1995). Effective physician-patient communication and health outcomes: A review. *Canadian Medical Association Journal, 152*, 1423–1433.

Stewart, M. (2001). Editorial: Towards a global definition of patient centred care the patient should be the judge of patient centred care. *British Medical Journal, 322*, 444.

Stewart, M., Brown, J. B., Weston, W. W., McWhinney, I. R., McWilliam, C. L., Freeman, T. R. (2003, 2nd ed.). *Patient-centered medicine: Transforming the clinical method* (2nd ed.). Oxford, England: Radcliffe Medical Press Ltd.

Stivale, C. J. (Ed.). (2005). *Gilles Deleuze: Key concepts.* Stocksfield, England: Acumen.

Strauss, A., Schatzman, L., Ehrlich, D., Bucher, R., & Sabshin, M. (1963). The hospital and its negotiated order. In E. Freidson (Ed.), *The hospital in modern society* (pp. 147–169). New York: Free Press of Glencoe.

Surowiecki, J. (2005). *The wisdom of crowds: Why the many are smarter than the few.* London: Abacus.

Swaro, A., & Adhiyaman, V. (2010). Autopsy in older medical patients: Concordance in ante- and post-mortem findings and changing trends. *Journal of the Royal College of Physicians of Edinburgh, 40*, 205–208.

Sweeney, K. (2006). *Complexity in primary care: Understanding its value.* Oxford, England: Radcliffe.

Sweeney, K., Toy, L., & Cornwell, J. (2009). Mesothelioma. *British Medical Journal, 339*, b2862.

Szasz, T., & Hollender, M. (1956). A contribution to the philosophy of medicine: The basic models of the doctor-patient relationship. *Archives of Internal Medicine, 97*, 585–592.

Szczeklik, A. (2005). *Catharsis: On the art of medicine.* Chicago: University of Chicago Press.

Tang, P. C., et al. (2003). *Patient safety: Achieving a new standard for care*. Washington, DC: Institute of Medicine of the National Academies, National Academy of Sciences/National Academies Press.

Tarkan, L. A. (2008, September 28). Problem for emergency room patients: Health illiteracy. *The Observer (The New York Times supplement)*, p. 6.

Tate, P. (2009). *The doctor's communication handbook* (6th Rev. ed.). Oxford, England: Radcliffe.

Taussig, M. (1992). *The nervous system*. London: Routledge.

Taylor, K. S., Lambert, T. W., & Goldacre, M. J. (2009). Career progression and destinations, comparing men and women in the NHS: Postal questionnaire surveys. *British Medical Journal, 338*, b1735.

Thomas, J., & Monaghan, T. (Eds.). (2007). *The Oxford handbook of clinical examination and practical skills*. Oxford, England: Oxford University Press.

Thoreau, H. D. (1995/1849). *Civil disobedience*. Harmondsworth, England: Penguin.

Tilly, C. (2007). *Democracy*. Cambridge, England: Cambridge University Press.

Tooke, J. (2008). *Aspiring to excellence: Findings and final recommendations of the independent inquiry into modernising medical careers*. London: Aldridge Press.

Tresolini, C. P. (Ed.) (2000). *Health professions education and realtionship-centered care: Report of the Pew-Fetzer Task Force on advancing psychosocial health education*. Retrieved from http://rccswmi.org/uploads/PewFetzerRCCreport.pdf

Truog, R. D., Browning, D. M., Johnson, J. A., & Gallagher, T. H. (2011). *Talking with patients and families about medical error*. Baltimore: The Johns Hopkins University Press.

Varpio, L., Hall, P., Lingard, L., & Schryer, C. (2008). Interprofessional communication and medical error: A reframing of research questions and approaches. *Academic Medicine, 83*(10 Suppl), S76–S81.

Verlander, G. (2004). Female physicians: Balancing career and family. *Academic Psychiatry, 28*, 331–336.

Veloski, J., & Hojat, M. (2006). Measuring specific elements of professionalism: Empathy, teamwork, and lifelong learning. In D. T. Stern (Ed.), *Measuring medical professionalism* (pp. 117–146). Oxford, England: Oxford University Press.

Verghese, A. (1998). *The tennis partner*. New York: HarperCollins.

Verghese, A. (2009). *Cutting for stone*. London: Chatto & Windus.

Vincent, C. (2001). Adverse events in British hospitals: Preliminary retrospective record review. *British Medical Journal, 322*, 1395.

Vincent, C. (2005). *Patient safety*. London: Churchill Livingstone.

Wadhwa, A., & Lingard, L. (2006). A qualitative study examining tensions in interdoctor telephone consultations. *Medical Education, 40*, 75.

Wagner, P., Hendrich, J., Moseley, G., & Hudson, V. (2007). Defining medical professionalism: A qualitative study. *Medical Education, 41*, 288–294.

Wahlstrom, O., Sanden, I., & Hammar, M. (1997). Multiprofessional education in the medical curriculum. *Medical Education, 31*, 425–429.

Waitzkin, H. (1984). Doctor-patient communication: Clinical implications of social scientific research. *Journal of the American Medical Association, 252*, 2441–2446.

Waitzkin, H., & Stoeckle, J. D. (1972). The communication of information about illness: Clinical, sociological and methodological considerations. *Advances in Psychosomatic Medicine, 8*, 180–215.

Warne, T., & McAndrew, S. (2005). *Using patient experience in nurse education*. Basingstoke, England: Palgrave McMillan.

Warriner, D. (2008). The inner consultation. *British Medical Journal, 337*, a1574.

Washburn, E. R. (2000). Are you ready for generation X? *Physician Executive, 26*, 51–57.

Wayne, S., Dellmore, D., Serna, L. Jerabek, R., Timm, C., & Kalishman, S. (2011). The association between intolerance of ambiguity and decline in medical students' attitudes toward the underserved. *Academic Medicine, 86*, 877–882.

Weber, M. (2002/1905). *The protestant ethic and the "spirit" of capitalism and other writings*. Harmondworth: Penguin.

Weingart, N. S., Wilson, R. M., Gibberd, R. W., & Harrison, B. (2000). Epidemiology of medical error. *British Medical Journal, 320*, 774.

Weiss, P. (2005). *The aesthetics of resistance*. Durham, NC: Duke University Press.

Wenger, E. (1998). *Communities of practice: Learning, meaning and identity*. Cambridge, England: Cambridge University Press.

Wershof Schwartz, A., Abramson, J. S., Wojnowich, I., Accordino, R., Ronan, E. J., & Rifkin, M. R. (2009). Evaluating the impact of the humanities in medical education. *Mount Sinai Journal of Medicine, 76*, 372–380.

West, M. A., & Borrill, C. S. (2002). *Effective human resource management and lower patient mortality*. Birmingham, England: University of Aston.

Westerstähl, A., Andersson, M., & Söderström, M. (2003). Gender in medical curricula: Course organizer views of a gender-issues perspective in medicine in Sweden. *Women Health, 37*, 35–47.

Weston, G. (2009). *Direct red: A surgeon's story*. London: Jonathan Cape.

White, J., Levinson, W., & Roter, D. (1994). "Oh, by the way …": the closing moments of the medical visit. *Journal of General and Internal Medicine, 9*, 24–28.

Whyte, S., Lingard, L., Espin, S., Ross Baker, G., Bohnen, J., Orser, B.A., et al. (2008). Paradoxical effects of interprofessional briefings on OR team performance. *Cognition, Technology & Work, 10*, 287–294.

Wilmer, H. A. (1968). The doctor-patient relationship and issues of pity, sympathy and empathy. *British Journal of Medical Psychology, 41*, 243–248.

Winnicott, D. W. (1971). *Playing and reality*. Harmondsworth, England: Penguin.

Winter, G. (2000). A comparative discussion of the notion of 'validity' in qualitative and quantitative research. *The Qualitative Report, 4*, 3–4. Retrieved from http://www.nova.edu/ssss/QR/QR4-3/winter.html

Winters, B. D., Aswani, M. S., & Pronovost, P. J. (2011). Reducing diagnostic errors: Another role for checklists? *Academic Medicine, 86*, 279–281.

Wispé, L. (1991). *The psychology of sympathy*. New York: Kluwer/Plenum.

Wolf, F. M. (2004). Commentary—Methodological quality, evidence, and research in medical education (RIME). *Academic Medicine, 79*, S68–S69.

Wolosin, R. J., & Gesell, S. B. (2006). Physician gender and primary care patient satisfaction: no evidence of 'feminization'. *Quality Management in Health Care, 15*, 96–103.

Wong, T. (2002). *Metaphor, metonymy and the two sciences*. The Science of Culture/The Culture of Science. Retrieved from http://serendip.brynmawr.edu/local/scisoc/brownbag0203/wong.html

Wykurz, G., & Kelly, D. (2002). Developing the role of patients as teachers: Literature review. *British Medical Journal, 325*, 818–821.

Xyrichis, A., & Ream, E. (2008). Teamwork: A concept analysis. *Journal of Advanced Nursing, 61*, 232–241.

Yardley, S., Littlewood, S., Margolis, S. A., Scherpbier, A., Spencer, J., Ypinizar, V., et al. (2010). What has changed in the evidence for early experience? Update of a BEME systematic review. *Medical Teacher, 32*, 740–746.

Young, M. (1993/1958). *The rise of the meritocracy, 1870-2033: An essay on education and inequality*. London: Thames & Hudson.

Author Index

A. Bleakley, *Patient-Centred Medicine in Transition: The Heart of the Matter*,
Advances in Medical Education 3, DOI 10.1007/978-3-319-02487-5,
© Springer International Publishing Switzerland 2014

Subject Index

Printed by Printforce, the Netherlands

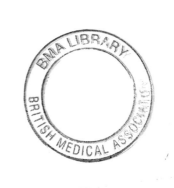